Career Development in Aca
Radiation Oncology

Ravi A. Chandra • Neha Vapiwala
Charles R. Thomas Jr.
Editors

Career Development in Academic Radiation Oncology

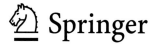 Springer

Editors
Ravi A. Chandra
Department of Radiation Medicine
Knight Cancer Institute, Oregon Health &
Science University
Portland, OR
USA

Neha Vapiwala
University of Pennsylvania
Philadelphia, PA
USA

Charles R. Thomas Jr.
Department of Radiation Medicine
Knight Cancer Institute, Oregon Health &
Science University
Portland, OR
USA

ISBN 978-3-030-71854-1   ISBN 978-3-030-71855-8   (eBook)
https://doi.org/10.1007/978-3-030-71855-8

This Springer imprint is published by the registered company Springer Nature Switzerland AG
The registered company address is: Gewerbestrasse 11, 6330 Cham, Switzerland

Foreword

Start by doing what is necessary, then what is possible, and suddenly you are doing the impossible… –St. Francis of Assisi

The quote above by St. Francis of Assisi in the thirteenth century encapsulates the essence of career development in academic radiation oncology. Our field is unique as it lies at the interface of multiple medical sub-specialties, including surgery, medical oncology, and radiology, while at the same time deeply rooted in cancer biology and medical physics. Mastery of the discipline requires the integration of key concepts and paradigms from these often-disparate fields, with a diverse array of both written and oral board exams being requisite for practice as an Attending in our specialty. This path can seem impossible to a radiation oncology trainee in the beginning of his/her career, but doing what is necessary, and then what is possible, will make the impossible a reality.

The chapters in this book provide a comprehensive roadmap with over 30 chapters from individuals who have successfully navigated this path, with pearls of wisdom and critical lessons for all of us in the field. Parts range from identifying and utilizing mentors to understanding the role of the department chair, and provide a glimpse into each stage of career development in radiation oncology. Written by luminaries in the field, this book also provides insights into how to balance career and personal life, how to avoid burnout, and strategies to branch out beyond academia into other areas and fields.

Success in academic radiation oncology extends far beyond the mastery of the literature, meticulous staging systems, contours, and dosing constraints. Much like running a marathon, the key is to learn from who is ahead of you, while helping those behind you. The chapters in this book provide a framework for this journey, and overall for a successful career in academic radiation oncology.

Ranjit S. Bindra
Department of Therapeutic Radiology
Yale School of Medicine
New Haven, CT, USA

Peter M. Glazer
Department of Therapeutic Radiology
Yale School of Medicine
New Haven, CT, USA

Foreword

Over the last two decades, radiation oncology became an extremely popular specialty among medical students, and residency slots were, consequently, very competitive. As in other popular specialties, medical students would leverage all their potential assets in order to secure a residency slot. Academic assets proved the easiest to measure and market. By 2018, those accepted to radiation oncology programs had the highest median board scores, the highest proportion of higher degrees (MPH, PhD, etc.), and the highest number of prior publications, when compared to other specialties. Although in the last couple of years the wave appears to have "crested" and the number of applicants is down, we do have a huge cadre of highly academic residents and junior faculty currently working their way through our training and career system. This is our own "baby boom." It is to this 15-year block of early career radiation oncologists that this book will prove exceptionally useful.

In a radiation oncology training, we spend much time teaching "to the test," meaning the ABR written and oral exams, and much time teaching "to the clinic," meaning pleasing referring doctors. We spend far less time teaching "to the career." Traditionally, academic-minded residents and faculty have found their way either by luck or by hitching themselves to a willing mentor. Mentorship is increasingly discussed these days, but less formally practiced. To make matters worse, mentors may have only a limited, or outdated, perspective on the many hurdles an early career radiation oncologist may face. The young academic may seek guidance elsewhere, perhaps from an ARRO (association of residents in radiation oncology) course, or a national workshop on, say, grant writing, but this is all piecemeal and random. As a senior radiation oncologist who blundered his way through the system by a mixture of chance and the generosity of my mentors, I appreciate how hazardous the current system of training is. I was able write a scientific paper, that skill was drummed in early, but no-one sat me down to explain, for example, how to think about job contracts, or when might be the right time to change job. No one explained to me how to be an organized and effective clinician, one who can please patients, referring physicians, and the members of the intra-disciplinary team simultaneously. No one taught me how to maintain academic connections while working at a peripheral hospital, nor how to resolve conflict among members of my team. Yet these are the human relation skills that, when cultured, make for the most effective researchers, teachers, and leaders.

Chandra and colleagues seek to address this deficiency. Their assumption is that, for the foreseeable future, a significant proportion of early career radiation oncologists will seek an academic path and can benefit from the collective wisdom of folks who have successfully trodden that road. They are correct in this, and they are also correct in their assumptions that future academics will not look like those of the past. Gone are the days when senior and successful radiation oncologists were all white men whose experience was forged in one of a limited number of Ivy League fires. The inclusion of chapters from the perspective of an underrepresented trainee, or from the perspective of someone trying to maintain academic connections while posted within a satellite network, is novel and powerful.

Radiation oncologists can no longer be "cookie-stamped" out of training programs underspiced and undercooked. This former process led to a high level of vulnerability and high rates of failure. An academic career was not so much a secure ladder to be climbed, as a tightrope to be crossed, with high instability and only the lucky few making it over the chasm. Those most successful were not necessarily the most talented or the most emotionally intelligent. In 2021, trainees deserve better and expect better. Their modern undergraduate and medical school teaching has already taught them the value of directed mentorship. To them, the laissez faire market of academic medicine seems savage and unjust. A book such as this, which brings together a mass of collective experience, will not substitute for the hands-on guidance of a strong mentor, or better still, a committed sponsor, but it will get trainees going. It teaches them where to target their energy and how to present themselves for success in whichever branch of our specialty they ultimately choose.

Boston, MA, USA   Anthony Zietman

Preface

It is with much anticipation that we present the first edition of *Career Development in Academic Radiation Oncology*.

There exists a longstanding crisis with respect to faculty development within academic medicine. Radiation oncology is not immune from the challenges that many faculty experience during their academic career journeys. Most training programs are simply unable to devote the resources and time required to consistently prepare radiation oncology residents and fellows for success in academic medicine. There are a number of unique career development skills that extend far beyond completing graduation requirements and passing the American Board of Radiology certification examinations. These skills are critical for career mobility and professional fulfillment, and historically have been either lacking or acquired on the job in varying degrees and formats. As such, we feel that this resource is urgently needed and long overdue.

We have assembled a novel text of over 30 chapters that are authored by nearly 60 established and emerging investigators within our illustrious specialty. These premier contributors comprise over several hundred collective years of experience navigating the terrains of academic medicine. Make no mistake, most of these contributors are already over-extended, but nevertheless were dedicated enough to find time to contribute their unique insight into this collection. The lived observations and experiences of the authors – together with evidence-based strategies when available – provide the framework for pragmatic approaches to assist the broad spectrum of faculty, including current and future, early career, and mid-career, within our specialty. Many of the approaches described will likely also be applicable to those within other academic medicine specialties, or in non-academic medicine. This work is divided into five parts:

Part 1 focuses on career planning, with dedicated chapters on foundations of career development, as well as a discussion of options within the specialty. Strategies for underrepresented-in-medicine (UIM) populations are also reviewed.

Part 2 attempts to provide both structure and nuance pertaining to the process of identifying, interviewing, and evaluating a faculty position.

Part 3 focuses on early career development. This is the largest part of the book since it represents the phase of highest risk for new faculty to get lost in the fog of the academic ecosystem and become underwhelmed, under engaged, which can contribute to premature attrition.

Part 4 attempts to provide a roadmap for mid-career and more senior members of the academy.

Part 5 includes a set of chapters that address important contextual, late-career, and transition issues within academic medicine, and are written by a diverse and well-balanced author list.

It is our opinion that this book should have been available decades ago. Our hope is that the pearls of wisdom shared herein by the diverse cadre of contributors will help cultivate academic careers of all ages and types. We wholeheartedly believe that this unique book will serve as a readily accessible resource and a highly valued set of actionable tools that can contribute to a successful career in academic radiation oncology.

We would like to thank all of the our authors for their efforts, as well as Margaret Moore, Janakiraman Ganesan, and the team at Springer for their generous contributions of time, talent, expertise, and discipline to ensure an outstanding final product.

Portland, OR, USA   Ravi A. Chandra
Philadelphia, PA, USA   Neha Vapiwala
Portland, OR, USA   Charles R. Thomas Jr.

Contents

Contributors

Kaled M. Alektiar, MD Department of Radiation Oncology, Memorial Sloan Kettering Cancer Center, New York, NY, USA

Carmen R. Bergom, MD, PhD, MPhil Department of Radiation Oncology, Washington University of Medicine in St. Louis, St. Louis, MO, USA

Scott V. Bratman, MD, PhD Radiation Medicine Program, Princess Margaret Cancer Centre, University Health Network, Toronto, ON, Canada

Department of Radiation Oncology, University of Toronto, Toronto, ON, Canada

Thomas Buchholz, MD Scripps MD Anderson Cancer Center, San Diego, CA, USA

Ravi A. Chandra, MD, PhD Department of Radiation Medicine, Knight Cancer Institute, Oregon Health & Science University, Portland, OR, USA

Daniel T. Chang, MD Department of Radiation Oncology, Stanford Cancer Institute, Stanford, CA, USA

Eric M. Chang, MD Department of Radiation Medicine, Oregon Health & Science University, Portland, OR, USA

Department of Radiation Oncology, University of California Los Angeles, Los Angeles, CA, USA

Bhishamjit S. Chera, MD Department of Radiation Oncology, University of North Carolina, Chapel Hill, NC, USA

Stephen G. Chun, MD Division of Radiation Oncology, The University of Texas, M.D. Anderson Cancer Center, Houston, TX, USA

Lauren Colbert, MD, MSCR The Department of Radiation Oncology, The University of Texas MD Anderson Cancer Center, Houston, TX, USA

C. Norman Coleman, MD Radiation Research Program, National Cancer Institute (NCI), Bethesda, MD, USA

International Cancer Expert Corps (Approved Outside Activity by NCI/NIH), Washington, DC, USA

Jennifer Croke, MD Radiation Medicine Program, Princess Margaret Cancer Centre, University Health Network, Toronto, ON, Canada

Department of Radiation Oncology, University of Toronto, Toronto, ON, Canada

Laura A. Dawson, MD Radiation Medicine Program, Princess Margaret Cancer Centre, University Health Network, Toronto, ON, Canada

Department of Radiation Oncology, University of Toronto, Toronto, ON, Canada

Curtiland Deville Jr., MD Department of Radiation Oncology and Molecular Radiation Sciences, Johns Hopkins University School of Medicine, Baltimore, MD, USA

Clifton David Fuller, MD, PhD The Department of Radiation Oncology, The University of Texas MD Anderson Cancer Center, Houston, TX, USA

Iris C. Gibbs, MD, FACR, FASTRO Stanford University, Stanford, CA, USA

Daniel W. Golden, MD, MHPE Radiation and Cellular Oncology, Pritzker School of Medicine, The University of Chicago, Chicago, IL, USA

Leonard L. Gunderson, MD, MS, FASTRO Department of Radiation Oncology, Mayo Clinic Arizona/Rochester, Scottsdale, AZ, USA

Daphne A. Haas-Kogan, MD Department of Radiation Oncology, Brigham and Women's Hospital, Dana Farber Cancer Institute, Boston Children's Hospital, Harvard Medical School, Boston, MA, USA

Bruce G. Haffty, MD Radiation Oncology, Rutgers Cancer Institute of New Jersey, New Brunswick, NJ, USA

Edward C. Halperin, MD, MA New York Medical College, and Provost for Biomedical Affairs, Touro College and University System, Valhalla, NY, USA

Kate Hardy, Clin PsychD Department of Psychiatry and Behavioral Sciences, Stanford University, Stanford, CA, USA

Kathryn E. Hitchcock, MD, PhD Department of Radiation Oncology, University of Florida College of Medicine, Gainesville, FL, USA

Sarah E. Hoffe, MD Department of Radiation Oncology, Moffitt Cancer Center and Research Institute, Tampa, FL, USA

Emma B. Holliday, MD Radiation Oncology, The University of Texas MD Anderson Cancer Center, Houston, TX, USA

David P. Horowitz, MD Department of Radiation Oncology, Columbia University Irving Medical Center, Herbert Irving Comprehensive Cancer Center, New York, NY, USA

Salma K. Jabbour, MD Rutgers Cancer Institute of New Jersey, Rutgers University, New Brunswick, NJ, USA

Lisa A. Kachnic, MD Department of Radiation Oncology, Columbia University Irving Medical Center, Herbert Irving Comprehensive Cancer Center, New York, NY, USA

Brian D. Kavanagh, MD, MPH, FASTRO Department of Radiation Oncology, University of Colorado, Aurora, CO, USA

Jennifer Yin Yee Kwan, MD Radiation Medicine Program, Princess Margaret Cancer Centre, University Health Network, Toronto, ON, Canada

Department of Radiation Oncology, University of Toronto, Toronto, ON, Canada

Nadia N. Laack, MD, MS Department of Radiation Oncology, Mayo Clinic, Rochester, MN, USA

Quynh-Thu Le, MD Department of Radiation Oncology, Stanford University, Palo Alto, CA, USA

Anna Lee, MD, MPH The Department of Radiation Oncology, The University of Texas MD Anderson Cancer Center, Houston, TX, USA

Jonathan E. Leeman, MD Department of Radiation Oncology, Brigham and Women's Hospital, Dana Farber Cancer Institute, Boston Children's Hospital, Harvard Medical School, Boston, MA, USA

Stanley L. Liauw, MD Department of Radiation and Cellular Oncology, University of Chicago, Chicago, IL, USA

Jonathan D. Licht, MD University of Florida Health Cancer Center, Gainesville, FL, USA

Fei-Fei Liu, MD, FRCPC, FASTRO Radiation Medicine Program, Princess Margaret Cancer Centre, University Health Network, Toronto, ON, Canada

Department of Radiation Oncology, University of Toronto, Toronto, ON, Canada

Nancy P. Mendenhall, MD Department of Radiation Oncology, University of Florida College of Medicine, Gainesville, FL, USA

University of Florida Health Proton Therapy Institute, Jacksonville, FL, USA

Timur Mitin, MD, PhD Department of Radiation Medicine, Knight Cancer Institute, Oregon Health & Science University, Portland, OR, USA

David T. Pointer Jr., MD Department of Gastrointestinal Oncology, Moffitt Cancer Center and Research Institute, Tampa, FL, USA

Valerie I. Reed, MD Division of Radiation Oncology, The University of Texas, M.D. Anderson Cancer Center, Houston, TX, USA

Jennifer Riekert, MBA New York Medical College, Valhalla, NY, USA

Sara T. Rosenthal, MBA MiraKind, Los Angeles, CA, USA

Mutlay Sayan, MD Radiation Oncology, Rutgers Cancer Institute of New Jersey, New Brunswick, NJ, USA

Roshan V. Sethi, MD Department of Radiation Oncology, Brigham and Women's Hospital, Dana Farber Cancer Institute, Boston Children's Hospital, Harvard Medical School, Boston, MA, USA

Monica E. Shukla, MD Department of Radiation Oncology, Medical College of Wisconsin, Milwaukee, WI, USA

Michael L. Steinberg, MD Department of Radiation Oncology, University of California Los Angeles, Los Angeles, CA, USA

Charles R. Thomas Jr., MD Department of Radiation Medicine, Knight Cancer Institute, Oregon Health & Science University, Portland, OR, USA

Ritchell van Dams, MD, MHS Department of Radiation Oncology, University of California Los Angeles, Los Angeles, CA, USA

Neha Vapiwala, MD, FACR University of Pennsylvania, Philadelphia, PA, USA

Paul E. Wallner, DO GenesisCare USA, Fort Myers, FL, USA
American Board of Radiology, Tucson, AZ, USA

Terry J. Wall, JD, MD TRI, PA, Kansas City, MO, USA

Joanne B. Weidhaas, MD, PhD, MSM University of California Los Angeles, Los Angeles, CA, USA

Christopher G. Willett, MD Department of Radiation Oncology, Duke University, Durham, NC, USA

Wendy A. Woodward, MD, PhD The University of Texas MD Anderson Cancer Center, Houston, TX, USA

Cheng-Chia Wu, MD, PhD Department of Radiation Oncology, Columbia University Irving Medical Center, Herbert Irving Comprehensive Cancer Center, New York, NY, USA

Sue S. Yom, MD, PhD, MAS University of California San Francisco, San Francisco, CA, USA

Part I
Career Planning

Career Options in Radiation Oncology

C. Norman Coleman

Three quotes, perhaps platitudes, are a useful way to start this book.

The first two have been attributed to various individuals. Yogi Berra, the major league catcher, is often the name associated with them. The third is a Chinese proverb:

> It's difficult to make predictions, especially about the future.

> The future ain't what it used to be

> If you do not change direction, you are likely to end up where you are headed

Subsections

- (**Disclaimer – this is personal opinion but based on interesting experiences**)
- Change is inevitable, and knowledge and information are expanding rapidly.
- Close doors very carefully.
- Conceptual leaps and disruptive change. Don't be fooled by bright-shiny objects.
- Current career options. Short-term opportunities to expand the denominator.
- Big teams can specialize. Competition should be for making progress not fighting it or each other.
- Radiation science has options beyond cancer care.
- Challenge conventional wisdom. When you feel too uppity, submit a grant!

C. N. Coleman (✉)
Radiation Research Program, National Cancer Institute (NCI), Bethesda, MD, USA

International Cancer Expert Corps (Approved Outside Activity by NCI/NIH),
Washington, DC, USA
e-mail: ccoleman@mail.nih.gov

© Springer Nature Switzerland AG 2021   3
R. A. Chandra et al. (eds.), *Career Development in Academic Radiation Oncology*, https://doi.org/10.1007/978-3-030-71855-8_1

- Careers and life are long. "Been there, done that" is an annoying construct for "What's next?".
- Physicians are a privileged lot with skills that are necessary. Content versus process.

Disclaimer: This Is Truly Personal Opinion But Based on Interesting Experiences

As are all chapters in this book, there is a good deal of personal opinion based on career and life experience. My perspective is from an era of medicine that saw the arrival of Medicare and government-funded programs, the determination of the structure and function of DNA, space flight, computers and transistors, television, ubiquitous car ownership, CT scans, medical subspecialty of oncology, radiology splitting into diagnosis and therapy, globalization of trade, and personal round-the-world travel. My training includes board certification in internal medicine, medical oncology, and radiation oncology with active clinical practice in medical and radiation oncology for 30 years. I have worked in labs for almost 50 years being a funded principal investigator for over 40. I've worked in academic practice in major teaching facilities and with visionary colleagues who actively established community outreach programs, often in underserved locales. For the past two decades, I have worked for the federal government where a good deal of our responsibility is to anticipate and plan for the future of the research of radiation oncology as a component of general oncology and the broader radiation sciences. The rapid change of generational perspective is recognized in that seminal events in one's life, for example, the terrorist attacks on the USA 20 years ago, may be distant historical events for those now entering medical school. COVID-19 struck during the time this chapter was written, and I am involved in managing disaster response as a nuclear/radiological expert. My family has traveled broadly with firsthand experience in a wide range of cultures, with a particular preference to listening, observing, and learning about differences and similarities. I have co-authored a book with my wife, a clinical social worker and trained mindfulness meditation teacher – technically unrelated but relevant to our professions – *Mindfulness for the High Performance World* (Springer Nature, 2019).

This chapter is my personal opinion that is not endorsed by the NCI or US government. I am a non-funded senior scientific advisor of a not-for-profit, the International Cancer Expert Corps, Inc (ICEC) which is an official "outside activity."

Change Is Inevitable, and Knowledge and Information Are Expanding Rapidly

Figure 1 makes it obvious for the need to have options in one's career. Even if it is the same general career, the content will change. Taken from a study of the National Academy of Sciences [1] is the graph showing the doubling time of information. The star is the date of the report with information-doubling time going from ~1 year to where it will be days as the "Internet of Things" takes hold. Information does not imply true knowledge or understanding, yet information can impact medical practice within days to weeks, as with diets of the day, pandemics, medical breakthroughs, testimonials of impact of something or other, and application of already-approved technology that might not require data, as seen with off-label use of drugs, application of radiation therapy techniques using existing linear accelerators, and nonregulated food supplements.

So, career options are essential in that there is a need to remain current to provide proper care to patients, and consequently not only will each individual's career have to adapt but it is likely that the configuration of practice will need to adapt numerous times in one's career due to the changing knowledge. Not only will change in a very positive way occur to advance cancer care based on scientific and conceptual advances, but it will also occur in the finance and structure of medical practice which may be a private sector, government program, or some amalgamation, required to reduce healthcare costs. In that this may well be detrimental to cancer care, there are career and skill options available to us that might minimize the care being diminished to patients for whom we are responsible.

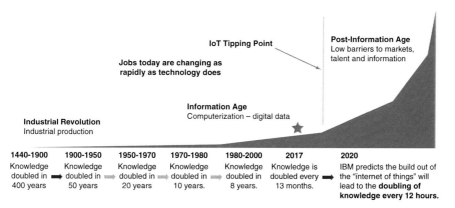

Fig. 1 Knowledge-doubling curve: The exponential increase in knowledge resulting from the growth of the "Internet of Things" (IoT). Used from source with permission. Star is the approximate time of the planning of this book. (Source [1]: https://www.nap.edu/catalog/25038/graduate-stem-education-for-the-21st-century)

An "assignment" I often suggested to incoming trainees is to look at an issue of the *New England Journal of Medicine*, the *International Journal of Radiation Oncology Biology Physics*, and *Science* from 10 and 20 years ago and see how much of that is "correct" and still an integral part of medical practice.

Close Doors Very Carefully

On more than rare occasion, an early-to-mid career colleague has noted that the expertise they had achieved early in their career, often in research or another discipline in college or graduate school, was surprisingly valuable as a radiation oncologist. To the contrary, other colleagues have lamented that they did not acquire sufficient skills in other medical disciplines through medical school electives or from choosing a PGY 1 year that did not provide sufficient breadth or responsibility for overall patient management. Some of the rotation choices have been due to the need for "auditioning" at a number of radiation oncology programs in order to secure a residency, losing valuable opportunities to absorb skills while still having the freedom of a student. Fortunately, some skills can be picked up later, such as returning to the lab and learning new techniques, by fellowship training or a sabbatical that might include general clinical responsibility.

Recognizing there is only so much one can actually do, one can remain connected to other areas of knowledge and skill by purposeful reading and educational opportunities beyond that "required" for one's career. If there is an area for which one is particularly interested or intrigued, it is wise to keep up as that might well reenter one's career (e.g., finance skills, political science, mathematics/statistics, policy, philosophy, art, law, or community outreach to the underserved/global health). The message here is hang on to and keep up with interests, no small feat during the decade or so of medical education and training, but surprisingly useful. Novel ideas frequently come from merging of concepts from seemingly disparate fields [2]. The other message is to read, read, read.

Conceptual Leaps and Disruptive Change. Don't Be Fooled by Bright-Shiny Objects

Aiming to avoid, hindsight embarrassment – if something looks, seems, or sounds dicey, wrong, or uncertain – it is likely dicey, wrong, and uncertain. Lab misinterpretation or even mistakes happen to studies of molecules and cells. That is bad for science and unwise for investors (e.g., the infamous Theranos story) if not corrected but usually not of great harm to patients. When the wrong questions are asked or experiments done poorly in preclinical animal studies, that is bad for the wasted creature and dangerous as it can be a step away from a clinical trial. A not-well-done clinical trial (poor design) or biased published clinical review or public statement can lead to a misapplication of a treatment, often as "off-label use" of a drug (i.e., use not formally approved by the FDA).

Radiation oncology has a particularly challenging situation as once our machines are approved, how they are specifically used is often unregulated, being subject to only to "guidelines" or reimbursement decisions or, as the final backstop, ethics. This happens all too often when groupthink applies new treatments to patients without reasonable data beyond a personal series [3]. It may be a fine treatment or nonsense so that data and ethics are essential. In the personal opinion style of this chapter, here are what I ask colleagues or advocates requesting that we go ahead with a new technology or drug:

1. Would you invest a substantial part of *your own 401 k* on this?
2. Would you agree to have this done to/for *your children*?
3. With 2–3 months to live, would you (or would you recommend to a patient to) travel a long distance to a center that advertises this treatment and spend 3 weeks and $100,000 on hope? (The *"what do I have to lose?"* Question may be answered with money, life, and time).
4. Is there well-done credible information as to *how does it actually work*?

One's career is peppered with dictums, suspect guidelines, and, as Eli Glatstein pointed out, "snake oil salesmen" [4]. Enthusiasm and creativity are most welcome linked to careful analysis and proper process to bring advances to patient care.

Current Career Options. Short-Term Opportunities to Expand the Denominator

When the issue of potential oversupply of radiation oncologists was raised, discussed more below, a group of experts in our field decided to reframe the issue [5]. Rather than too many (numerator) over need (denominator), the approach taken was "it's the denominator, stupid!" The paper published in 2019 described ten potential new career paths that will require radiation oncologists in areas that have opportunity now and into the future (Fig. 2).

Some of the career options are full-time, such as industry, frontier medicine, and government service. The others can be hybrid positions, including clinical radiation oncology with varying amount of time for the other activity, likely 40–80% of a full-time equivalent (FTE) doing clinical work and the remainder of the time in the "other" activity. One can readily envision dividing one person's requirement for providing clinical care among two or more people. Or one person may do a portion of the 100% for clinical care and the remainder "paid for" by external support from grants, contracts, foundations, agencies, or direct charitable donation. But, paying a salary nowadays is often tied to billable relative value units or other

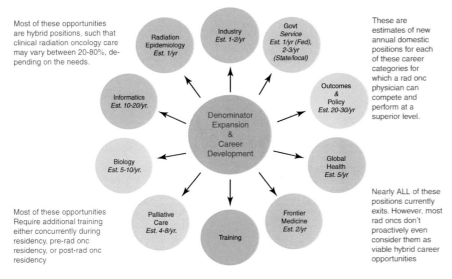

Fig. 2 Expanding the scope of radiation oncology careers. The circles each represent existing careers considered in this paper that are evolving and carry potential for new dimensions. They are a mixture of hybrid positions that can be additive to clinical radiation oncology practice (e.g., outcomes and policy), positions that could require additional formal training (e.g., epidemiology or palliative care), and full-time opportunities (e.g., government service and industry). The number of opportunities per year is an estimate based on current experience and ongoing early expansion; creation (i.e., new positions that need to be filled) of even 20 full-time equivalents annually (10–15% of graduates) could have a substantial impact on radiation oncology. Some areas, such as global health, could require many more individuals per year and offer the opportunity for fully or partially retired radiation oncologists to increase years of work, serving as mentors for program building in underserved communities globally and domestically and opening or accelerating opportunities for those earlier in their career. (Reprinted with permission from Vapiwala [5])

institution-imposed metrics of what is valued and supportable. While conditions of employment vary, some people may only request a partial salary; however, as discussed next, it is possible for these "other pathways" in Fig. 2 to be considered an *integral part* of a position if what that does is seen as valued for the institution, department, or practice.

Big Teams Can Specialize. Competition Should Be for Making Progress Not Fighting It or One Another

Having the time and opportunity to expand one's horizon and skills seems like a luxury, but it should not be. This investment in people can reduce physician burnout, which may pay for itself simply by having folks work longer and/or at least having people enjoy their careers and add breadth and depth to their lives. Seemingly eons ago I chaired a program in Boston that built a substantial network of academic and community hospitals, creating a community network from a novel model academic program established by my predecessor, Dr. Sam Hellman, called the Harvard Joint Center for Radiation Therapy. Our community outreach models (not satellites!!) were staffed by full-time Harvard faculty whose primary assignment was a clinical facility in the community, each person with a day per week for truly academic time, including time in Boston as they so chose [6]. The advent of the hospital wars and network tussles changed that, but the fact that one could have a range of talent and venues within a large-sized faculty with a common goal of establishing a top rate department with superb care and research as the overarching goals demonstrates one can work with the collegial side of clinicians, although possibly less so for administrators (whose salaries are earned by the doctors yet they control medical practice).

Healthcare in America has its problems patently obvious during the COVID-19 crisis. Therefore, collaborative models with the balanced sharing of personnel, resources, time, and ideas might be possible and acceptable by demonstrating a value proposition to the community practice members and administration. The complex world of radiation oncology involves not only site-specific and often surgical expertise and includes very complex and expensive technology so that when over-proliferation occurs, it is obvious. Duplication of technology and highly specialized treatments such as particle radiotherapy, many programs of which have been economic disasters due to over-proliferation, are best shared. Possibly new models (or resurrection of successful approaches in the prehospital war era) lend itself to experiments. Such a concept is in Fig. 3 [7].

Like any well-constructed team, sharing of the expertise enables both more breadth and depth. Many practices are being acquired by academic departments, enlarging the integrated talent pool. Certainly, cooperation even among so-called competitors is conceivable. The blue trapezoid indicates that more can be obtained by partnering than by spending time duplicating efforts and technology by competing, although hospital systems seem to have business models built on their doctors doing the latter. What this approach could create are novel career paths, innovative resource-conserving partnerships, and much bigger impact. Clearly, as seen during the COVID-19 epidemic, our US healthcare system is much more interdependent than recognized so that lessons learned from the pandemic might well call for new models with shared "expensive" radiation oncology being a pilot or pioneer. Perhaps this can be a goal for the administration/policy experts in our field.

Radiation Science Has Options Beyond Cancer Care

And, there's more!!

A few years ago, when the term "personalized medicine" was renamed by a senior leader as "precision medicine," we math and physics types were somewhat amazed, although one wonders if the distinction between precise and accurate was on purpose realizing how far off the mark oncology was or just a catchy name. The

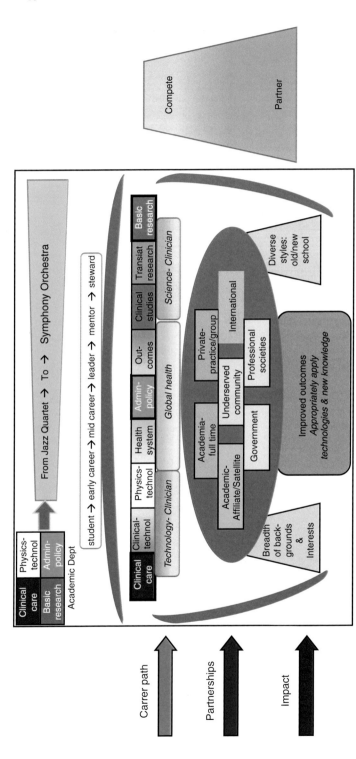

Fig. 3 Inside the box, the traditional four pillars of an academic department are indicated in the boxes on the upper left (red, white, green, and blue). The phases of a career are below the title, going from trainee to steward as experience, knowledge, and wisdom expand. To meet emerging challenges, the four classic pillars require new expertise, included in the five additional boxes. New positions for formal interdisciplinary linkage (three boxes with italics (technology clinician, science clinician, and global health) are proposed, for which 20–30% of dedicated time is supported by the enterprise: a clinician who keeps the group up to date with emerging technologies, one who does so with emerging science, and one committed to global health. Their responsibility is for the enterprise to be on the leading edge. The oval contains the players. Our field's diversity and breadth (gray trapezoids) provides a plethora of skills. Outside the box are three arrows that this model can enhance, career path, partnerships, and impact, and how professionals can interact with one another – compete versus partner. The goal is improved outcomes for our patients and the global community and a model for the medical profession. (Modified from [7])

original wasn't so bad. A group of us who look at horizons for our field (from NCI and CERN) were preparing a chapter for a book on particle therapy and were using the descriptor "at the crossroads" when we realized that radiation oncology sciences are much different than other medical disciplines. Figure 4 uses the rotary for the intersection of four crossroads, with the different colors showing a pair. The concept that struck us is reflected in the complex title: *Accurate, Precision Radiation Medicine: A Meta-Strategy for Impacting Cancer Care, Global Health, and Nuclear Policy and Mitigating Radiation Injury From Necessary Medical Use, Space Exploration, and Potential Terrorism* [8]. As we note, even in the absence of cancer care, what radiation oncology touches on reflects broad aspects of society from healthcare systems, cancer care, terrorism, nuclear power (and global climate change), health disparities, complex technology, space exploration, environmental contamination, and fundamental relationship between physics and biology.

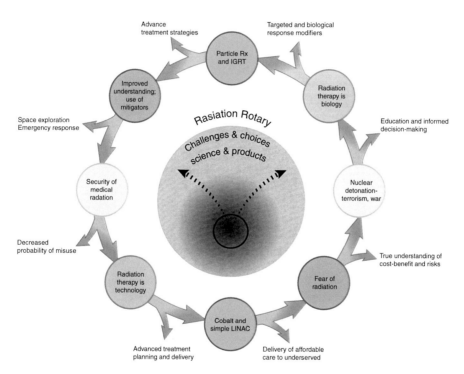

Fig. 4 The radiation rotary. There are a number of crossroads facing the field of radiation sciences, best addressed as part of a rotary. Four sets of issues are illustrated, with both sides of a particular issue in circles of the same color: (1) cancer care (blue); (2) global collaboration (orange); (3) nuclear policy (yellow); and (4) mitigating radiation injury (purple). Talent and ideas entering the rotary face challenges and choices that will lead to unique collaborations, new knowledge, and products that, in turn, will impact greater society in general. The scope of talent and opportunities is large. Even in the more limited context of cancer treatment, there is a wide range of expertise needed to carry out the work intended in the radiation rotary, including specialized chemistry, physics, biology, and medical skills. Abbreviations: IGRT, image-guided radiation therapy; linac, linear accelerator. (Reprinted from [8])

Figure 1 illustrates that having growth potential for one's talents and skills is welcome and necessary. Figure 2 includes career options generally within medical careers, and Fig. 4 contains an array of opportunities for radiation oncologists to use their skills, even well beyond clinical radiation oncology. To do the latter may require diverging from or leaving one's career; however, given the technological nature of radiation oncology with expensive equipment and the need for us to know oncology, immunology, physics, basic science, and health policy, the novel means of collaboration as in Fig. 3 might make it possible to do a lot more within your career than you may have realized when you opened this book.

Challenge Conventional Wisdom. When You Feel too Uppity, Submit a Grant!

Being filled with optimism and boundless opportunities is a great approach to a career. Of course, the routine aspects of a career are required with attention to detail. Of the fears one should never lose in a profession that is responsible for people's lives is that of insufficient knowledge, even more challenging based on the timeline in Fig. 1. The practice model in Fig. 3 allows for a big enough team to be able to have team members educate one another and have the best treatments available for every locale in their practice.

From time to time, people get a bit carried away with their idea or finding. Some are sufficiently talented in thinking and communicating that success often follows success. Since it is not likely that all disease will be eradicated without toxicity in our careers, some sense of humility in our knowledge and skills is particularly wise. The advice in this section as the cure for being uppity is to submit a grant. Any of your colleagues who have had a few trips through this will nod approvingly. Subject your ideas to detailed scrutiny and listen to the comments and suggestions. Some will be infuriating and some will be wrong but take the time to learn and remember your "era" of science will makes it mark but better will follow.

But all that being said, it is easy to take rejection or criticism personally. Having a paper rejected or grant not funded are both more likely to occur than being serially successful. So, presumably by the fact you're reading this book you made it to medical school, you have passed a substantial screening procedure and have been given an opportunity to use your mind and be creative. Despite setbacks, remember the three quotes from the beginning of the chapter, and don't ever stop being creative and inquisitive.

Careers and Life Are Long. "Been There, Done That" Is an Annoying Construct for "What's Next?"

The chapters in this book have a superb set of authors and topics. That the hub and spoke of career-enhancing opportunities in Fig. 2 came about because of a feeling/concern of oversupply of radiation oncologists was soon followed by a decline in resident applicants. Nothing like a crisis to sharpen attention and make changes (I believe a concept raised by Sir Winston Churchill).

In a book about radiation oncology careers, these are worth examining:

1. Was the wrong message conveyed? Was there a general oversupply or a focal oversupply?
2. If the issue is supply, is it one of fixing the numerator to make it smaller or the denominator to make it bigger? Or possibly redefining what is included in radiation oncology?
3. Were the resident education, training, and experience unsuitable?

Being a specialty attentive to the issues of trainees having created by the force of the trainees the Association for Residents in Radiation Oncology as part of the American Society for Radiation Oncology (ARRO/ASTRO), the specialty properly surveyed the residents with the following list of 14 specific concerns (Fig. 5).

The top concerns were the topic of the Kahn paper, and the bottom concerns are an interpretation of mine. In some sense it can be a bit of a career timeline from top being trainee, middle mid-career leaders, and bottom, senior stewards. All the points are appropriate and, as with the hub-and-spoke chart of Fig. 2, providing terrific career-long options and steps to make important contributions in addition to being a superb physician from trainee to steward in Fig. 3.

Physicians Are a Privileged Lot with Skills That Are Necessary. Content Versus Process

Returning to the beginning quotation "If you do not change direction, you are likely to end up where you are headed" and having practiced three medical subspecialties, from close to the beginning of radiation and medical oncology as their own specialties, and from 20+ years in government, one can lose perspective on the very privileged roles we serve in society. As seen now in COVID-19 and I experienced in Japan, the physicians are highly trusted. This is especially so in situations where major judgments must be made based on partial information, as is required for emergency medicine and surprisingly so for oncology as the final tumor profile, gene sequence, and metabolic (and microbiome) status are not known at the time a treatment decision must be made.

Can (should) we build bottom up and top down?

Item	Overall Rank	Rank Distribution	Score	No.of Rankings
Job Market	1		1,958	156
ABR Written Examinations: Radbio and physics	2		1,692	146
Residency Expansion	3		1,316	144
oral Boards	4		1,316	134
Maintaining/declining reimbursement in the era of hypofractionation	5		1,273	145
Variability in Training in Residency	6		1,059	122
Fellowship expansions	7		1,035	126
Other specialties' awareness and understanding of radiation oncology	8		846	120
Assessing technical competence in providing radiation for practitoners far out of training	9		750	115
Trainee specific funding available for research	10		711	112
Gender Inequity in Radiation Oncology	11		690	113
Medical Student interest in the field/ exposure	12		680	114
Parental Leave polocies	13		575	107
Racial Diversity/ Inequity in Radiation Oncology	14		544	103

Top Concerns of Radiation Oncology Trainess in 2019: Job Market, Board Examinations, and Residency Expansion

Bottom Concerns for 2020+ : low because they aren't concerns and are okey? Or just not as bad as others?

← Lowest Rank   Highest Rank →

Fig. 5 Radiation oncology trainee responses to "Please rank in order any issues that concern you as a future radiation oncologist." The chart is from the paper; the side comments are added. (Modified from Kahn et al. [9])

Experience in government and policy is that there are many people who know process, some having decision-making and analytical skills, but when the topic is health of people, it is the content - complex knowledge of disease, people, and treatment that matter. Often process folks outnumber content folks in policy working groups. There are a very limited number who are skilled at both. Communication and listening skills are essential, and for our specialty to make the contributions, we must have a broad scientific, technological, and sociological background as well as a sufficient number of us expert in medical reimbursement, healthcare policy, and politics.

Regarding privilege, I'll end with a short anecdote from my time as a department chair at Harvard when our faculty was arguing about salary, one even likening themself to being like a "free agent" in sports. A colleague and friend who grew up in the UK in a very working-class neighborhood finally spoke up and reminded us "We are in the TOP 1% in salary in the USA." Our privilege and responsibility given to us by being physicians and the access we are given to very personal life stories from our patients and families as oncologists in our life-and-death business is in itself an enormous reward. Having freedom to grow and flourish throughout a career is another compensation. One of my middle-age Hodgkin disease patients who had been very successful in business and who was then having inexorable disease progression remarked how fortunate I was as … "I wish, like you, I had had a calling."

We Are Cancer Doctors and Radiation Is Scary

Finishing with the truly personal opinion motif of this chapter, radiation oncology is an interesting specialty as it involves complex technology; fundamental interaction of physics with biology; molecular mechanisms of disease; perturbations in tumor, normal tissue, and the immune system by radiation; patient care for a wide variety of diseases; normal tissue injury that impacts energy policy and space flight; and an essential component of cancer care globally from the most expensive technology to basic linear accelerators in poor countries and poor isolated regions in our own resource-rich country. What we do for our living was better stated to me as a comment to a presentation regarding the ongoing nuclear power plant disaster in Japan: "he works on the 2 most frightening things in the world, cancer and radiation!". We have a specialty that is small enough so that we can truly be familiar with a large proportion of us globally. That the editors and authors had the forethought to even write such a book speaks to how we in radiation oncology are stewards of our specialty and its members.

You are students and trainees with 4–5 decades to go. There will always be the need to anticipate change, guide transitions, and find dilemmas that can use a second (or tenth) opinion. And, there are societal, social, and economic problems that will need constant attention, some so difficult that they are largely ignored. The obvious example is yet again the price of inequality seen during the COVID-19 pandemic. Passion for a cause is good. But, I suggest taking on some problem or injustice you may have already encountered and that you despise, for example, inequality of access to healthcare and education, ignorance in decision-making by using political gain over knowledge, simplistic solutions to a complex problem, unabated climate change, etc., and aim to help solve it as long as it may take. Having forward-looking actions in desperate times – a patient with cancer, a world with potential nuclear war, or a pandemic that requires experimentation and thinking – enables one to be a part of or even a driver of a solution as a trusted professional seeking to help others in times of life crisis.

Final advice: (1) Read, read, read. (2) Join the American Association for the Advancement of Science (AAAS), subscribe to the paper journal, and look at all the pages in each issue. (3) Relish a career that has so many opportunities to learn and to serve others.

For Discussion with a Mentor or Colleague

- How can I find a mentor who can think both within the context of radiation oncology and beyond into our role in greater society?
- How can I sequence and balance my career and family realizing that it is really impossible to do it entirely correctly?
- How should I respond when I have a great idea and I am told by an attending, administrator, or supervisor "it can't be done?"

References

1. Graduate STEM education for the 21st Century. Available at: https://www.nap.edu/catalog/25038/graduate-stem-education-for-the-21st-century. Accessed 11 Apr 2020.
2. Dyer J, Gregersen H, Christensen CM. The innovator's DNA: mastering the five skills of disruptive innovators. 1st ed. Boston: Harvard Business Review Press; 2011.
3. Coleman CN, Ahmed MM. Implementation of new biology-based radiation therapy technology: when is it ready so "perfect makes practice?". Int J Radiat Oncol Biol Phys. 2019;105(5):934–7. https://doi.org/10.1016/j.ijrobp.2019.08.013.
4. Glatstein E. The return of the snake oil salesmen. Int J Radiat Oncol Biol Phys. 2003;55(3):561–2. No abstract available. PMID: 12573740.
5. Vapiwala N, Thomas CR Jr, Grover S, Yap ML, Mitin T, Shulman LN, Gospodarowicz MK, Longo J, Petereit DG, Ennis RD, Hayman JA, Rodin D, Buchsbaum JC, Vikram B, Abdel-Wahab M, Epstein AH, Okunieff P, Goldwein J, Kupelian P, Weidhaas JB, Tucker MA, Boice JD Jr, Fuller CD, Thompson RF, Trister AD, Formenti SC, Barcellos-Hoff MH, Jones J, Dharmarajan KV, Zietman AL, Coleman CN. Enhancing career paths for tomorrow's radiation oncologists. Int J Radiat Oncol Biol Phys. 2019;105(1):52–63. https://doi.org/10.1016/j.ijrobp.2019.05.025. Epub 2019 May 22. Review. No abstract available. PMID: 31128144.
6. Linggood R, Govern F. Coleman CN. A blueprint for linking academic oncology and the community. J Health Polit Policy Law. 1998;23(6):973–94. PMID: 9866095.
7. Coleman CN. Masters of our destiny: from Jazz quartet to symphony orchestra. Int J Radiat Oncol Biol Phys. 2016;96(3):511–3. https://doi.org/10.1016/j.ijrobp.2016.07.006. No abstract available. PMID: 27681746.
8. Coleman CN, Prasanna PGS, Bernhard EJ, Buchsbaum JC, Ahmed MM, Capala J, Obcemea C, Deye JA, Pistenmma DA, Vikram B, Bernier J, Dosanjh M. Accurate, precision radiation medicine: a meta-strategy for impacting cancer care, global health, and nuclear policy and mitigating radiation injury from necessary medical use, space exploration, and potential terrorism. Int J Radiat Oncol Biol Phys. 2018;101(2):250–3. https://doi.org/10.1016/j.ijrobp.2018.02.001. No abstract available. PMID: 29726348.
9. Kahn J, Goodman CR, Albert A, Agarwal A, Jeans E, Tye K, Campbell SR, Marcrom S, Colbert LE. Top concerns of radiation oncology trainees in 2019: job market, board examinations, and residency expansion. Int J Radiat Oncol Biol Phys. 2020;106(1):19–25. https://doi.org/10.1016/j.ijrobp.2019.07.006. Epub 2019 Oct 21. No abstract available. PMID: 31648872.

Foundations for a Successful Career

Neha Vapiwala and Thomas Buchholz

Introduction

Key attributes for career success in the world of academia are not dissimilar to those critical for personal success. While a solid educational background and technical expertise are certainly requisite, they form the foundation upon which other factors create a ladder for continued advancement. Traditional educational models and curricula for healthcare training are very focused on the "hard skills," the basic how-to's, and know-how's of one's trade. The literature suggests, however, that it is the so-called "soft skills" or leadership attributes that comprise 75% of career success. Too often, careers can get side-tracked because inadequate attention is paid to these relationship skills. In this chapter, we will review the myriad competencies that contribute to professional and personal success in academic environments and beyond. Some represent natural tendencies and habits of mind, while others may be skills to be acquired. In all cases, these are traits that can be developed and strengthened over time.

Getting Started: Identifying Opportunities

Establishing a successful career starts with earning a reputation for capability and reliability. When first establishing this reputation – whether for a new position or a new institution – showing up and demonstrating a willingness, if not downright

N. Vapiwala (✉)
University of Pennsylvania, Philadelphia, PA, USA
e-mail: vapiwala@pennmedicine.upenn.edu

T. Buchholz
Scripps MD Anderson Cancer Center, San Diego, CA, USA
e-mail: Buchholz.Thomas@scrippshealth.org

© Springer Nature Switzerland AG 2021
R. A. Chandra et al. (eds.), *Career Development in Academic Radiation Oncology*, https://doi.org/10.1007/978-3-030-71855-8_2

eagerness to take on the necessary tasks can leave an indelible impression. The appeal of the actual tasks may need to take a backseat in these beginning stages, when your attitude and energy are what others are monitoring – the oft-used but still relevant concept of being a "true team player." Having the skill set and resourcefulness to get the job done is requisite, however, since it's not the eagerness but the follow-through that ultimately translates to trustworthiness. A *curriculum vitae* with many abstracts but lacking in manuscripts can be more concerning than one with a limited but comparable number of both; enthusiasm is great, but execution is critical. A solid work ethic and willingness to roll up one's sleeves for the task at hand are foundational to a reputation for capability and reliability. In cases where the tasks at hand entail new collaborations and team interactions, open and early communication regarding the individual roles and responsibilities of team members can lead to successful outcomes for the group. Listening more than leading is the name of the game in these earlier days, when you may be the newest member on the team.

There are a host of opportunities that can be sought out early in a professional career. One pathway toward success is to find leadership opportunities in areas of less interest to others. Rather than immediately competing to be a principal investigator on a cooperative group phase III trial, for example, new junior faculty can instead volunteer for a variety of lower-profile but high-yield tasks, such as organizing a monthly grand rounds lectureship series (fantastic way to network with senior invited speakers), developing quality or clinical efficiency initiatives, and/or reshaping the medical student clinical rotation. Another successful strategy is to look at the portfolio of leadership responsibilities of your mentor or your chair and volunteer to take over some of the less glamorous responsibilities. Successful senior faculty members are often overwhelmed with institutional and national responsibilities and are eager to pass along some of the less visible but still important leadership tasks.

Another attribute of early career success is the willingness to say yes. Junior faculty are often given the advice to focus, which allows one to define a niche in a subspecialty area of study and build a reputation of excellence within a specific domain. Therefore, the recommendation to always be receptive to opportunities, even if they come at the expense of time and opportunity costs, may seem counterintuitive. Numerous career benefits can often be found in a variety of areas that may not seem to obvious when first presented. For example, service on an institutional review board (IRB) or grant review panel requires a lot of time and effort. However, the skills learned during this service are invaluable to understanding how to efficiently write a protocol or a grant. In addition, the network of experienced colleagues you meet in such committees can lead to new collaborations. Other examples include leading a journal club or a multidisciplinary conference that focuses on a controversial clinical topic. Such efforts can lead to new research protocols or a review paper on a timely topic. Finally, volunteering to review papers for peer-reviewed medical journals gives junior faculty insights into how to successfully publish. In addition, when appropriate, you can volunteer to write an accompanying editorial and begin to establish an authoritative voice within your field. To be invited to review papers is not that challenging. Editors are always interested in finding reviewers that can be counted on to provide timely and thoughtful reviews. You can also enlist senior faculty colleagues to contact section editors and offer your name as a potential reviewer. Finally, there is little harm in directly reaching out to editorial boards and expressing this interest yourself.

As your leadership team and institution become more familiar with your positive attitude and consistent work ethic, the opportunities and invitations to collaborate should increase, permitting further reinforcement of your can-do attitude and also ultimately placing you in a position where you can gradually but steadily become more selective. In turn, true academic success will be measured not just by the projects you lead, but by the various opportunities you pass along to more junior or more qualified colleagues and ultimately those you create for others.

Developing Skill Sets for Success: Clinical, Research and Publishing, Communication

Strong people skills still require a solid foundation in the craft in order to translate to recognition and respect. From a clinical standpoint, radiation oncologists not only need to master oncologic principles for all cancer types, adult and pediatric, but they must also integrate radiation biology, medical physics, diagnostic imaging, histopathology, and three-dimensional anatomy – a daunting list. Further, the proficient radiation oncologist is also well-versed in the surgical and medical oncology literature so as to contribute meaningfully to the multidisciplinary cancer care team. The knowledge base is important, but resourcefulness is critical. No matter what path your career takes you, being highly respected as a clinician and having respect as a radiation oncologist should be a cornerstone of your professional identity.

Given continually emerging and evolving data, the ability to efficiently curate what matters from the overwhelming amount of available content is an added survival advantage. Learning how to multitask, if not already a natural inclination, can be particularly useful in our current environment of constant digital access to each other and the resulting expectations of 24/7 availability and rapid turnaround. While it's important to focus on singular tasks when the occasion calls for it (i.e., when speaking to a patient), and to unplug regularly from a well-being standpoint, it's rare to find a successful academic physician who isn't emailing while walking, reading while on conference calls, working on the laptop while watching TV.

Academic careers often offer the chance to subspecialize in one or more particular areas of interest. Sub-specialization permits you to gain content expertise, develop relationships with national colleagues and close working relationships with multidisciplinary team members, and establish greater efficiencies in clinical work.

Once the clinical foundation is established, there are academic skill sets that are also fundamental to early success in a junior faculty's career path. Formal instruction and/or hands-on practice in protocol, grant, and/or manuscript writing is essential. As mentioned, serving on review committees such as the IRB, grant review committees, and manuscript reviews teaches you invaluable lessons about scientific design, feasibility, and biostatistics. Translating these skills into your own original work requires additional effort. This is an area where mentorship from an experienced and successful academic colleague can be helpful. In addition to clinical excellence, most academic radiation oncology careers include conducting and publishing original research. With respect to the conduct of original research, we have found the following tenets to be of importance:

1. Develop a collaborative co-investigator team at the very onset of a research project, rather than during or toward the end. When starting an academic project, it is advisable to write a 1- to 2-page proposal highlighting the background, methods, and timeline of the project. Defining authorship roles at the onset often avoids controversies later. Written project descriptions also help you to find out if someone else in the institution may be working on the exact or similar subject. This can help to avoid a challenging political situation later.
2. Follow through on all of your projects to completion and keep your collaborators involved and informed. It is not uncommon for junior faculty to have too many pending works, with too few converted into peer-review publications.
3. Choose mentees wisely – working with students and residents can be tremendously rewarding and also requires substantial time and effort. Prior to taking on too many mentees, junior faculty should first become very comfortable with their own ability to complete projects and manage time.
4. Develop an effective biostatistical collaborator – this helps to assure the integrity of the final product and is a very important key to success.

A second and equally important academic and clinical skill is learning how to effectively communicate. Communication is a cornerstone of being a good doctor. Seeing patients even when not convenient, reporting back to referring doctors, and explaining your thought process are integral skills for building a reputation as a go-to radiation oncologist. These communication skills can be practiced and refined throughout one's career, from standardized patient encounters in medical school to oral examinations for radiation oncology board certification to workshops for practicing oncologists (e.g., Health Literacy and Communication Strategies in Oncology, sponsored by the National Cancer Policy Forum in collaboration with the Roundtable on Health Literacy, July 15–16, 2019, Washington, DC). The impact of low health literacy among patients on compliance and eventual outcomes is sobering. Thus, the ability to both compassionately and effectively communicate some of the highly enigmatic and technical aspects of radiation therapy delivery in a manner that is accessible to patients and loved ones can be transformative. It can make you the oncologist that patients want to see. Master the art and the science, and you can become the physician to whom others send their family members.

Communication skills are also critical with respect to presenting original research or giving a seminar/grand rounds. Professional communication is a skill that can be taught and should be learned. Effective communicators are noticed. When attending meetings, rate the presentations you hear and decide what characteristics made them compelling or boring. If provided with an opportunity to give a lecture, take time to make sure it will be remembered by the audience. Once you gain a reputation as an excellent speaker, numerous additional opportunities will come your way. Most promotion committees like to see evidence of a national reputation of excellence, so seek out opportunities to be included in scientific forums and use these opportunities to make a positive impression.

A final attribute that determines success concerns the ability to develop effective relationships. It is important to recognize colleagues' perspectives, their history within the organization, and their personal goals. Acknowledge how they may have built a foundation that now allows for junior faculty opportunities. Relationships with multidisciplinary colleagues are critical for both academic and clinical success. Too often a misunderstanding about authorship credit can lead to a long-standing competitive rather than collaborative environment. Find ways to become an integrated team member who focuses on overarching mission goals such as providing outstanding clinical care or contributing to practice changing research, rather than solely on one's own career success. Individuals who can combine this attribute with a personal effectiveness at clinical and academic success are those most likely to gain leadership opportunities.

Becoming a Leader

As a career progresses, faculty who have achieved initial success are often given leadership opportunities. Many skills that lead to early career success, such as effective communication, efficient work habits, and effective ability to develop relationships, overlap with skills necessary for being an effective leader. However, leadership skills encompass a greater portfolio that may require additional training. An oft-overlooked technical skill that is important throughout one's career is meeting etiquette and management. A natural and unavoidable extension of our clinical, research, administrative, and volunteer committee responsibilities, meetings are a science of their own and require structure and planning. Too often, attendees of departmental or institutional meetings will attend them wondering what the purpose of the meetings is, sit through them feeling distracted and overwhelmed with other more pressing tasks, and/or leave the meetings thinking they were a waste of time. Whether in-person or virtual and whether you are attending or leading, meetings can serve an important purpose if organized and conducted properly. Clear meeting agendas provided with notice, involvement of only key players, respect of operating norms, and conclusion of every meeting with summary points and/or action items are just a few general steps that can help combat the aforementioned negative perceptions. There are a variety of resources for effective meeting management that one can use to hone these skills, as a natural extension of being a good colleague .

Effective communication also applies to the meeting management skills. In every meeting, being mindful of one's title and position and how it may influence others' willingness to speak is important. Encouraging meeting attendees to contribute requires creation of a safe space; stimulating discussion, allowing for dissenting opinions, and developing consensus moving forward are strategies that lean heavily on one's listening skills, reputation for openness, and ability to keep biases (philosophical, political, and interpersonal) in check.

As noted, leadership opportunities can bring new challenges to one's careers. It is important that leaders are open to continually learning from others – regardless of their rank and age – and to sharing their own didactic and experiential knowledge. Both are at the heart of being a respected leader. Many institutions offer faculty leadership academies that teach fundamentals of leadership including faculty management, strategic planning, and business operations and finance.

As leaders develop, they should also begin to focus on mentorship. Leaders are responsible for group success more than individual success. During the transition to leadership, it is important to understand that individuals find success in very diverse ways. Whether it's a formal lecture or bedside teaching, cognizance of different learning styles and adaptation accordingly can make the difference between connecting with the learner versus not. Mentorship requires common traits from both the mentor and mentee – commitment, mutual respect, clear expectations with follow-through, willingness to both give and receive feedback, and content expertise. A mentee with a strong track record in these areas is likely to make a smooth transition to mentor, to one who listens, guides, and creates opportunities and connections. In the mentor role, you may serve in different capacities to different mentees, or to the same mentee at different times, tailoring to what is needed. Being recognized as a mentor is in many ways the pinnacle of success and fulfillment in academia. Promoting success around you elevates everyone.

Institutional Considerations

There are other key attributes for a strong foundation and success in academic medicine that are more external-facing. If and as one advances up the career ladder to leadership positions such as departmental program director, vice chair, chair, or dean, there is an accompanying and increasing need for thoughtful and nimble decision-making. Defining your team's mission, vision, and core values is the crucial first step. This process should be done with engagement of the entire team such that they feel co-ownership. The mission, vision, and core values serve as a foundation for decision-making and strategic planning. Leaders should use these to help define a culture and then work with the team to define expectations and accountability. For example, most teams would agree that they wish to work in a professional environment, free of intimidation, harassment, and anger. Setting this expectation with the group prior to any incidents rather than in reaction to an incident helps to establish a culture and makes any subsequent potentially uncomfortable conversation with members who haven't adhered to these expectations a bit easier. Expectations should also be communicated in a fair and transparent fashion concerning clinical productivity metrics, academic accountability, and other performance measures.

Identifying, engaging, and building consensus among these team members are necessary for buy-in and viability and often requires a large investment of time and resources. When done well and regularly, however, building consensus can serve to reinforce your leadership. While some directions and decisions will not be up for discussion, to the extent that plurality of input united by singularity of purpose can drive the agenda, trust in the leader can be earned and engendered. Establishing a culture of trust rests on demonstrating respect for the individuals on the team, while establishing and communicating clear and transparent expectations and metrics, both verbally and in writing. Transparent and fair processes require more than communication; leaders should continually check their biases, assumptions, and personal actions to minimize, if not eliminate, discrimination of individuals and ideas. Taking a further step to understand the perspectives of your team members, to periodically walk in the shoes of your direct reports – or at least imagine doing so – can further reinforce your accessibility and openness. Addressing inefficiencies and low-hanging fruit to enable your team members to function better at and outside of work can reap endless dividends.

Just like the personal skills discussed above, there are some essential "hard skills" of leadership that should be acquired. Management skills and business acumen have historically been foreign concepts in medical training, but are increasingly a focus in today's healthcare environment. As an academic leader, you are expected to manage a large-scale business and are accountable for finances. Identifying and recruiting good people with administrative and financial expertise to complete your leadership bench will enable realization of the agreed-upon mission, vision, and core values. Of course, this doesn't just apply to the leadership bench. Surrounding yourself with the best people – easier said than done – and recognizing and rewarding them are integral to ultimate success.

Summary Points

- Soft skills, such as interpersonal and communication skills, are a critical component of career success for a successful academic radiation oncologist.
- Early in one's career, developing a reputation for dependability and a "can-do" attitude are critical in creating opportunities for future success.
- As one advances into levels of higher leadership, a focus on building in the areas of team building and vision setting is important, as is an emphasis on mentorship and building in to other team members.
- Indeed as one advances higher, an emphasis on a different skill set is required.

For Discussion with a Mentor or Colleague

- What are some soft skill areas where I could stand to develop and that you've found especially important in your career to date?
- What sorts of experiences should I obtain to develop myself for future leadership roles and advancement?
- Are there specific individuals you'd suggest I speak with locally and nationally for mentorship?

Suggested References

1. Green A, Hauser J. Managing to change the world: The nonprofit manager's guide to getting results paperback: John Wiley & Sons; 2012.
2. McNamara C. Field guide to leadership and supervision in business and field guide to leadership and supervision for nonprofit staff: Authenticity Consulting, LLC; 2010.

Strategies for Applicants Belonging to Underrepresented Groups

Curtiland Deville Jr. and Charles R. Thomas Jr.

Introduction

The path to radiation oncology for students and trainees from demographic groups that are underrepresented in radiation oncology, such as women and/or racial and ethnic minority groups that are historically underrepresented in medicine (URM), may be long and challenging and at times may seem insurmountable. Moreover, career advancement and professional development within radiation oncology may seem similarly difficult for underrepresented trainees, junior and mid-level faculty, and practicing physicians, given the disproportionate underrepresentation and systemic bias encountered. The purpose of this chapter is to reveal the barriers, obstacles, and deterrents to training and career advancement and to elucidate the successful strategies to specialty entry and professional development so that you may thrive in your future careers as academic radiation oncologists.

Physician Workforce Trends

Having an awareness of the physician workforce data is paramount to your success given the overwhelming isolation, hypervisibility, and otherness that you may experience at times in your academic progression. Women, Blacks, Hispanics, American

C. Deville Jr. (✉)
Department of Radiation Oncology and Molecular Radiation Sciences,
Johns Hopkins University School of Medicine, Baltimore, MD, USA
e-mail: cdeville@jhmi.edu

C. R. Thomas Jr.
Department of Radiation Medicine, Knight Cancer Institute, Oregon Health & Science
University, Portland, OR, USA
e-mail: thomasch@ohsu.edu

© Springer Nature Switzerland AG 2021   25
R. A. Chandra et al. (eds.), *Career Development in Academic Radiation
Oncology*, https://doi.org/10.1007/978-3-030-71855-8_3

Indians, Alaska Natives, Native Hawaiians, and other Pacific Islanders remain disproportionately underrepresented in radiation oncology relative to other medical specialties [1]. While URM and female representation of residents continues to improve in medical school and graduate medical education, the rate of increase had been less for women and largely unchanged for URM groups in radiation oncology [2, 3]. The male predominance of the field also acts to exacerbate the disparities in Black representation, given the increased proportions of Black women entering medical school [4]. Limited data are available regarding the representation of other demographic groups in radiation oncology, such as disabled [5], veterans, sexual and gender minorities [6], religious minorities, disadvantaged background (e.g. lower socioeconomic status), first generation, immigrants, and international medical graduates [7]. However, future attention to these specific groups is warranted to ensure specialty diversification that mirrors both US society and the broader medical school, graduate medical education (GME), and practicing physician pools and to ensure that other structural and systemic barriers are removed for all of those interested in the field. While the concepts discussed in this chapter largely focus on women and URM groups, they may still be extrapolated to other demographically underrepresented groups.

Several imperatives support a diverse workforce. Increasing workforce diversity has been tasked by accrediting bodies such as the Liaison Committee for Medical Education and the Accreditation Council for Graduate Medical Education (ACGME). The clinical imperative is illustrated by data showing that minority providers are more likely to practice in underserved communities [8], that physician-patient race concordance improves communication effectiveness and trust for minority patients [9], and that medical school with more diverse medical student bodies produce students that feel more comfortable managing patients from diverse backgrounds [10]. The business rationale demonstrates that diverse teams produce better innovation, profits, and products. Finally, the moral imperative obliges the elimination of longstanding systemic biases and structural barriers that have produced a medical school pipeline that historically lacks representative diversity. In the next sections, potential barriers to diversification will be reviewed.

Exposure and Access

For most medical students, exposure to radiation oncology may occur as an elective, very late in their medical school curriculum when the opportunity to seek out radiation specific rotations and research experiences may be limited. Early exposure experiences have generally shown benefit in introducing the specialty and providing skills to students earlier in their training. The participation of radiation oncology faculty in early medical school program, such as basic science lectures, may help address these limitations. Similarly, interest groups in oncology and radiation oncology, specifically, can provide meaningful early and continue longitudinal opportunities to learn about the field, technology, and career options [11].

For many other medical students, the opportunity to be exposed to radiation oncology may never occur without outside intervention or intentional and deliberate efforts. Many medical schools, including disproportionately those with greater URM representation, do not have affiliated radiation oncology residency programs and/or departments [12]. Meanwhile, in an analysis of radiation oncology residents in 2013, the majority (80%) of residents attended medical schools with affiliated radiation oncology programs and 30% stayed at their home institution [13]. For students at schools without affiliated residency programs and departments, this statistic highlights the need to seek out exposure and training opportunities with longitudinal mentorship outside of their home institution. Virtual rotations in radiation oncology created during the coronavirus disease 2019 (COVID-19) pandemic may help to reduce this gap and provide increasing access opportunities [14].

Interest and Deterrents

While there is not clear data to support any theories of pervasive disinterest in radiation oncology by women and/or URMs and/or other demographic groups, previously suggested barriers and themes include their limited involvement in science, technology, engineering, and math (STEM) sciences, a perceived lack of specialty engagement in health equity and health disparities, a perceived lack of opportunities to make a difference (social justice) and educate patients, radiation exposure, limited diversity and inclusion (male and/or non-URM predominance of the field), and physics requirements. To address these specifically, students can be reassured that the physics requirements of the field are not far beyond or different from the premedical requirements for medical school. The relative lack of specialty diversity highlights the need for students from diverse demographic backgrounds to enter the specialty so that its future physicians can mirror the diverse populations that they serve. Moreover, since physician workforce diversity is considered a means to address health equity, as a trainee from a historically underrepresented group in radiation oncology, you may heed the lack of workforce diversity as a call to action. There are increasing specialty interest, research initiatives, and leaders addressing cancer health disparities and inequities in their work. You may in fact be part of this growing group of a radiation oncologists that intersect with health services research, health disparities research, global health, health policy, medical education, and/or administrative medicine. The opportunities to make a difference, engage in social justice, and educate patients are therefore innumerably present.

Preparation, Mentorship, and Sponsorship, and Network-Building

URM and female trainees and physicians with an interest in radiation oncology, must be appropriately mentored, sponsored, and prepared to ensure their successful entrance and progression in the field. The relative lack of diversity among academic faculty and leaders in radiation oncology highlights the extreme attrition of individuals from underrepresented groups, as well as the challenges in finding sensitive and capable mentors and sponsors. For example, a study examining gender trends in radiology authorship over a 35 year period found that 23% of female first authors versus 14% of male first authors published with a female senior author and suggested a tendency for men to publish with men and women to publish with women [15]. Another analysis assessing the factors that predicted for a specialty having lower representation of women in graduate medical education included the percentage of female faculty members, such that for every 1% increase in female faculty, female trainees increased 1.45% ($p < 0.001$) [16]. Yet factors requiring strong mentorship are highly rated in the path to successfully matching in radiation oncology. In the annual program director's survey from the Association of American Medical Colleges for Radiation Oncology, program directors rated demonstrated involvement/interest in research and commitment to the specialty as more important than grades in the radiation oncology clerkship, USMLE Step 1 scores, and honors in clinical clerkships, while also highly rating letters of recommendation [17].

As a student hoping to match into radiation oncology, these criteria can be used to develop a point of attack and strategy; however, it also emphasizes the need for access to the field and sustained mentorship to ensure a successful specialty match. Such activities are costly and perpetuate societal economic inequities as discussed in viewpoint piece by radiation oncologists entitled, *The Hidden Costs of Medical Education and the Impact on Oncology Workforce Diversity* [18]. The authors note that black medical students often graduate with the highest median educational debt including the greatest proportion with debt above $200,000, and that away rotations, application fees, interview travel expenses, paid or unpaid gap years, and research positions that are made requisite by a competitive environment in order to become the most desirable candidate can ultimately limit and exclude those who can't afford these advantages. Nonetheless, while the specialty works to address these financial impediments and structural barriers, an awareness of these inevitably necessary activities can present an opportunity for interested medical students and trainees to plan and search accordingly. There are increasing numbers of enrichment programs that will be discussed in the sections that follow, which act to provide funded experiences to students to engage in research. As is well-discussed in an article entitled, *Achieving gender equity in the radiation oncology physician workforce*, mentoring programs are particularly efficient ways of addressing multiple barriers faced by underrepresented groups in allowing access to opportunities to which they might not otherwise be privy, yet there is also a growing recognition of the importance of sponsorship in addition to mentorship in promoting access to opportunities to demonstrate their abilities and achieve success particularly during the path to career progression during training and early practice [19]. While mentors may help their mentees develop a career vision and instill important lessons, such as resilience and persistence, sponsors may serve more as advocates for their protégé's career growth and advise them more specifically on loopholes and pathways to navigate of which they may not be aware.

Bias

It is important to acknowledge that students and trainees from underrepresented groups who are adequately exposed, interested, mentored, and prepared may still experience conscious and unconscious bias along their path to radiation oncology. Unconscious bias refers to ways that humans unknowingly draw upon assumptions about individuals and groups to make decisions about them; it occurs involuntarily, automatically, and beyond one's awareness and often contradicts conscious values and positive intentions [20]. Several tools assist to allow an individual to assess their own biases, such as the Implicit Association Test [21], and increasingly departments, institutions, and organizations are incorporating such tools into their staff training and search committee processes with varying degrees of success and buy-in. An increasing body of literature serves to expose the types of interpersonal and systemic biases that trainees, faculty, and practicing physicians may encounter. The resume study which replaces only the names at the top of the resume demonstrates the classic example of unconscious bias. In one such example, the exact same resume was sent to US academic STEM faculty members for a lab manager position where only the first name was altered as John or Jennifer [22]. Despite equivalent resumes, both male and female faculty rated the female candidate as being less competent, less hireable, less mentorable, and offered her significantly less salary. While this issue of the gender pay gap and wage inequity is well documented in medicine and other fields, the impact on additional accumulated wealth and subsequent generational wealth is less often acknowledged [23]. Similar results have been found for racial and ethnic minorities [24], and thus it begs the question, if equally qualified women and URMs are perceived as having less aptitude, how may their educational and career opportunities be limited?

Much how cell phone footage increasingly captures encounters with interpersonal and systemic bias, the medical literature increasingly captures the systemic bias in seemingly unbiased metrics and honors. USMLE Step 1 scores have been converted to pass/fail to account for such bias and largely unvalidated use in serving as an initial screen of residency applicants. As another example, in a study of *Racial Disparities in Medical Student Membership in the Alpha Omega Alpha (AΩA) Honor Society*, which examined 4655 US med student ERAS applicants from 123 allopathic US med schools who applied to 12 Yale residency programs in 2014, after controlling for USMLE Step 1 scores, research productivity, community service, leadership activity, and Gold Humanism membership, Black and Asian medical students remained less likely to be AΩA members than White medical students. In another study of an educational continuous quality improvement process at the University of California San Francisco, School of Medicine, the authors examined data for the classes of 2013–2016 to determine whether differences existed between URM and non-URM students' clinical performance (clerkship director ratings and number of clerkship honors grades awarded) and honor society membership – all of which influence residency selection and academic career choices – and found differences that consistently favored non-URM students [25]. Whereas the size and magnitude of differences in clerkship director ratings were small, URM students received approximately half as many honors grades as non-URM students and were three times less likely to be selected for honor society membership. Much like the salary pay gap yields larger disparities in accumulated wealth over time, the authors use these findings to illustrate the amplification cascade, a phenomenon in which small differences in assessed performance lead to larger differences in grades and selection for awards. This amplification cascade ultimately raises concerns about opportunities for URM students to compete successfully for competitive residency programs, such as radiation oncology, and later, potentially enter academic careers.

The potential impact of bias on career advancement is, similarly, increasingly documented. In a now-landmark analysis of RO1 funding, examining the probability of NIH R01 award by race and ethnicity between 2002 and 2006, applications from Black scientists were significantly less likely to receive an R01 award than those submitted by white scientists, even after controlling for educational background, country of origin, training, previous research awards, and employer characteristics [26]. In subsequent analyses and years, the disparity was noted to be greater for Asian and Black women PhDs and Black women MDs [27], and topic choice alone accounted for >20% of the funding gap after controlling for multiple variables, including the applicant's prior achievements [28]. In the latter study, it was noted that Black applicants tend to propose research on topics with lower award rates at the community and population level, as opposed to more fundamental and mechanistic investigations which tend to have higher award rates, demonstrating systemic bias and preferences determining the importance of scientific research. Other causes of attrition in academia and barriers to faculty diversity and career advancement for practicing physicians include absent institutional and executive commitment to diversity and inclusion; the minority tax/majority subsidy [29], which are terms used to describe the additional and usually unrewarded work of promoting diversity and inclusion that fall disproportionately to URM physicians; social isolation and exclusion; burnout; overt discrimination, harassment, and bias; and undervaluing of activities that do not meet traditional metrics of academic promotion, such as community outreach and engagement [30]. Sexual harassment more specifically can include sexual coercion, unwanted sexual advances, and/or gender harassment – defined as both verbal and nonverbal behaviors that systematically objectify, humiliate, disparage, or convey hostility toward women and gender minorities; numerous studies have documented the negative effects of all three forms of sexual harassment on the physical, psychological, and professional well-being of individuals (e.g., reduced productivity, decreased organizational commitment, increased rates of anxiety and depression, and greater turnover) [31].

Interventions

Fortunately, academic medical centers, societies, and organizations are increasingly acknowledging the need to strategically address workforce diversity and the impediments and deterrents to training. Statements such as the American College of Radiology's (ACR) white papers on *Improving Diversity, Inclusion, and Representation in Radiology and Radiation Oncology* [32] and the *American Society for Clinical Oncology (ASCO) Strategic Plan for Increasing Racial and Ethnic Diversity in the Oncology Workforce* [33] demonstrate this commitment. Students, trainees, and faculty may feel reassured that the moral arc of diversity and representation is long but seemingly continues to bend toward justice and equity in representation. Nonetheless, in the short term, your strategic efforts and preparation are warranted to maximize your likelihood of success.

Students

Although you may have already been exposed to and be interested in radiation oncology, if you are early in your medical school (or pre-med) training and career, you should seek out continued, extracurricular exposure opportunities in radiation oncology beyond your medical school curriculum, as they will likely be limited or non-existent. As previously noted, a large proportion of medical schools do not have affiliated radiation oncology residency programs and/or academic departments. Even those that do may have limited visibility and inclusion in the academic and clinical curriculum. Examples of high-yield extracurricular development include the following:

1. Interest groups – seek out interest groups in radiation oncology and/or oncology at your medical school or neighboring medical schools (if feasible and permitted). If one does not exist at your medical school, you may consider creating an interest group with institutional support and resources. Partnering with existing interest groups may help to leverage resources and expertise and ensure long-term sustainability and efficacy.
2. Shadowing/observership – Even if you are already committed to radiation oncology as a specialty, exposing yourself to the breadth and depth of the field can still be helpful. Exploring different disease sites (e.g., gynecology oncology and breast cancer) and specialty niches like brachytherapy, stereotactic radiation, global health, or immunotherapy can lead to unique linkages (i.e., network building) and further set yourself apart from the rest of the applicant pool.

3. Seek out shared interests – reach out to radiation oncologists with varied interests that you might share, such as health equity, global health, rural health, indigenous populations, cross-cultural care and cultural humility, and vulnerable populations. This may also facilitate more natural partnerships with shared research interests. Having this type of intentionality with networking connections and activities will assist you in cv-building and in the long run, when it comes time to submit your residency application and request effective letters of recommendation.

4. Student membership – apply for student membership in national organizations (e.g., ASTRO, ASCO, ACR, and AACR), which may often be free or at a reduced cost for medical students. This will provide access to lectures, meetings, mentorship and fellowship programs, and other educational content in the field.

5. Research fellowships – as described above, research experiences are highly valued and ranked by program directors during the residency selection process, so it will behoove all applicants to gain some experiences in some category of research, such as basic science, translational, clinical, and/or health services research. Most national organizations and societies now have pipeline and enrichment programs for underrepresented minorities and/or women to gain such experience, acknowledging the barriers and biases to doing so. Increasing evidence in the literature demonstrates that robust programs, which provide meaningful research opportunities, skills development, and opportunities for sustained mentorship, such as the Nth Dimensions program in Orthopedic Surgery for women and URMs [34], and the Diverse Surgeons' Initiative in surgical subspecialty training for URM residents [35], are more likely to facilitate a successful applicant match in the specialty. While performing these programs is not a prerequisite to matching, they strongly increase the likelihood of a successful match for those that do participate in them. Examples of programs funding and facilitating research in oncology include the ASTRO Minority Summer Fellowship Award [36], the ASCO Medical Student Rotation for Underrepresented Populations [37], the ACR Pipeline Initiative for the Enrichment of Radiology (and Radiation Oncology) [38], and the American Society of Hematology (ASH) Minority Medical Student Award Program [39].

6. Travel grants – similar to dedicated research funding opportunities, several academic departments and societies have travel grants to attend their annual meeting or to perform away rotations. These can generally be found on their department or society website. These are often changing, so you may also ask the radiation oncology residency program director or coordinator directly if such funding exists for underrepresented individuals. Examples of such programs include the AACR Minority [40] and Women [41] in Scholar in Cancer Research Awards and the Duke University School of Medicine Visiting Clinical Scholars Program [42].

7. Mentorship and sponsorship strategies – some of the aforementioned pipeline and enrichment programs will match you with a preidentified mentor, while most others will provide funding for a research project that you have developed with a pre-identified mentor. Identifying a mentor and research project can be

challenging regardless of whether you are located at a medical school with or without an affiliated residency training program.

(a) How to identify a mentor:

As discussed above, seek out faculty working in areas that interest you, both geographically and with respect to clinical and research interests. You may reach out to them via email with a very brief introduction and statement of interest in pursuing a research project in their area of expertise and preferably attach your curriculum vitae (cv). If possible, solicit recommendations from past and present peers and residents regarding faculty that are supportive of student trainees and have a track record of ethical collaboration and timely published research with students. Doing a PubMed search of their name and research will give you a quick sense of their track record in working with students and trainees. The residency program director and/or chief resident may similarly be willing to speak with you or communicate via email and facilitate connections with appropriate faculty. Be proactive and persistent. It may take several attempts and email exchanges before you make a productive connection and fit.

(b) How to identify research project:

When searching for a research project and mentor, it is important to be realistic and selective. While your faculty mentor will have abundant and often endless time to complete their work, as a student, your time windows are narrow and often minimally flexible. A research project conducted during an 8-week window – with the goal of submitting an abstract and moving on to publication of a full manuscript – will be facilitated by having a clearly delineated timeline and with weekly goals. It is important to have honest and clear communication with your mentor to state your goals and expectations, including as to whether the project will have you as a first or middle author. While middle author opportunities can certainly be worthwhile and useful for your cv, you may also advocate for follow-up opportunities that will yield the coveted first author position understanding that this position requires that you actively see the project through to fruition. Some research projects may occur in stages, and you may also lay out a timeline with your mentor to begin a portion of the data collection and analysis during a certain calendar block (e.g., summer break) and complete it in another (e.g., research elective).

8. Gap year – relatedly, a gap year may provide time to gain additional research skills and/or an additional degree, such as a master's degree in public health, health services research, and business administration, that can also help you stand apart. Some of the aforementioned pipeline and enrichment programs may also be applied for a research year. Talk to your research mentors or advisory deans about funding opportunities, which may or may not be readily posted or obvious to support a year of funded research and/or a master's degree.

The strategies above should provide extensive opportunities to adequately gain exposure, access, interest, research experience, mentorship, and sponsorship to prepare you to apply in radiation oncology. In preparation for the residency application review and interview process, itself, it is worth noting that *holistic review* is gaining relevance especially with the changing of USMLE Step 1 to pass/fail. This may include more attention to parameters such as (1) research scholarship, (2) academic achievements, (3) demonstrated compassion, (4) commitment to radiation oncology, (5) diversity of perspective, background, and life experiences, (6) interpersonal skills, and (7) demonstrated leadership [43]. The interview process itself may include novel components such as validated assessments of emotional intelligence and behavioral-based interviewing techniques, which seek to standardize the assessment of candidates within noncognitive domains with the goal of selecting those with the best fit the institution's residency program [44]. Speaking to past and current applicants can provide insight into the types of interview techniques and questions that are being utilized by different programs. Preparing for the interview process can also be useful regardless of whether you consider yourself to be an introvert or extrovert. Create lists of interview questions and practice asking yourself these questions and responding to them out-loud to prepare for the interview date. It may be helpful to practice with a medical student colleague (or trusted resident) even if they are going into another specialty and asking each other questions. This will instill confidence in your responses and show areas of weakness or discomfort that can be strengthened. Potentially relevant for underrepresented groups, cultural nuances like eye contact and excessive deference to authority may be candidly reviewed and assessed so that they are not misinterpreted. Ask your trusted mentors and sponsors to review your personal statement and cv prior to submission of your residency application. Their feedback is invaluable given that they have likely participate on selection committees for such applications and can provide critical insight and constructive feedback. You may similarly ask them to ask you interview practice questions to prepare.

Finally, although it may not seem like it, the most empowered state you will have is the transition from medical school to residency and residency to attending. When selecting programs to apply to and rank, it is important to consider the comprehensiveness and strengths of the program with respect to diversity of clinical training, research opportunities, and educational support staff and resources. Certain programs may have particular strengths in physics vs. radiation biology vs. certain technologies and modalities, etc. As a student, programs with the broadest diversity of experiences will likely strengthen your overall training and options for future employment. Some residency programs may have clear statements, efforts, and cultures supporting diversity and inclusion, while others may have nonexistent cultures of inclusiveness. When finalizing your rank list, thoughtfully assessing the program fit with your goals and needs will set you up to be more likely to succeed and thrive as a resident both inside and outside of the clinic.

Trainees

In order to best prepare yourself for your future job search, as a trainee, you should focus on strengthening your clinical skills across a variety of disease site and treatment modalities. As your clinical interests evolve, you may seek out collaborative research opportunities with faculty members specializing in that area. The advice above to students on how to select a research mentor and mentored projects also applies to trainees. Setting realistic goals, explicit expectations, and clear timelines from the outset will ensure productivity in the form of abstract presentations, manuscript publications, and opportunities for grant funding.

Minimizing burnout and optimizing work life balance with positive support systems and outlets become increasingly important during the course of residency training. This is particularly important for underrepresented groups given the inevitable micro- and macroaggressions, isolationism, hypervisibility, and stereotype threats that may ensue [45]. If relatable mentors and sponsors do not exist within your department, it will likely be necessary to seek support systems outside of your department, institution, and/or even specialty. Societies such as the Association of American Indian Physicians, the National Medical Association, the National Hispanic Medical Association, and the GLMA: Health Professionals Advancing LGBTQ Equality (previously known as the Gay & Lesbian Medical Association), and/or the American Association for Women Radiologists (AAWR) may provide valuable mentorship and networking opportunities which also fill this void. Similarly, institutional cohorts such as a minority or women's housestaff committee may similarly provide necessary emotional support and identification of culturally specific events and resources that may exist within the institution to mitigate bias, harassment, and other such challenges. Many of the pipeline and enrichment programs and travel grants listed in the student section are similarly available to trainees, such as the AACR MICR (Minorities in Cancer Research) and WICR (Women in Cancer Research) awards, as well as the ASCO Resident Travel Award for Underrepresented Populations [46]. The National Institutes of Health (NIH) and the Centers for Disease Control and Prevention Diversity supplements may serve as a resource to fund your support on a faculty member's existing NIH grant; these funds are available for administrative supplements to enhance the diversity of the research workforce by recruiting and supporting students, postdoctorates, and eligible investigators from diverse backgrounds, including those from groups that have been shown to be underrepresented in health-related research [47].

As you emerge from the early years of residency training and begin your search for potential faculty positions, remember that one of the most empowered states that you will have in selecting and negotiating your future work environment and career is the transition from residency to attending. In the latter years of residency, you should begin to build your network of mentors, sponsors, and allies. While few in number, the radiation oncology department chairs from the Black diaspora are always willing to engage you. Some candidates may be very clear on the type of career they envision: tenured faculty physician scientist at an NCI designated cancer center vs. community-based radiation oncologist at an academic-affiliated facility. Most others will likely fall somewhere in the middle and not have specific clarity on their desires even as they near the end of residency. As a senior resident it would behoove you to call on your immediate network of faculty members and colleagues who inevitably have contacts at institutions and geographic locations that suit your interest. Radiation oncology is indeed still a relatively small field where a brief email connection from a mutual colleague or acquaintance can open doors and windows that might not have opened otherwise. The reality is that a large proportion of academic positions may not be broadly or obviously posted in expected locations like society websites. Many opportunities may present informally after repeated inquiries and conversations. This again highlights the needs for trainees from backgrounds that are historically underrepresented to be proactive in utilizing available networks to form linkages with radiation oncologists leading search and selection committees.

More detailed considerations to aid in your academic job search are discussed in other chapters of this textbook, including how to effectively evaluate positions and ultimately negotiate your contract and efforts. Still a few job evaluation and negotiation tips to highlight for underrepresented and historically disenfranchised groups include the following:

- Exploring, investigating, and understanding the variety of academic tracks at each institution to which you may apply, e.g., tenure track vs. non-tenure track and clinician education vs. clinical associate.
- Thoroughly evaluate academic departments from the perspective of ethics, equity, and staff support.
- Review offered contracts with an attorney familiar with medical employment contracts.
- Discuss and broadly explore grant and funding options with your mentors and sponsors, as well as the department chairs. Understand how these fund your time and effort specifically. Since the NIH has documented the inequity in the process of peer review and awarding of grants for Black faculty, specifically at the R01 level, it is critical for URM faculty to be able to avail themselves of nontraditional funding mechanisms, such as private foundation grants, especially those created to alleviate this kind of funding inequity [48].
- Senior trainees and new faculty members should seek out resources and venues specifically for navigating isolation, hypervisibility, stereotype threat, and institutional racism. Investigate whether specific funding is available (and hopefully encouraged) for tailored professional development for underrepresented groups. Departments and/or health systems should provide support for URM-specific local and national funding opportunities. These may include programming from groups such as the NMA, the Association of Black Radiation Oncologists, as

well as offerings such as Executive Leadership in Academic Medicine (ELAM) Program for Women [49], the AAMC Minority Faculty Leadership Development Seminar [50], and the NIH/National Medical Association Travel Award [51].
– Ask the human resources and/or administrative contacts whether pay scales and compensation have been reviewed for equity [52].
– Engage in implicit bias and anti-bias training to understand how bias permeates decision-making environments to empower your own participation in search and selection committees in your work environment.

Summary

Although unique challenges are encountered by underrepresented students, trainees, and junior faculty members on the educational and career development path to academic radiation oncology, they need not be insurmountable. Increasing evidence reveals the barriers, obstacles, and deterrents to training and career advancement and elucidates the successful strategies to specialty entry and professional development as addressed in this chapter. As future, diverse radiation oncologists, there are increasing numbers of tools, resources, and strategies to ensure that you may thrive in your careers, despite the inevitable challenges endured. These should continue to aid in the development of a diverse workforce in academic radiation oncology that reflects the diversity and needs of the patients it serves to achieve enduring health equity.

References

1. Deville C, Hwang W, Burgos R, Chapman CH, Both S, Thomas CR. Diversity in graduate medical education in the United States by race, ethnicity, and sex, 2012. JAMA Intern Med. 2015;175(10):1706–8.
2. Ahmed AA, Hwang WT, Holliday EB, Chapman CH, Jagsi R, Thomas CR Jr, Deville C Jr. Female representation in the academic oncology physician workforce: radiation oncology losing ground to hematology oncology. Int J Radiat Oncol Biol Phys. 2017;98(1):31–3.
3. Chapman CH, Hwang WT, Deville C. Diversity based on race, ethnicity, and sex, of the US radiation oncology physician workforce. Int J Radiat Oncol Biol Phys. 2013;85(4):912–8.
4. Deville C Jr, Cruickshank I Jr, Chapman CH, Hwang WT, Wyse R, Ahmed AA, Winkfield KM, Thomas CR Jr, Gibbs IC. I can't breathe: the continued disproportionate exclusion of black physicians in the United States radiation oncology workforce. Int J Radiat Oncol Biol Phys. 2020;108(4):856–63.
5. Hill C, Deville C, Alcorn S, Kiess A, Viswanathan A, Page B. Assessing and providing culturally competent care in radiation oncology for deaf Cancer patients. Adv Radiat Oncol. 2020;5(3):333–44.
6. Lightfoote JB, Fielding JR, Deville C, Gunderman RB, Morgan GN, Pandharipande PV, Duerinckx AJ, Wynn RB, Macura KJ. Improving diversity, inclusion, and representation in radiology and radiation oncology part 1: why these matter. J Am Coll Radiol. 2014;11(7):673–80.

7. Ahmed AA, Hwang WT, Thomas CR Jr, Deville C Jr. International medical graduates in the US physician workforce and graduate medical education: current and historical trends. J Grad Med Educ. 2018;10(2):214–8.
8. Marrast LM, Zallman L, Woolhandler S, Bor DH, McCormick D. Minority physicians' role in the care of underserved patients: diversifying the physician workforce may be key in addressing health disparities. JAMA Intern Med. 2014;174(2):289–91.
9. Alsan M, Garrick O, Graziani G. Does diversity matter for health? Experimental evidence from Oakland. Am Econ Rev. 2019;109(12):4071–111.
10. Saha S, Guiton G, Wimmers PF, Wilkerson L. Student body racial and ethnic composition and diversity-related outcomes in US medical schools. JAMA. 2008;300(10):1135–45.
11. LaRiviere MJ, Santos PMG, Jones JA, Lukens JN, Vapiwala N, Swisher-McClure SD, Berman AT. Introducing multidisciplinary oncology management to the medical student. Adv Radiat Oncol. 2019;5(2):289–91.
12. Mattes MD, Bugarski LA, Wen S, Deville C Jr. Assessment of the medical schools from which radiation oncology residents graduate and implications for diversifying the workforce. Int J Radiat Oncol Biol Phys. 2020;S0360–3016(20):31259–61.
13. Ahmed AA, Holliday EB, Ileto J, Yoo SK, Green M, Orman A, Deville C, Jagsi R, Haffty BG, Wilson LD. Close to home: employment outcomes for recent radiation oncology graduates. Int J Radiat Oncol Biol Phys. 2016;95(3):1017–21.
14. Kahn JM, Fields EC, Pollom E, Wairiri L, Vapiwala N, Nabavizadeh N, Thomas CR Jr, Jimenez RB, Chandra RA. Increasing medical student engagement through virtual rotations in radiation oncology. Adv Radiat Oncol. 2020;6(1):100538.
15. Piper CL, Scheel JR, Lee CI, Forman HP. Gender trends in radiology authorship: a 35-year analysis. AJR Am J Roentgenol. 2016 Jan;206(1):3–7.
16. Chapman CH, Hwang WT, Wang X, Deville C. Factors that predict for representation of women in physician graduate medical education. Med Educ Online. 2019 Dec;24(1):1624132.
17. Results from the 2020 National Resident Matching Program. https://public.tableau.com/profile/national.resident.matching.program#!/vizhome/PDSurvey2020-Final/Desktoptablet. Accessed 11 Oct 2020.
18. Vapiwala N, Winkfield KM. The hidden costs of medical education and the impact on oncology workforce diversity. JAMA Oncol. 2018;4(3):289–90. https://doi.org/10.1001/jamaoncol.2017.4533. PMID: 29302685.
19. Holliday EB, Siker M, Chapman CH, Jagsi R, Bitterman DS, Ahmed AA, Winkfield K, Kelly M, Tarbell NJ, Deville C Jr. Achieving gender equity in the radiation oncology physician workforce. Adv Radiat Oncol. 2018;3(4):478–83.
20. Allen BJ, Garg K. Diversity matters in academic radiology: acknowledging and addressing unconscious bias. J Am Coll Radiol. 2016;13(12 Pt A):1426–32.
21. Project Implicit. http://implicit.harvard.edu/implicit/. Accessed 11 Oct 2020.
22. Moss-Racusin CA, Dovidio JF, Brescoll VL, Graham MJ, Handelsman J. Science faculty's subtle gender biases favor male students. Proc Natl Acad Sci U S A. 2012;109(41):16474–9.
23. Rao AD, Nicholas SE, Kachniarz B, Hu C, Redmond KJ, Deville C, Wright JL, Page BR, Terezakis S, Viswanathan AN, DeWeese TL, Fivush BA, Alcorn SR. Association of a simulated institutional gender equity initiative with gender-based disparities in medical school faculty salaries and promotions. JAMA Netw Open. 2018;1(8):e186054.
24. Ginther DK, Haak LL, Schaffer WT, Kington R. Are race, ethnicity, and medical school affiliation associated with NIH R01 type 1 award probability for physician investigators? Acad Med. 2012;87(11):1516–24.
25. Teherani A, Hauer KE, Fernandez A, King TE Jr, Lucey C. How small differences in assessed clinical performance amplify to large differences in grades and awards: a Cascade with serious consequences for students underrepresented in medicine. Acad Med. 2018;93(9):1286–92.
26. Ginther DK, Schaffer WT, Schnell J, Masimore B, Liu F, Haak LL, Kington R. Race, ethnicity, and NIH research awards. Science. 2011;333(6045):1015–9.

27. Ginther DK, Kahn S, Schaffer WT. Gender, race/ethnicity, and National Institutes of Health R01 research awards: is there evidence of a double bind for women of color? Acad Med. 2016;91(8):1098–107.
28. Hoppe TA, Litovitz A, Willis KA, Meseroll RA, Perkins MJ, Hutchins BI, Davis AF, Lauer MS, Valantine HA, Anderson JM, Santangelo GM. Topic choice contributes to the lower rate of NIH awards to African-American/black scientists. Sci Adv. 2019;5(10):eaaw7238.
29. Ziegelstein RC, Crews DC. The majority subsidy. Ann Intern Med. 2019;171(11):845–6.
30. Deville C Jr, Cruickshank I Jr, Chapman CH, Hwang WT, Wyse R, Ahmed AA, Winkfield KM, Thomas CR Jr, Gibbs IC. I can't breathe: the continued disproportionate exclusion of black physicians in the United States Radiation Oncology Workforce. Int J Radiat Oncol Biol Phys. 2020;S0360–3016(20):31413–9.
31. Beeler WH, Cortina LM, Jagsi R. Diving beneath the surface: addressing gender inequities among clinical investigators. J Clin Invest. 2019;129(9):3468–71.
32. Lightfoote JB, Fielding JR, Deville C, Gunderman RB, Morgan GN, Pandharipande PV, Duerinckx AJ, Wynn RB, Macura KJ. Improving diversity, inclusion, and representation in radiology and radiation oncology part 2: challenges and recommendations. J Am Coll Radiol. 2014;11(8):764–70.
33. Winkfield KM, Flowers CR, Patel JD, Rodriguez G, Robinson P, Agarwal A, Pierce L, Brawley OW, Mitchell EP, Head-Smith KT, Wollins DS, Hayes DF. American Society of Clinical Oncology strategic plan for increasing racial and ethnic diversity in the oncology workforce. J Clin Oncol. 2017;35(22):2576–9.
34. Mason BS, Ross W, Ortega G, Chambers MC, Parks ML. Can a strategic pipeline initiative increase the number of women and underrepresented minorities in orthopaedic surgery? Clin Orthop Relat Res. 2016;474(9):1979–85.
35. Butler PD, Britt LD, Green ML Jr, Longaker MT, Geis WP, Franklin ME Jr, Ruhalter A, Fullum TM. The diverse surgeons initiative: an effective method for increasing the number of under-represented minorities in academic surgery. J Am Coll Surg. 2010;211(4):561–6.
36. https://www.astro.org/Patient-Care-and-Research/Research/Funding-Opportunities/ASTRO-Minority-Summer-Fellowship-Award. Accessed 11 Oct 2020.
37. https://www.asco.org/research-guidelines/grants-awards/funding-opportunities/medical-student-rotation-underrepresented-populations. Accessed 11 Oct 2020.
38. https://www.acr.org/Member-Resources/Medical-Student/Medical-Educator-Hub/PIER-Internship. Accessed 11 Oct 2020.
39. https://www.hematology.org/awards/medical-student/minority-medical-student-award-program. Accessed 11 Oct 2020.
40. https://www.aacr.org/professionals/meetings/aacr-travel-grants/aacr-minority-scholar-in-cancer-research-awards/. Accessed 11 Oct 2020.
41. https://www.aacr.org/professionals/meetings/aacr-travel-grants/women-in-cancer-research-scholar-awards/. Accessed 11 Oct 2020.
42. https://medschool.duke.edu/about-us/diversity-and-inclusion/office-diversity-inclusion/pipeline-programs/visiting-clinical. Accessed 11 Oct 2020.
43. Odei B, Das P, Pinnix C, Raval R, Holliday E. Potential implications of the new USMLE step 1 pass/fail format for diversity within radiation oncology. Adv Radiat Oncol. 2020; https://doi.org/10.1016/j.adro.2020.07.001.
44. Tatem G, Kokas M, Smith CL, DiGiovine B. A feasibility assessment of behavioral-based interviewing to improve candidate selection for a pulmonary and critical care medicine fellowship program. Ann Am Thorac Soc. 2017;14(4):576–83.
45. Deville C Jr. The suffocating state of physician workforce diversity: why "I can't breathe". JAMA Intern Med. 2020;31
46. https://www.asco.org/research-guidelines/grants-awards/funding-opportunities/resident-travel-award-underrepresented-populations. Accessed 11 Oct 2020.
47. https://grants.nih.gov/grants/guide/pa-files/PA-20-222.html. Accessed 11 Oct 2020.

48. Doll KM, Thomas CR Jr. Structural solutions for the rarest of the rare - underrepresented-minority faculty in medical subspecialties. N Engl J Med. 2020;383(3):283–5.
49. https://www.aamc.org/professional-development/affinity-groups/gfa/faculty-vitae/spotlight-elam. Accessed 11 Oct 2020.
50. https://www.aamc.org/professional-development/leadership-development/minfac. Accessed 11 Oct 2020.
51. https://www.niddk.nih.gov/research-funding/research-programs/diversity-programs/travel-scholarship-awards/nih-national-medical-association. Accessed 11 Oct 2020.
52. Chapman CH, Gabeau D, Pinnix CC, Deville C Jr, Gibbs IC, Winkfield KM. Why racial justice matters in radiation oncology. Adv Radiat Oncol. 2020;5(5):783–90.

Part II
Applying to Faculty Positions

Informational Interviews/Interviewing for a Position

Roshan V. Sethi, Daphne A. Haas-Kogan, and Jonathan E. Leeman

Introduction

Interviewing is in many ways the central component of the job application process. The process can consume a great deal of time, particularly as interviews are often conducted during the senior year of residency when applicants still have active clinical responsibilities. However, these encounters should be viewed primarily as a remarkable opportunity to interact with many of the leaders in the field at diverse institutions. The interview season, which can sometimes stretch across several months, is perhaps the only time when the budding radiation oncologist will meet such a broad swath of the field. Many of these connections persist beyond the process of interviewing, regardless of the outcome.

Interviewing should also be viewed as a two-ended process, designed to allow both interviewer and interviewee to assess mutual compatibility [1, 2]. Both should keep an open mind about the possibilities of arrangements not previously considered, including different disease sites and practice locations. Overall, applicants should strive to consider interviewing as a genuine open-ended exploration of a relatively small and intimate specialty.

Preparing for the Interview

Preparation for all interviews should begin with identifying personal priorities, which are frequently focused on the following: location, diversity of faculty/staff, patient population, compensation/benefits, academic potential, disease site, main

R. V. Sethi · D. A. Haas-Kogan (✉) · J. E. Leeman
Department of Radiation Oncology, Brigham and Women's Hospital, Dana Farber Cancer Institute, Boston Children's Hospital, Harvard Medical School, Boston, MA, USA
e-mail: dhaas-kogan@bwh.harvard.edu

© Springer Nature Switzerland AG 2021
R. A. Chandra et al. (eds.), *Career Development in Academic Radiation Oncology*, https://doi.org/10.1007/978-3-030-71855-8_4

campus versus satellite, research opportunities, protected time, startup funds, involvement with residents/medical students, collegiality/personality of the department and relationships with surgeons or medical oncologists, involvement with cooperative groups, and technology such as protons, MR-linac, or advanced brachytherapy.

Most interviews will touch upon the applicant's reasons for interest in a particular department. Every department has a particular attitude and culture. It can be helpful to review the department website, and the research work of each faculty interviewer you are scheduled to meet or call. In addition, many department chairs and prominent faculty are now active on Twitter, where a good sense of academic inclinations and personal interests can be obtained. Touching base with former residents who now work in that department or who have interviewed with that department in the past can also be helpful.

If an applicant is strongly interested in a particular position, it may be helpful to speak with professional connections in advance and consider asking them to place a phone call or email highlighting your strengths and unique attributes. The radiation oncology community is relatively small, and personal recommendations can have considerable sway.

It can also be helpful to rehearse questions to common, expected questions, and to look back at previous interview experience (medical school, residency, etc.), reflecting on what worked and what did not. Develop your own set of potential questions for interviewers. Ideally these demonstrate your interest and show that you have done research and know something about the department/position. Familiarize yourself with the interview schedule in advance. Be prepared with respect to logistics (travel/lodging) to avoid unnecessary stress, confusion, or tardiness. Try to avoid travel close to the time of the last interview so as not to create additional stress. Most institutions have an interview coordinator who helps organize the interviews and visit. Remember to treat everyone you interact with as a potential interviewer or evaluator, including administrators, as they can also provide important feedback.

Interview Formats

The process often begins with a phone interview, conducted as a preliminary step to gauge mutual interest and fit. These phone calls are often short (15–20 minutes) and can be conducted with multiple faculty members.

A common next step is an in-person interview at the annual meeting of ASTRO, something of a tradition in radiation oncology. These interviews take place at the convention center—and nearby hotels and restaurants. The process of scheduling these interviews with multiple institutions can be quite involved, and it is helpful to start planning at least a few weeks in advance. Most schedulers are familiar with the competing demands of this process and will offer a great deal of flexibility. These interviews can assume various formats including one on one, panel, or multiple individual interviews in a row with faculty from the same institution. An interview may even be as informal as a casual invitation to an institutional event.

This process has the advantage of extreme efficiency, allowing you to very quickly meet with members of institutions from geographically disparate parts of the country. It can also be stressful—it's often the case that applicants have to rush across the convention center due to the timing of back-to-back interviews. The stress, however, should be taken in stride. There is a certain exhilaration in meeting so many people from so many institutions in the span of a few hours. You will continue to see these people at the annual meeting for perhaps the rest of your career; in a way, you are making connections and friends as much as you are finding a job.

The next step is often an on-site interview, when an applicant is invited for a single- or multiday visit to the campus. The purpose is more comprehensive vetting by multiple faculty members and staff. Flight and accommodations are generally paid for by the program. The agenda, also set by the institution, may include informal meals with the faculty, which should be treated as a version of an interview. If you have clinical, research, or academic interests outside of radiation oncology, for example, global health or other complementary fields of interest, you might consider asking the visit organizers to include meetings with individuals relevant to and informed about your broader interests. Such meetings are an excellent venue to explore potential for collaborations across the institution. There is also often time set aside for exploration of the city or talks on housing options. Some centers even arrange for a consultation with a real estate agent.

At academic centers, the on-site visit may also require the presentation of a so-called job talk, which is the summary of one of your significant research projects. These talks follow the format of a typical scientific presentation lasting approximately 45 minutes to leave time for questions. Try to distill your slides to the most critical findings in table or graph format. Limit text, except as a "headline" summarizing the major point or message of each slide. If possible, aim for the content of each slide to communicate only a single point. If the research is narrow or very technical, try to focus on the broad application of your data. Know your findings well enough to do very little reading off the slide. Be flexible with audience questions, which might crop up during the presentation of your slides instead of at the end. Finally, avoid presenting multiple studies unless they are closely related. The overall purpose of the "job talk" is to communicate your research interests and style. The content of the scientific study rarely matters as much as the evidence of an inquisitive and engaged mind. In formatting the job talk, it is important not just to describe the work that you have done but ideally to provide a vision of what you plan to do next with your background and training and how you could contribute specifically to the department.

Successfully Performing During the Interview

An interviewer may be considering a variety of factors including medical knowledge, quality of training, self-sufficiency, leadership potential, convergence of interests with the department/institution, and the likelihood that the applicant will stay in the posted position for a long time.

The interviewee's most important priority is to answer in a way that is truthful, natural, and unforced. Avoid the overly constructed or shaped narrative. Often interviewees are encouraged to advance a personal "brand," a philosophy that unites their research activities into a single niche focus. This can be difficult for applicants who have taken a more wide-ranging approach to research—even though exploring multiple fields is a perfectly valid strategy, particularly at the beginning of a career. It may be worth embracing the sprawl, if there is one. Attempting to shape or explain your work can introduce a hint of artifice and decrease the likelihood of a genuine connection. After an interviewee has left the office, most interviewers do not remember the particulars of an applicant's research or the details of their background. What lingers most strongly is the interviewee's demeanor, confidence, curiosity, and the genuineness of their interests. Avoid supplication or curating yourself—instead consider speaking with confidence, conviction, and a certain kind of directness when it feels appropriate.

It is also important to make the interview as conversational as possible. While it is helpful to rehearse answers to common questions, try to deliver these answers in a way that does not feel overly rote or mechanical. Be flexible, pivoting quickly as the conversation changes. The inevitable small talk can sometimes be as important as the formal portions of the interview—most faculty care about collegiality in their evaluation of an applicant's candidacy. Nevertheless, striking the right tone can often feel difficult and varies widely depending on the interviewer, as some will assume a formal posture from the beginning. Mutual connections are common in radiation oncology as it is such a small field and they are frequently brought up during interviews casually. It reflects well to always speak positively of others in the course of conversation.

Ideally, the interviewer will study your CV and background prior to the interview. But, given the demands of the interview process, it should be assumed that many will not be familiar or may not recall the particulars among the multiple CVs they have read. Practice summarizing the highlights in a way that takes a big picture view without getting overly bogged down in details. The applicant should not be afraid to describe "failures" as often as successes, as these together form a more complete and human picture of the applicant. If there are weaknesses in the application (real or perceived), these should not be avoided or overly explained, which often calls greater attention. Most physicians have "failed" during the long journey of training, and the acknowledgment of this failure can be liberating and human. The overall goal of an interview, after all, is connection—and connection is best forged by truth and openness.

Similarly, try not to feel overly punitive thoughts if you say something you regret. Applicants often feel these mistakes out of proportion to their actual effect, which is diluted by the general impression of the interview. It is also often the case that an applicant will misread the affect of an interviewer, usually by projecting their own fears. An interviewer may appear impassive or bored or even irritated—it may instead be the case that their expression assumes the form of your anxiety. For example, in the famous Kuleshov experiment, subjects were shown a shot of Tsarist matinee idol Ivan Mosjoukine assuming an expressionless posture. When this shot was alternated with images that carried emotional pungency, the experimental subjects felt the actor was conveying pensiveness, sorrow, or other emotion in reaction to the accompanying image. But it was the same basic shot of his expressionless face each time.

The task of the interviewee is therefore to project him or herself into a darkened audience regardless of the response. Do not allow yourself to panic because of a momentary impression, and know that your impressions can be inflected by anxiety.

Some applicants are more introverted than others, and feel particularly at sea during the interview process, which requires more purely social interaction than the applicant may typically encounter. It is normal to feel "drained" after a day of interviews. Take advantage of breaks when they occur. You do not always have to be "on"—as mentioned, the least contrived version of yourself may be the most successful.

It is also important to be consistent between interviews without "selling" a different story to different interviewers or institutions based on what one may expect they are looking for. Such inconsistencies can frequently backfire after interviewers have had a chance to regroup and discuss the applicant. Furthermore, there is a high likelihood that an interviewer may reach out to an applicant's mentors or associates to learn more about the applicant's performance, interpersonal skills, and aspirations. As a result, a disingenuous approach to this process is unlikely to succeed, whereas honesty and straightforwardness are more likely to achieve a mutually desired outcome.

It is natural to feel most focused on earning the approbation of the interviewer. But it is equally your goal to evaluate the program. Ask questions that will help your decision should you have a decision to make, which is more likely than not. If something offensive occurs during the interview—if, for example, you are asked an inappropriate question about your plans with child rearing or gender/sexual orientation—you should try as much as possible to confide the experience in the relevant leadership. This may be difficult due to the power dynamic, particularly at places where the applicant is keen to gain a position. In some cases, you may want to disclose the experience to the leadership at your own program in the hope that it can be indirectly communicated. But most leadership will be receptive, and reporting inappropriate episodes can help prevent these experiences for other applicants.

Post-Interview

We recommend writing thank-you notes to each interviewer within a week after the interview. These notes should be brief, warm, and personalized to some degree; try to avoid language that gives the appearance of a template letter and express genuine enthusiasm if you feel it. It's now perfectly acceptable to send these notes by email. ASTRO's membership site has a useful directory if you don't have contact information.

Take care to maintain positive relationships even if the position does not work out, and try to accept a rejection notice or lack of follow-up cordially. If you are considering multiple offers or close to accepting another, err on the side of honesty and clarity in your post-interview communications. There is a good chance you may interact with your interviewers in other contexts in the future.

Interview Considerations in the Time of COVID

Due to the social distancing and travel limitations brought on by the COVID pandemic, it is possible more interviews will be conducted via video technology and that this technology will remain the predominant form of interview even after the pandemic subsides. Video interviews have particular advantages (convenience, lower cost, safety) as well as disadvantages (interpersonal connection is more challenging, difficult to ascertain body language or visual cues, no department tour or sense of physical department, no experience of the location or city).

Consider general ways to improve your impression over video. This includes making sure you are not backlit, testing AV setup and internet connection prior to the interview, and wearing professional clothes despite the informal feeling of these conversations. Silence computer notifications that can interrupt these sessions.

Conclusion

The interview process ultimately requires that both applicant and interviewer make fairly consequential decisions based on a relatively narrow interaction, a short impression that may or may not be relevant. The best way to cope with the limitations of this process is to accept them; both interviewer and interviewee should try as much as possible not to generalize a limited experience. At the same time, the interview is a critical process that produces an often intangible feeling that comes from interacting with our colleagues and understanding what drives them and where they are most likely to be happy and succeed.

For Discussion with a Mentor or Colleague

- From your perspective, which departmental and institutions would best suit my career goals and my personal characteristics?
- Could we continue to collaborate as I move to my first position?
- If I wanted to stay at the institution at which I trained, how should I best go about exploring this option?
- What have been the "rose, thorn, bud" of your career, and how have these changed the trajectory of your career and the choices you made about where to practice and how to focus your career?
- If you could do one thing differently in your career, what would it be?
- When you interview candidates for residency/jobs, what are some of the qualities you look for? Is there anything you dislike? What are some of the questions you ask?
- What are your thoughts on the best format and style of a job talk presentation?
- What communication and follow-up you do you consider appropriate after an interview?
- How can one succeed in achieving work/life balance?
- How can I best evaluate prospective mentors at a new institution?
- How do I go about maintaining positive relationships with those at my current institution after I have left for a new position elsewhere?

References

1. Harolds JAPA. Tips for a physician in getting the right job, Part IX. Clin Nucl. Med. 2014;39(4):336–8. https://doi.org/10.1097/RLU.0000000000000354.
2. Bradley KE, McClain R, Berger JS, Andolsek KM. Successfully navigating the physician job interview. J Grad Med Educ. 2019;11(5):611–2.

Preparing Your CV and Cover Letter

David P. Horowitz, Cheng-Chia Wu, and Lisa A. Kachnic

Introduction

A curriculum vitae (CV) serves an important role for any job seeker, whether a medical student applying for residency positions, an academic physician trying to move up the promotion and tenure ladder, or a physician moving to a field outside of clinical medicine. The CV is a document of professional training, licensure, and accomplishments. Beyond standard divisions such as academic/private practice and clinical/basic science research, multiple career paths are available to radiation oncologists such as palliative care, global health, and informatics [1]. A properly crafted CV is therefore essential, and enables the radiation oncologist to tell a compelling story about his or her career path and goals.

For junior physicians who are completing residency, the end of residency training and entering the job market may be the first time a formal CV is required. All activities related to work and professional development should be included. Important differentiators that are often overlooked in the CV are committee work, involvement with quality-improvement or quality-assurance projects, and medical student teaching and mentoring. These items should also be briefly described, so that one who is reading the CV easily understands the nature and the outcome of the work. Residents and fellows should have a trusted mentor review the CV for help with crafting and polishing [2]. As a document of one's professional accomplishments, the CV must be unquestionably accurate.

D. P. Horowitz · C.-C. Wu · L. A. Kachnic (✉)
Department of Radiation Oncology, Columbia University Irving Medical Center,
Herbert Irving Comprehensive Cancer Center, New York, NY, USA
e-mail: Dph2119@cumc.columbia.edu; Cw2666@cumc.columbia.edu;
lak2187@cumc.columbia.edu

© Springer Nature Switzerland AG 2021
R. A. Chandra et al. (eds.), *Career Development in Academic Radiation Oncology*, https://doi.org/10.1007/978-3-030-71855-8_5

The format of the CV should be consistent with the goal of the document—to clearly and concisely convey a person's professional history. Attention to detail, such as proper grammar and spelling, consistency in font and upper vs. lower case usage, justification and alignment, as well as ordering of dates in time, is warranted. A single font and size should be used throughout the document. The font size should be large enough to be easily legible, 11 or 12 point, unless otherwise required. It should be meticulously reviewed to ensure no spelling or grammatical errors are present. A footer with the physician's name and page number should be included on all pages. If the CV is written in a non-native language, consider having it proofread for grammatical correctness and clarity or seek professional help with crafting it. As a frequently changing record, the CV is often in an easily editable format such as a Microsoft Word document. However, when sending it electronically, it is advisable to use a format such as PDF, which reduces risk of formatting errors between computers.

Proper CV structuring from early in one's career—based on one's home institutional format—helps to avoid unnecessary delays when preparing for advancement, and allows for recognition of potential deficiencies that will need to be addressed prior to promotion [3, 4]. Many radiation oncologists pursue academic medicine pathways, and career progression from assistant to associate or full professor occurs at one of the fastest rates among academic medical specialties, again emphasizing the need of a properly structured CV [5].

Not all portions of the CV are equally important, and their relative importance depends on the position for which one is applying. A CV highlighting the strengths of an academic clinical physician may not be appropriate for a lab-based physician scientist or a private practice physician. As such, this chapter will discuss the components of a structured and polished CV, as well as cover letter, from the perspective of an academic clinical, private practice, academic research, and industry job candidate.

Cover Letter

A first page cover letter is typically independent of the rest of the CV. It conveys information about the position being sought, and provides a brief introduction to the applicant. Importantly, the cover letter allows for the applicant to state why he or she is applying for the job, and provide a career statement of relevant experience detailing why she or he may be especially qualified for the position. As the first document a prospective employer sees, the cover letter must be meticulously edited. It should be tailored to the position being sought, which indicates an understanding of the needs of the employer and that the applicant has put due consideration into how he or she can be successful in the job. It is also an opportunity to highlight key points in the CV to identify an applicant's strengths, and why the applicant is specifically interested in the institution or practice offering the job. For example, succinctly describe how the applicant's strengths harmonize with strengths of the

Thomas Goat, MD, PhD
Professor & Chair
Department of Radiation Oncology
Patriots University
PUMC 6
Superbowl, MA 11111

May 30, 2020

Dear Dr. Goat,

I am writing to express my strong interest in a faculty position in your Department of Radiation Oncology at Patriots University beginning in July of 2021. I am a rising PGY-5 resident at Sunshine University and will be Chief Resident in the upcoming academic year.

As a resident, I received broad clinical training at Sunshine with exposure to a diversity of cases and treatment modalities including protons, SBRT, Gamma Knife SRS, LINAC-based SRS, and brachytherapy. While I have a particular interest in gastrointestinal cancers, my research and clinical interests are widely applicable, and I am comfortable in treating any disease site based upon the needs of your department.

My primary academic interests are related to optimizing outcomes for gastrointestinal malignancies. I am currently in the process of submitting two trials to our IRB based on my preclinical laboratory and machine learning work. The first is combining dual checkpoint inhibition with radiosurgery in borderline resectable pancreas cancer, and the second is performing a small pilot of on-line adaptive radiation for locally advanced anal cancer.

Patriots University has a reputation for excellence in clinical acumen and research, and I know it to be a world class cancer center. I am hopeful that I would be able to collaborate with investigators at your Institute of Immuno-oncology, such as Drs. Gronk and Slater, in carrying out my trial interests.

I would be grateful for the opportunity to discuss any potential career opportunities at Patriots University with you and your colleagues. Please do not hesitate to contact me should you have any additional questions. Thank you so much for your time and consideration.

Sincerely

Michaela Pence

Michaela Pence, MD
Sunshine University
Department of Radiation Oncology
(011) 111-1111 (cell)
MPence@sunshine.edu

Fig. 1 Example cover letter for a resident entering the academic clinical job market

institution or practice. This demonstrates that the applicant is not just sending out form letters for a certain type of position. For an example of a suitable cover letter for a senior resident entering the radiation oncology job market in search of an academic position, see Fig. 1.

Resume vs. CV vs. Biosketch

While a resume is generally a 1–2-page document that is tailored to the particular job to which a person is applying, a CV is a comprehensive record of all professional achievements, skills, and experiences, and may span tens of pages. The applicant should not try to restrict the number of pages in their CV, unless the job she or he is applying for specifically denotes a page limit. The CV is further distinguished from the National Institutes of Health (NIH) biographical sketch or "biosketch," which is used when applying for NIH grants. The biosketch allows applicants to describe the significance of their contributions to science, as well as provide details about their research experience relative to the proposed project. The NIH biosketch begins with a description of one's training and then contains a personal statement highlighting experience and qualifications for the particular grant for which one is applying. Further, the biosketch contains a "Contributions to Science" section in which applicants may list up to five significant contributions, each around a half-page in length, and each with up to four publications. This should show the investigator's personal impact, and demonstrate to reviewers that he or she is the most qualified investigator to do the work contained within the grant [6]. The National Center for Biotechnology Information services "My NCBI" and "SciENcv" are useful for building one's biosketch [7, 8].

Academic Clinical Position

The precise format of the CV will be dictated by one's institutional guidelines. However, the CV of an applicant for an academic position with a largely clinical focus should keep in mind the tripartite mission of most academic medical centers—patient care, research, and education. Residents entering the job market for the first time will naturally have CVs that differ in size and scope than practicing academic physicians, and the graduating resident CV will feature education and training prominently. Publications, grant support, and involvement with local, regional, or national committees should be highlighted, as these serve as significant differentiators. For a sample of an academic clinical CV for a senior radiation oncology resident, please see Fig. 2. Physicians already in practice will likely have additional sections included in their CVs, as described below.

Commitment to patient care must be demonstrated through a description of clinical training and particular skills one has (especially with relation to modalities such as proton therapy, brachytherapy techniques, boutique platforms such as Gamma Knife or MRI-guided linear accelerators, etc.). While fellowships are relatively uncommon in radiation oncology, the skills learned during fellowship training (if pursued) should be particularly highlighted as they serve as important differentiators. Clearly demonstrating an interest in a particular area of radiation oncology or disease subsite is also important, as large departments with subspecialized services want physicians who will fill the clinical need at hand. For newly graduating residents, this can be a challenge unless one's research is particularly focused on a disease site. Nonetheless, it is important to demonstrate an interest and ability in treating particular disease sites, as well as understanding how one's research interests complement or expand upon the needs of the department.

Academic productivity must be described clearly and comprehensively, as this is perhaps the primary determinant of advancement within an academic department. Publications (original data, peer-reviewed) should be listed in either chronological or reverse-chronological order (as dictated by one's institution). Publications in which one was first author, senior author, or corresponding author should be considered for inclusion separately from middle-author publications, which have less of an impact on advancement. For the publications list, the format can be simplified so

Michaela Pence, MD
1 Rainbow Circle, Kansas, MS 11111
MPence@sunshine.edu
Cell 001-111-1111

RESIDENCY

Sunshine University Radiation Oncology, Kansas, MS   7/2017 – 6/2021
- Chief Resident: 2021

Sunshine University Hospital, Kansas, MS   7/2016 – 6/2017
Preliminary Intern Year
- Medicine Resident

EDUCATION

Sunshine University School of Medicine, Kansas, MS   8/2012 – 6/2016
- Medical Doctorate

Sunshine University, Kansas, MS   9/2008 – 6/2012
- Bachelor of Science Degree in Biology
- Graduated Summa Cum Laude with 3.99 GPA and designation as Scholar of the University

LEADERSHIP & SERVICE
- 2019 – Member, Association of Residents in Radiation Oncology (ARRO) Governance Subcommittee
- 2018 – Junior Editor, *Practical Radiation Oncology*
- 2018 – Lecturer, Sunshine University School of Medicine (SUSM) Radiation Oncology Clerkship
- 2017 – Member, Quality Assurance Committee, Sunshine University Department of Radiation Oncology
- 2015 – 2016 Chair, Sunshine University Radiation Oncology Student Interest Group
- 2012 – 2016 Member, Sunshine University Radiation Oncology Student Interest Group

HONORS & AWARDS
- 2019 American Society for Radiation Oncology (ASTRO) Best Science Abstract Award
- 2018 Radiological Society of North America (RSNA) Travel Grant
- 2012 Scholar of the University: Sunshine University
- 2008 – Phi Beta Kappa: Sunshine University

PEER REVIEWED PUBLICATIONS
1. **Pence M**, Klaw I, You A. Development and Implementation of an Adaptive Radiation Delivery Protocol for Anal Cancer. *Int J Radiat Onc Biol Phys*. In Press, 2020.
2. **Pence M** & Klaw I. Machine Learning Predictors for Sexual Dysfunction following Pelvic Radiation. *J Clin Oncol* 2019. PMID: 11111111
3. Fauci M, Klaw I, **Pence M**. Hypofractionated Image-guided Radiation Delivery for Pancreas Cancer in Combination with Checkpoint Inhibition Delays Disease Progression. *J Clin Oncol* 2019. PMID: 22222222
4. Fauci M, Klaw I, **Pence M**, You A. Damper1 Promotes Treg Cell Generation in Combination with Radiation in a Pancreatic Cancer PDX Model. *Nature* 2018. PMID: 33333333
5. **Pence M** & Klaw I. Machine Learning Predictors for Near Misses in a Radiation Oncology Clinic. *Int J Radiat Onc Biol Phys* 2018. PMID: 44444444
6. **Pence M** & Klaw I. Role of Daily Team Huddles in Preventing Adverse Events in a Radiation Oncology

Fig. 2 Example CV for a resident entering the academic clinical job market

MANUSCRIPTS IN PREPARATION
1. **Pence M**, Klaw I, You A. Development and Implementation of an Adaptive Radiation Delivery Protocol for Pancreas Cancer SRS.
2. Fauci M, Klaw I, **Pence M**, You A. Deciphering the Role of Damper1 in Immune Checkpoint Blockade.

PRESENTATIONS AND ABSTRACTS
1. Fauci M, Klaw I, **Pence M**, You A. Damper1 Promotes Treg Cell Generation in Combination with Radiation in a Pancreatic Cancer PDX Model. *Oral Presentation and Awarded Best Science Abstract at the 2019 ASTRO Annual Meeting, Chicago, IL.*
2. **Pence M** & Klaw I. Machine Learning Predictors for Sexual Dysfunction following Pelvic Radiation. *Oral Presentation and Travel Grant Awardee at the 2018 RSNA Annual Meeting, Chicago, IL.*

RESEARCH SUPPORT
- **RSNA Research Resident Grant (P.I. Pence)**   2017 – 2018
  $50,000
  Sexual Toxicity Detection in Pelvic Malignancies Receiving Radiation with Artificial Intelligence
  Used machine learning, leveraging EPIC and Aria, to determine clinical, dosimetric and biomarker determinants of sexual dysfunction in patients who underwent curative pelvic radiation for endometrial, cervical, anal and rectal cancers. These data informed a clinical trial which I am currently submitting to the IRB.

- **Sunshine University Institutional Resident Grant (co-P.I. Pence)**   2017 – 2018
  $25,000
  Damper1 Promotes Treg Cell Generation in Combination with Radiation in a Pancreatic Cancer PDX Model
  In collaboration with the Institute of Genetics, used their PDX pancreatic cancer model to perform small animal irradiation radiosurgery in combination with Treg manipulation to assess immune response, tumor response and progression-free survival. These data informed a clinical trial which I am currently submitting to the IRB.

CLINICAL SKILLS
- Proton therapy (including pediatrics)
- SBRT (stereotactic body radiation therapy)
- LINAC Based SRS (stereotactic radiosurgery)
- Gamma Knife frame and frameless SRS
- IMRT (intensity-modulated radiation therapy) and VMAT (volumetric modulated arc therapy)
- Motion management including 4D-CT and breath-hold techniques
- Electron therapy for skin malignancies
- Total body irradiation (TBI)
- HDR intracavitary and interstitial brachytherapy for gynecologic malignancies
- LDR seed implants for prostate cancer
- Treatment planning and delivery using: Aria, RayStation, and Eclipse
- Electronic Medical Record: EPIC

REFERENCES

Ima Klaw, MD, PhD	John B. Goode, MD	Ambeneatha You, MD	Michelle Fauci, PhD
Professor & Chair	Professor	Associate Professor	Associate Professor
Department of Rad Onc	Program Director	QA Director	Vice Chair of Research
Sunshine University	Department of Rad Onc	Department of Rad Onc	Department of Rad Onc
Research Mentor	Sunshine University	Sunshine University	Sunshine University
IKlaw@sunshine.edu	JGoode@sunshine.edu	AYou@sunshine.edu	MFauci@sunshine.edu
101-111-1111	102-222-2222	103-333-3333	104-444-4444

Fig. 2 (continued)

that the key information is quickly visible: (1) the author list in abbreviation (last name, initial) with your name bold and underlined, (2) title of the article, (3) the journal and the year of publication in bold, and (4) the PMID number. The inclusion of this information will allow the interviewer quick understanding of the candidate's contribution to the work, impact, and quick access to search the article. Submitted publications, invited publications/reviews, book chapters, abstracts, and invited presentations should have their own designations. In the abstract section, it may be worthwhile to list abstracts that were accepted for publication separately. This is a good indicator for productivity and the ability to bring a project into completion. Grant support for academic clinicians is highly desirable, and provides the best way to have protected research time. One should craft one or two sentences to describe each grant award. Particularly for those with an interest in clinical trial design and translational research, demonstration of involvement with professional societies and collaborative groups is also a valuable avenue for professional advancement.

With the multifaceted mission of the academic medical center, administrative leadership and academic service are important for developing and highlighting on one's CV. Demonstration of commitment to, and results of, service within the medical center and the department can be conveyed with short descriptions of activities and responsibilities.

Teaching of resident physicians and medical students is also an important aspect of work within an academic medical center. Education and mentorship of students and junior physicians should be quantified and described, with brief descriptions of publications and grants obtained with mentees. Lectures, bedside teaching, and work on teaching services should be denoted. For physician educators, description of any education research is important, especially novel programs developed and presentations or publications that resulted from these programs.

As an example, the Columbia University Irving Medical Center CV template is as follows:

1. Date of preparation of CV
2. Personal data:

    (a) Name—Include any other names you may have used
    (b) Contact information
    (c) Birthplace
    (d) Citizenship

3. Academic appointments, hospital appointments, and other work experience
4. Education
5. Training
6. Explanation of any gaps in work/training/education

7. Licensure and board certification
8. Honors and awards
9. Academic service
10. Professional organizations and societies

    (a) Memberships and positions
    (b) Consultative
    (c) Journal reviewer
    (d) Editorial board
    (e) Study sections

11. Fellowship and grant support
12. Educational contributions

    (a) Direct teaching/precepting/supervising
    (b) Advising and mentorship
    (c) Educational administration and leadership
    (d) Instructional/educational materials used in print or other media
    (e) Community education

13. Report of clinical and public health activities and innovations

    (a) Practice or public health activities
    (b) Clinical or public health innovation
    (c) Clinical or public health administration and leadership
    (d) Additional clinical or public health service activities

14. Patents and invention
15. Publications

    (a) Peer-reviewed research publications in print or other media
    (b) Other peer-reviewed publications in print or other media
    (c) Reviews, chapters, monographs, and editorials
    (d) Books/textbooks for medical or scientific community
    (e) Meetings/invited oral and poster presentations
    (f) Case reports
    (g) Letters to the editor
    (h) Other media
    (i) Thesis
    (j) Other non-peer-reviewed publications in print or other media
    (k) Non-authored publications

16. Invited and/or peer-selected presentations at regional, national, or international levels

Private Practice

Private practice constitutes the majority of jobs in radiation oncology, and there is no one-size-fits-all approach to an optimal CV for private practice. A single- or two-physician practice will have different needs than a large group with subspecialized services. As with academic clinicians, a demonstrated commitment to patient care is essential. Skills developed during training and technological proficiency are valuable to highlight, as well as special skill sets such as brachytherapy and radiosurgery. While proficiency in a second or third language is an asset regardless of practice type, it can be especially valuable in this situation.

Administrative leadership is an important attribute to highlight in one's CV, which serves one well within the practice, hospital, and community. Involvement in the oncology community and outreach are addition aspects that are valuable to describe within an applicant's CV.

Many practices are actively involved with research protocols, and an interest and ability to develop new collaborative protocols is encouraged. Prior research productivity therefore should not be downplayed, and it also demonstrates an ability to see tasks through to completion. However, a CV laden with grants and publications may not carry the same weight as within academia, and care should be taken that one's CV does not prioritize research activities at the expense of clinical ability. Additional information may include treatment planning software and electronic medical record systems one is familiar with, additional training certificates or medical licenses, and second or third languages one can speak fluently.

Important key points to include on the private practice CV include:

1. Technology/skills one knows or is able to do
2. Type of training in residency
3. Special skill sets: Brachytherapy, SRS, and SBRT and second or third language
4. Involvement in oncology community/outreach
5. Administrative and leadership experience

Academic Research Position

An academic laboratory research scientist position is a very unique job opportunity that differs from clinical radiation oncology and private practice, as the commitment from the hospital and the academic center is substantial. As such, the approach to the CV must be clear in terms of the research direction, productivity, mentorship, and, most of all, track record for securing funding. The vision for one's career trajectory should also be included. Leading up to the submission of the CV, it is important to also have a brief research proposal written and ready to submit along with the CV. The written research proposal can be argued to be as critical as the CV itself. It gives the academic institute an insight of your research interest, your understanding of finance and budgeting, and an estimate of what you are asking for to achieve research success. Typically, the proposal is written in an NIH format. An NIH-R21 format would be reasonable. Information regarding NIH grants can be found at https://grants.nih.gov/funding/index.htm. The inclusion of a brief one paragraph personal statement can also be beneficial to help provide a brief snapshot of your research and an introduction to your written proposal. For a comprehensive description of sections of the CV, please review the CV template example in the above academic clinical section.

In your academic research CV, it is important to pay special attention to the "Fellowship and Grant Support" section. Remember to identify the funding agency, the amount of money received over a set period of time, and the role of the applicant. This demonstrates a track record for successfully securing funds. For applicants coming out of residency, it may be useful to identify if one participated in writing a grant for their mentor, as it demonstrates experience for obtaining funding. Depending on the percentage of research in comparison with clinical requirements, additional skills may be important to include such as clinical trial design and IRB submission.

Other important key points to emphasize on the academic research CV include:

1. Research interest and path
2. Productivity
3. Research skill sets
4. Prior collaborations
5. Track record for mentorship

Industry

The field of radiation oncology is exciting due to its evolving footprint. In addition to the aforementioned paths, alternative careers are available including those in pharmaceutical companies and government. The specific requirements for a CV may be different for such positions. However, the fundamental interest is the same and can be broken down into those who are interested in a laboratory career, a role in clinical trial design and execution, or administration.

The most important aspect of the industry CV is a clear understanding of the position being applied for and what the job entails. This narrative must be reflected in your CV. For pharmaceutical roles, ideal candidates are physicians with clinical trial experience in designing, executing, monitoring, and analyzing trials, as well as working with the FDA (Food and Drug Administration). Previous experience with being a principal investigator on a clinical trial, or having a leadership role in clinical trial administration, may be helpful. The CV for pharmaceutical employment is similar to an academic position in which a track record of productivity is key. Similar headings as those described in the CV template example in the above academic clinical section are used. Additional skills that may be beneficial include biostatistics and programming. More important than the CV are the cover letter and the interview process itself. The applicant needs to demonstrate an understanding of the position, as well as background information regarding the company.

Important key points to emphasize on the industry CV include:

1. Personal and institutional background
2. Demonstration of productivity
3. Practical skills: protocol writing or leading clinical trials
4. Administrative and leadership experience

Summary

Your cover letter and CV should provide a compelling and comprehensive review of training, skills, accomplishments, and career goals. It should be structured in a manner that emphasizes one's strengths, and allows for the reader to conclude that the candidate has the abilities to succeed in the job at hand. The CV should therefore be tailored to the position being applied for, and informed by an understanding of the requirements of the job.

Bullet Point

1. Understand the job being applied for and the needs for the private practice, academic clinical or physician-science setting, or sector of industry.

For Discussion with a Mentor or Colleague

- C/M: Do you know someone in the practice/department?
- M: Does my CV tell the right story about me?
- M: What are gaps in my CV that are preventing me from getting the job/promotion that I want?
- M: Is everything in the CV structured correctly? Is everything spelled correctly and is it grammatically correct?

Bibliography

1. Vapiwala N, Thomas CR Jr, Grover S, et al. Enhancing career paths for tomorrow's radiation oncologists. Int J Radiat Oncol Biol Phys. 2019;105:52–63.
2. Darves B. Creating a physician CV that shines, 2018.
3. Goldstein AM, Blair AB, Keswani SG, et al. A roadmap for aspiring surgeon-scientists in today's healthcare environment. Ann Surg. 2019;269:66–72.
4. Hughes BD, Butler PD, Edwards MA, et al. The Society of Black Academic Surgeons CV benchmarking initiative: early career trends of academic surgical leaders. Am J Surg. 2020;219:546–51.
5. Odei B, Martin C, Gawu P, et al. Do US radiation oncologists progress through the academic ranks at the same rate as physicians of other medical specialties? Int J Radiat Oncol Biol Phys. 2019;105:S15–6.
6. Health NIo: Biosketch format pages, instructions and samples. 2019.
7. Information NCfB: My NCBI, 2020.
8. Information NCfB: SciENcv: science experts network curriculum vitae, 2020.

Evaluating Your Contract/Medical Legal Considerations

Terry J. Wall

Introduction

Contract evaluation for an academic practice differs from the evaluation when contemplating entry into private practice largely because there are often less opportunities to negotiate certain terms (which are often fixed by nearly immutable institutional human resource policies) and by freedom from concern about certain commercial issues such as buy-ins to professional entities after a period of employment. Issues related to physician entry into private practice are not covered in this chapter.

Arguably the most important aspect of contracting for physician employment is to strive to have every representation that was critical to your selection of a particular job (both things that you wanted and things that you wanted *to avoid*) to be legally enforceable promises. A legally enforceable promise occurs if you and the institution sign a contract and every critical representation is contained within that document, per se, or is specifically denominated within that contract as being "incorporated by reference." Nothing that cannot be found within "the four corners of the written contract" is a legally enforceable contractual promise. Representations made, for example, in e-mails or conversations or "letters of intent" that are not included specifically in the written contract are typically not legally enforceable. The law refers to such representations as "parol evidence" and, with certain exceptions, does not consider such evidence when adjudicating a contract dispute. This does not mean that performance of a "noncontractual promise" will not be forthcoming by virtue of good faith or honor, but it does mean that the "power of the state" through the court system is not available to ensure that you get what you thought that you had bargained for. In fact, there is a substantial likelihood that all "critical representations" may not be offered to you in the form of legally enforceable promises, but

T. J. Wall (✉)
TRI, PA, Kansas City, MO, USA

© Springer Nature Switzerland AG 2021
R. A. Chandra et al. (eds.), *Career Development in Academic Radiation Oncology*, https://doi.org/10.1007/978-3-030-71855-8_6

you will need to know that. That possibility is why a critical inquiry during your interview process is to ask new faculty if there were representations made to them whose fulfillment was not forthcoming and what dispute resolution mechanisms are available within the institution. Not all written documents signed by two parties are legally enforceable contracts, which is why you will want to review proffered documents with an attorney who is licensed in the state where the academic institution is located.

Another important aspect of contracting with an institution, even one of size and repute, is to avoid assuming that everything that is offered is reasonable and "it's OK to just go ahead and sign" on the faith that "big institutions don't do irrational things." You actually do need to pay attention to the details. For example, I have reviewed a proposed contract from one of the nations' most respected radiation oncology departments, chaired by a chairman of deserved good repute, which actually contained the phrase "the terms of this contract can be modified at any time by (the institution)." The chair obviously didn't draft that contractual term and probably wasn't even aware of it! As another example, I was a consultant to the medical staff of a billion-dollar health system whose intellectual property policy, applicable to both independent and employed physicians, claimed ownership of all physician-generated intellectual property, even if it derived from "a thought" the physician had while on system property! In short, you need to read the proffered documents, understand their contents, and have them reviewed by your own legal counsel.

A Few Preliminary Thoughts

About Your Presence on Social Media Speaking of being on guard, you should also be on guard for self-inflicted wounds; take a careful look at your online presence. Potential employers (although with some risk to themselves) may elect to visit your social media sites. A study of medical students and residents at the University of Florida (fortuitously, no radiation oncology residents were included in the study) found that 63% of Facebook accounts were open to the entire public, and in a random subset given more thorough assessment, 70% of pages showed students consuming alcohol, and several profiles contained images of lewd or drunken behavior, and also contained photographs of patients from a mission trip overseas, an obvious breach of confidentiality [1]. Another study showed that 18% of blogs by healthcare providers carried negative descriptions of patients, and 17% contained sufficient information that specific patient identification was likely possible (a violation of federal statute) [2]. Your potential institution may not be impressed. A future consideration in this regard is that patients who learn things about your personal life that they may not like are arguably more likely to sue you, if disgruntled about some aspect of their care.

There Is No Perfect Job Obviously, any institution that is hiring will present their practice in its best light. If you begin the job search with an absolute conviction of the truth of the statement: "There is no perfect job," it will be easier for you to ask the questions that enable you to find out why the job under consideration is not the perfect job. A good mental attitude in life is: "Run to the problem."

Distinguish Understanding the Terms of an Offer from the Process of Bargaining for Its Terms You can ask a million questions but you can't make a million demands. *Being inquisitive* about the practice, seeking to understand the exact extent and details of the offer by asking questions, etc., will be taken as a sign of your interest in the practice, your attention to detail, your intelligence and curiosity. *Negotiating for terms* will be taken as a surrogate of what kind of team player and colleague you will prove to be.

You absolutely must ask probing, detailed, and incisive questions to achieve a perfect understanding of "what the offer is.[1]" If, for example, they don't mention, say, disability insurance, you should ask about it. Make it clear that your inquiry is not a demand; it's just a question about what the offer contains.

The negotiation part is tricky. Two things are clear: your bargaining power is greatest at the outset, before you are hired. It is also probably true that if you get everything you asked for, you probably didn't ask for enough. That being said, negotiations provide ample opportunities for getting off on the wrong foot. You certainly have an obligation to be a good steward of your education and to get a rightful return on your investment. However, you don't want to seem pushy, grasping, or unreasonable.

Be Forearming with Knowledge of the Academic Market The Association of Residents in Radiation Oncology (ARRO) performs annual surveys of the salary, benefits, and recruiting experiences of former residents who have just joined academic practice and presents that data annually (The "Dr. Wall Survey") at the ASTRO meeting. The survey provides information on potential contractual benefits, such as signing bonuses, moving expenses (these, by the way, are now considered taxable income), educational allowances, time off, salary, insurance policies, family leave, retirement benefits, and the like. You should be familiar with that data (and should participate in completing those surveys when the opportunity arises!).

Who should do the negotiations, you or your attorney? I believe that the clearly better answer is you—after receiving proper legal advice. For one thing, *like any relationship in life, there will always be tensions to resolve* in a practice relationship, and you might as well get an idea, early on, of how the institution/your chair handles conflict. Zealous advocacy has its role in professional life, but I believe your lawyer more profitably remains in the background giving advice and counsel behind the scenes. If the institution does not take ownership of an item of contention

---

[1] The same is true of asking these types of questions about the professional side of the practice—how a given diagnosis is managed in the practice, etc., but our scope of inquiry here is about the medical/legal aspects of entering practice.

("Oh, our lawyer told us we had to have that in the contract"), then it may be appropriate to have opposing counsel confer directly.

In addition to your own personal employment Academic practitioners may wish to secure contract provisions giving them the right to at least interview any nurses or employees whom they will directly supervise and to make recommendations on their hiring, firing and disciplining.

The Process of Analyzing a Practice Offer

Evaluate All Phases of Your Academic Life at the Outset Your eventual goal, presumably, is to be promoted and become tenured and not to just have a job with no possibility of advancement. If tenure or promotion is never going to be an option, you need to know that before you commit to a period of employment.

It is easy to be mesmerized by the employment phase, with its sudden rise in income from residency and its benefits. And yet you don't want to work hard for a few years, and then come up against some draconian terms that should either have been renegotiated before employment (when your bargaining power is greatest) or a least have been better understood from the start. Your starting salary is a small thing: the trajectory of your career is the big thing. Keep things in perspective.

What is reasonable? I think that your employment contract should contain language about the criteria and processes determining retention, promotion, and tenure.

Hire a Lawyer; Get a Contract

Contract law is very much a creature of state law, so your advisor needs to be a lawyer who practices law in the jurisdiction where you will be practicing medicine.

What kind of lawyer? Preferably someone in civil practice already versed in employment law in the healthcare setting. How to find such a lawyer? There are many avenues of successful referral. The Martindale-Hubbell Company has a legal directory, online at www.lawyers.com, where you can search by jurisdiction and see the area of law in which the attorney concentrates and some of their sample clients. There are specialty organizations such as the American College of Legal Medicine, the National Health Lawyers Association, and other concentrations of expertise in health law whose members may practice in your jurisdiction. State and local medical societies are also a good source of referrals. The American College of Radiology (ACR) has an attorney referral service—which is a state-by-state, "specific topic" list of attorneys recommended by an ACR member who has used them and was pleased with their services.

You need to be represented by your own attorney; you cannot rely on the institution's legal department to represent your interests.

With any luck, the contract that you sign will go in a drawer and never see the light of day again. But the PROCESS of writing everything down is an essential discipline to achieve a more complete "meeting of the minds," to protect against fading memories, and to document the relationship to third parties. The *process* of drafting the contract not only establishes mutual expectations but sets the tone of the relationship.

What Should Be in the Contract? It bears repeating: anything that was important to you in accepting the job. And that means things that you wanted, and it means things that you wanted to *avoid*. Insist on the discipline of achieving important mutual understandings with sufficient particularity that they are capable of being reduced to an enforceable, written document. In addition to salary and benefits, academic practitioners need representations about research facilities and protected time for academic work.

Legal Entities The presence of multiple legal entities within a practice is generally less of an issue for academic practitioners than for those in private practice However, it is possible, for example, that faculty income may derive from a separate corporation than the nominal institution. Be sure to ask about the presence of (and your potential relationship within) any legal entities involved in the practice other than the "named" institution that you think that you are joining.

Specific Contract Provisions

Just as there is no perfect job, there is no perfect contract. Here are some important features to be concerned with:

Scope and Definition of Duties You should expect your potential employer to be explicit in what they expect of you. Remember, if a promise was made to you that was important to you in your decision to join the group, that promise should be incorporated into your contract. Your "scope and definition of duties" may include a limitation on outside income. Be sure to have representations regarding "nonclinical duties" that can erode into research time, such as committee assignments. You should know what, if any, "quality metrics" will be used to assess your clinical and research performance.

Trojan Horses and Supremacy Clauses Many contracts will contain language indicating that you will comply with all policies of the practice or hospital as they may be implemented from time to time. If there is a particular issue of interest to you, such as the ownership of intellectual property, you may want specific contract language, rather than "standard policy" to apply. In order to avoid a potential hassle, in all cases there should be a clause explicitly indicating that if any such present or future policy conflicts with a specific term of the contract, then the specific contract language should prevail and reign "supreme." There are good legal arguments that might come to your aid if your contract lacks such a clause, for example, an argument that the contract is illusory and therefore unenforceable if readily changeable by one party, but explicit language in a contract beats a good argument in court every time.

Choice of Law and Choice of Venue Clauses   Likely contained in the seemingly mindless "standard boilerplate" at the end of the contract, you will likely find a statement that the contract will be governed by the law of one state or another. If it's not the state in which you practice, beware! Sometimes these clauses are inserted to allow contract language to operate that would otherwise be unenforceable. For example, California courts hate restrictive covenants, while courts in other states, like Ohio and Missouri, are happy to enforce them. If you practice in California, but your contract is to be interpreted under the laws of Missouri, you could be in trouble.[2] When conflict erupts, these situations can lead to a "race to the courthouse" with the first party to file a suit in a disagreement gaining an important advantage just because they get to select the jurisdiction in which the matter is adjudicated, the so-called "first to file" rule.

Incorporating Exhibits "by Reference"   Many contracts may have "exhibits" that specify duties, fringe benefits, or the like. Make sure that the contract itself contains the "magic" legal words "incorporating by reference" those exhibits, and specifying that the exhibits can only be changed by written mutual consent. Make certain to review any exhibits in detail, especially if they become part of the contract by reference.

Term of Employment   Typically, this will be a term for a specific time, after which one hopes for an offer of tenure or promotion. The employment agreement should specify the conditions under which you can be "let go" before the expiration of that term and dismissal, in my view, should only be "for cause." Those are two little "magic" words in the law. There are basically two types of employment: *employment at will* (where, broadly speaking, you can be let go at any time, for any or no reason) and termination only "for cause." Graduating residents should seek contracts that only allow termination "for cause." (If you are an employee at will, there should at least be parity in the amount of notice each party has to give before a termination—if they can fire you today, they shouldn't require 3 months' notice before you can leave.)

What types of things are appropriate to be listed as causes for termination? Typically these should only be things like your inability to be licensed in the state, inability to get a DEA license, inability to be credentialed, inability to legally submit charges to Medicare and Medicaid, or because you are dead.

---

[2] This trick by the drafting attorney doesn't always work; *see, e.g., Bunker Hill Int'l Ltd. v. Nationsbuilder Ins. Servs,* 3099 Ga. App. 503 (Ga.Ct.App. 2011), but who needs the hassle?

Employment at will is exactly what it says, but perhaps more pointedly should be called "unemployment at will." While some courts have intervened to prevent "at will" firing of physicians on the basis of a "public policy" interest in the continuity of healthcare[3], the general rule is that physicians employed "at will" can, in fact, be fired at any time, for any reason, or for no reason.

Attorney Fees The contract may obligate you to pay attorneys' fees in the event of dispute, a potentially huge liability. You should resist any "one-sided" attorneys' fee provisions—consider accepting a provision that the prevailing party gets their attorneys' fees from the loser, or that you get your attorneys' fees covered if the agreement (particularly a restrictive covenant) is declared unenforceable.

The Restrictive Covenant Not to Compete

A "restrictive covenant not to compete" is an agreement wherein an employee, as a requisite of employment, agrees not to compete with their employer POST TERMINATION. These covenants may restrict a physicians' ability to practice: within a certain geographic area, for a certain period of time, may restrict performance of certain medical procedures or, commonly, restrict some combination of all of these elements.

These covenants are often accompanied by consents to injunctive relief, which would allow the institution to go to court in a matter of hours or days (rather than possibly waiting months or years to get into court) to obtain a temporary restraining order, which is generally followed in a few days by the "restricted physician" having to "show cause" why a permanent injunction against their practice should not be entered. Once the injunction is issued, the physician risks punishment if they continue to breach the noncompete clause [3].

I believe that restrictive covenants are acceptable if they ONLY apply DURING one's employment—it is not unreasonable for an employer to prevent your competing with them while you are their employee. But post-termination restrictions have serious ethical problems [4], because they interfere with the sanctity of the doctor/patient relationship, which is the sine qua non of our identity as members of a profession. Our colleagues in the legal profession have taken higher ground—law firms cannot, by law, have restrictive covenants in the employment contracts of their associates.[4]

---

[3] *See, e.g., LoPresti v. Rutland Regional Health Services, Inc. 2004 WL 2365402 (Vt. Oct 22, 2004)* Where Rutland Health Services attempted to fire an "at will" physician employee, Dr. LoPresti, for his referral of patients to specialists outside the Rutland group, because Dr. LoPresti felt that the Rutland specialists were inferior to physicians in another group. The Supreme Court of Vermont found that public policy would forbid Dr. LoPresti's firing on that basis.

[4] Rule 5.6 of the Model Rules of Professional Conduct, American Bar Association. In disapproving restrictive covenants in physician contracts, the Supreme Court of Tennessee put it this way: "We see no practical difference between the practice of law and the practice of medicine. Both profes-

Here's how the AMA ethical guidelines put it:

> (c)ovenants not to compete restrict competition, can disrupt continuity of care, and may limit access to care. Physicians should not enter into covenants that unreasonably restrict the right of a physician to practice medicine for a specified period of time or in a specified geographic area on termination of a contractual relationship; and do not make reasonable accommodation for patients' choice of physician.[5]

It is undeniable that these covenants can sever the doctor/patient relationship, interfere with a patient's right to see the physician of their choice, and, conversely, interfere with a willing physician's ability to continue to minister to their patient's needs. It is also undeniable that the only reason for these covenants is strictly economic. Patients are neither chattel nor merchandise, and the trust between a physician and their patient should not be up for sale. The AMA has put it more eloquently:

> The practice of medicine and its embodiment in the clinical encounter between a patient and a physician, is fundamentally a moral activity that arises from the imperative to care for patients and alleviate suffering. The relationship between patient and physician is based on trust and gives rise to physician's ethical obligations to place patients' welfare above their own self interest…[6]

Given that strong stance, one might legitimately wonder why the AMA has not outright said that restrictive covenants are unethical (like the lawyers have).[7] Indeed, they have done so in the case of restrictive covenants between residents and their training institutions.[8]

These covenants cause real pain and disruption in the lives of physicians and their patients. And they are, regrettably, upheld in many states. States vary widely in their willingness to enforce these agreements. Appellate courts in Missouri upheld a restrictive covenant with a radius of 350 miles (larger than the geographical

---

sions involve a public interest generally not present in commercial contexts. Both entail a duty on the part of practitioners to make their services available to the public. Also, both are marked by a relationship between the professional and patient or client that goes well beyond merely providing goods or services." *Murfreesboro Medical Clinic, P.A. v David Udom,* 166 S.W.3d 674, at 682 (2005).

[5] American Medical Association Council on Ethical and Judicial Affairs,11.2.3.1 (2016).

[6] Council on Ethical and Judicial Affairs Report 1-A-01 (June 2001)

[7] A complete ethical ban on restrictive covenants was, in fact, in place between 1933 and 1960, at which time various waffling formulations replaced the complete ban. It has been suggested that a stronger stance by the AMA on restrictive covenants has been chilled (despite resolutions to categorically condemn them having been introduced in the House of Delegates) after the AMA entered into a consent decree with the Federal Trade Commission in 1975 over allegations that the AMAs' stand on the corporate practice of medicine violated Section 5 of the Federal Trade Commission Act. *See* Leichter, P., *A Bitter Pill to Swallow: The Negative Impact of Non-Compete Clauses in Physician Employment Contracts,* Thesis for Masters of Law, submitted to the George Washington University Law School, May 17, 2015, and *In re American Medical Association,* 94 F.T.V. 701 (1979), *modified and enforced American Medical Association v Federal Trade Commission,* 638 F.2d 443 (2nd Cir.,1980), *aff;d* 455 U.S. 676 (1982).

[8] AMA Council on Judicial Affairs 11.2.3.1

size of Missouri).[9] Just over the border, the Kansas Supreme Court struck down a 25-mile limit as unreasonable.[10] The Supreme Court of Arizona, in a case involving a brachytherapist, struck down a five-mile restriction as unreasonable.[11]

Some states have placed limitations on, or have outright barred, restrictive covenants in physician contracts, and this reportedly includes Colorado, Delaware, Massachusetts, Alabama, California (by both statute and judicial decision!), Hawaii, Florida, Montana, Oklahoma, and North and South Dakota,[12] although some of these states allow "liquidated damages"[13] (but not "specific performance"[14]) for breach of a restrictive covenant. Texas requires that a liquidated damages clause be present in any physician contract that contains a restrictive covenant.[15] In Tennessee, by case law, physician restrictive covenants are banned except where specifically authorized by a Tennessee statute.[16]

Elsewhere, judicial relief may be possible from a restrictive covenant under one of the two doctrines. One is called the "rule of reasonableness" wherein courts will use a multipronged analysis looking at different parties' interests. The other doctrine applicable in some states is called the "blue pencil" test, where the court will simply strike out the words they find unreasonable, although they will generally not insert language or "rewrite" the contract. Unfortunately, in order to benefit from either doctrine, a physician would have to go to court to contest the operation of the restrictive covenant.

So, what to do if you are offered a contract with a restrictive covenant? First, appeal to the "better angels" of the institutions' nature, pointing out the ethical problems. If that doesn't work, think carefully about what the institution is saying, which is, essentially: "We think you will like practicing here, we think you are likely to be successful, we have the greatest control over whether you will be happy here or not, and we have reason to think that you may want to leave our department

---

[9] *Mid-States Paint and Chemical Co. v. Herr*, 746 SW 2d 613 (Mo App. 1988)

[10] *Graham v. Scirroco* 69 P.3d 194 (Kan. Ct. App. 2003)

[11] *Valley Medical Specialists v. Farber*, 194 Ariz. 363, 982 P.2d 1277, 1999

[12] See, e.g., Cal Bus. And Prof. Code §(West 1987), Mont. Code Ann §(1995); N.D. Cent. Code §(1987), Okla. Stat. Ann tit. 15 §217 (West 1993), MASS ANN Laws Ch. 112 §12x, Colo. Rev. Stat. §8-2-113(3), Del. Code Ann. Tit, 6 §2707 (2005).

[13] "Liquidated damages" are contract provisions that specify an amount of damages that are agreed to in advance if a specific section of a contract is breached by a party.

[14] "Specific performance" is a legal "term of art" that means being required to *actually do* what the contract says you will do, as opposed to "getting off" by paying damages for not performing according to the contract. In other words, in these jurisdictions, the law will allow you to practice despite the covenant, but if your contract states that you will pay liquidated damages if you breach the covenant, you will still have to pay those damages.

[15] Tex. Bus. and Com. Code Ann §15.50(b)

[16] For a state-by-state survey of the enforceability of restrictive covenants, up to date as of December 2012, see Horton, R., *Restrictive Covenants in Physician Employment Relationships*, April 2013 Member Briefing, American Health Lawyers Association. However, you should secure local counsel in the jurisdiction of your future practice for specific legal advice if you are presented with a contract containing a restrictive covenant.

at some point and compete with us." Why might that be? Ask yourself, also, how responsive are they likely to be to concerns you encounter in the practice, if you are hemmed in by a restrictive covenant?

If the institution will not abandon the restrictive covenant, an alternate strategy is to offer a "non-solicitation" clause whereby you agree not to solicit your former patients if you leave. (If they find you independently, you can still see them.) Agreeing to a reasonable "liquidated damages clause" is another alternative to a restrictive covenant that they might accept.

If you decide to go ahead and accept a restrictive covenant, at least try to negotiate decreases in time, distance, and activity restrictions, and/or bargain for a "severance" package to be included with the restrictive covenant, in order to cover your costs of relocation.

Nondisclosure Agreements You will also likely be asked to sign a confidentiality agreement (which may seek to lock up, in perpetuity, all patient information, including contact information) and agreements whereby you agree not to solicit either the practice's patients or their personnel, if you leave. It is considered unethical for a physician to be prohibited from informing a patient of their departure, and patients should be given their physician's forwarding address.[17]

Intellectual Property and Outside Income

It is essential for physicians entering academic practice that there be a clear understanding of how intellectual property is defined, and the parameters that determine who owns intellectual property that the physician may develop. Intellectual property may include articles that you write, devices you invent, or processes that you develop. Broadly written clauses could interfere with nonmedical and "after-hours" development of intellectual property.

The Bayh-Dole Act[18] and other federal law[19] give universities the right to take title of any inventions developed with federal funding, but university technology transfer offices have the ability to grant the researcher the right to commercialize

---

[17] *See*, e.g., Opinion 7.01 of the AMA Council on Ethical and Judicial Affairs, which reads, in relevant part: "The interest of the patient is paramount in the practice of medicine, and everything that can reasonably and lawfully be done to serve that interest must be done by all physicians who have served or are serving the patient. A physician who formerly treated a patient should not refuse for any reason to make his records of that patient promptly available on request to another physician presently treating the patient." Opinion 7.03 of the same document provides, in relevant part: "The patients of a physician who leaves a group practice should be notified that the physician is leaving the group. Patients of the physician should also be notified of the physician's new address and offered the opportunity to have their medical records forwarded to the departing physician at his or her new practice. It is unethical to withhold such information upon request of a patient."
[18] 35 US Code § 200–212
[19] 37 CFR § 401

their invention: a great potential benefit of an academic career, if you have an entrepreneurial streak!

Insurance Issues Space requirements in this chapter preclude an opportunity to discuss insurance issues in detail. However, your contract should specify who is responsible for "reporting endorsement" malpractice coverage, commonly known as "tail coverage" if you leave the practice. You must never allow a period of time to exist when you are not covered by a malpractice policy. Also, if life insurance is offered as a "benefit," be sure that you can name the beneficiary; sometimes the institution is the beneficiary!

Hospital-Based Physicians and Their Relationship to the Hospital

If you are employed by an academic institution, it's important to remember that such a relationship may not give you the guarantees of due process that you would expect as an independent, non-employed member of the hospital medical staff. If questions about quality or behavior arise, you might not have the luxury of review by your peers, because your hospital administrator can just fire you, especially if you are an employee "at will." Employment contracts will typically require you to surrender your medical staff privileges if you are no longer an employee.

The Requirement for Fair Market Value in Dealings Between Physicians and Institutions It may be worth noting that it is illegal (under fraud and abuse legislation) to enter into any agreement with the hospital that calls for such things such as salary, rental of office space, equipment, or services to be provided on terms other than their *fair market value*.

Benefits

A few general comments might be in order regarding "pension and profit sharing." It is rare in this day and age to have a "defined benefit plan" (also known as a "pension") whereby you are guaranteed a benefit, like healthcare, when you retire. Most all benefit plans are now "defined contribution plans" such as 401(k), 403(b) (the nonprofit entity's analog to a 401(K)), money purchase plans, or profit-sharing plans. Both employer and employee may contribute to these plans, in amounts that are capped by the relevant law, called ERISA.[20] Various "vesting schedules" will determine how many years you must practice with an institution before you can take the institution's contribution with you when you depart. Consult the ARRO

---

[20] Formally, the Employee Retirement Income Security Act, 29 U.S.C.A. §1001, *et seq.*

Table 1 Potential "benefits" to be included in a contract

Signing bonus
Performance incentives
Moving expenses (the amount for its taxable nature)
Educational/meeting allowance
Time off
Maternity/paternity leave
Retirement accounts and their vesting schedule
Malpractice insurance and "tail" coverage
Disability insurance
Long-term care insurance
Life insurance
Health insurance
Opportunity to "commercialize" discoveries/inventions
Right to interview and comment on hiring of personnel you supervise
"Protected" research time

survey and Table 1 for a description of various other benefits that may be offered by an academic practice.

In Conclusion

- Ask a lot of questions to understand what is contained in the offer of academic employment, and compare that to ARRO data of what other academic positions are offering.
- Strive to have all of what your regard as critical elements of the position reduced in writing to legally enforceable promises.
- Review all documents yourself and also with an attorney licensed to practice in the jurisdiction where you will practice medicine.
- Be particularly vigilant about rules governing the development and ownership of intellectual property.
- Resist signing, or seek to modify, a restrictive covenant.
- Use legal guarantees and insurance to maximize your flexibility in future employment and to minimize risk.

For Discussion with a Mentor or Colleague

- Ask new faculty members what, if any, representations about their position are at variance with their actual experience.
- What are the timetables and criteria for advancement and tenure?
- How are disputes resolved within the department?
- What rules govern nonmedical duties, such as committee assignments, etc.?
- How is research time "protected?"

References

1. Thompson L, et al. The intersection of online social networking with medical professionalism. J Gen Intern Med. 2008;23(7):954.
2. Lagu T, et al. Content of weblogs written by health professionals. J Gen Intern Med. 2008;22(10):1642.
3. Loeser D. The legal, ethical, and practice implications of noncompetition clauses: what physicians should know before they sign. J Law Med Ethics. 2003;31:283.
4. Wall T. Ethics in the legal and business practice of radiation oncology. Int J Rad Oncol Biol Phys. 2017;99:265.

Changing Jobs

Jennifer Croke, Ravi A. Chandra, and Laura A. Dawson

Introduction

In a rapidly changing medical system, most physicians will not stay in their first job for the course of their entire careers. Whether motivated by a desire to change career paths (e.g., academia versus private/community practice or industry, urban versus rural, etc.), to accommodate family or for other personal reasons, to pursue leadership opportunities, and/or to overcome burnout, a substantial number of physicians face the prospect of changing their position or trajectory at one or more junctures in their career. Having flexibility in medical career paths and the types of practice (part-time or shared practice) is (appropriately) becoming more acceptable in academia, private/community practice, and industry. Thus, it is expected that more radiation oncologists will contemplate making career changes in the future. In fact, studying and working at one institution for one's entire career can be limiting, and being exposed to more than one practice can open one's eyes to different approaches and more diversity, hopefully leading to improved patient care, as well as better job satisfaction. The goal of this chapter is to provide guidance on how to approach these career transitions.

J. Croke (✉) · L. A. Dawson
Radiation Medicine Program, Princess Margaret Cancer Centre, University Health Network, Toronto, ON, Canada

Department of Radiation Oncology, University of Toronto, Toronto, ON, Canada
e-mail: Jennifer.Croke@rmp.uhn.ca; Laura.Dawson@rmp.uhn.ca

R. A. Chandra
Department of Radiation Medicine, Knight Cancer Institute, Oregon Health & Science University, Portland, OR, USA
e-mail: chandrav@ohsu.edu

© Springer Nature Switzerland AG 2021
R. A. Chandra et al. (eds.), *Career Development in Academic Radiation Oncology*, https://doi.org/10.1007/978-3-030-71855-8_7

Why Make a Change?

Although there are advantages to making a career change, it is important to reflect, do background work, speak to those who have worked and are working where you may want to be, and not be hasty in making a change. It is natural in a career to go through dips and lulls, e.g., a "7-year itch" to do something different. It is important to reflect upon why one is considering changing jobs, and to consider if a job change is in fact the best solution.

Sometimes the reason for a change is clear, especially in personal situations mandating a move, (e.g., a partner's job leading to relocation or a move to be closer to aging family members). In other circumstances, the reason for a change may be to actively seek a new opportunity, perhaps due to a desire to change geography (or even country), salary, or job function (switching from private practice to academics, or vice versa; pursuing a teaching role or a potential leadership role at another institution). For others, their current job may not have turned out as they expected or may have changed (e.g., due to changes in leadership and/or department priorities) in a substantial enough way to prompt consideration of a job change. It is recommended to investigate strategies regarding how to improve one's present job before deciding to make a change for these reasons. It is important to explore one's own priorities and goals, and whether they can be fulfilled. Sometimes, one's value to a department may be higher than one realizes, and with changes in the job (salary, part-time, promotion, leadership, etc.) and genuine support, the present job may be adjusted enough to improve satisfaction enough to stay. One's own values and priorities ideally should be well aligned with those from leadership of the practice. If there are not, then a change may be the best solution.

The job market within radiation oncology has become increasingly more competitive. As a result, some new graduates may accept a position that was not their perceived "dream job" (e.g., not focusing on their desired clinical sites, not preferred geography, salary lower than expected, etc.) [1, 2]. As time goes on, a more desirable position may open up, causing one to consider a job transition. Again, it is worth reflecting and giving substantial thought into whether such a change is advantageous, not only for you professionally but also for your family and personally. Many radiation oncologists have thrived in positions that they would not have thought were "ideal," treating sites they never expected too, and finding substantial fulfillment in their career. Note that author LAD never expected to have a career treating hepatic malignancies, and now after 20 years, she could not imagine not treating patients with hepatic malignancies. There are advantages to being open-minded.

Although no rules exist, when prospective candidates have moved every few years or many times throughout their career, their commitment and team-playing ability may be questioned. The job market within radiation oncology continues to evolve; however, given these considerations and the logistical complexity of moving a medical practice, the threshold to relocate should be appropriately high.

Is a move necessary? The answer to this question may be obvious at first, especially if external forces (e.g., family/friends) are prompting the move. In such cases, it is worth considering whether your current job will enable flexibility to accommodate temporary external circumstances. Consider whether a temporary period of leave or a modified clinic schedule may be alternative solutions.

Some individuals are looking to transition because they are dissatisfied with their current employment situation. In such cases, it is critical to reflect and explore upon reasons why: is it an acute response to situational events or chronic unhappiness? If it is due to insufficient leadership, a toxic culture, or a negative change in salary structure, then consider whether these reasons are permanent or temporary. Similarly, market dynamics within a region can also change over time. Are there opportunities to make changes within your job to improve career satisfaction? For example, is it possible to change your schedule, hire a scribe or midlevel, or pursue additional training/roles with an organization? Furthermore, seeking advice from mentors is strongly recommended as mentorship has been shown to positively influence professional and personal development, lessen burnout, and facilitate job retention [3]. Furthermore, it is important to consider how a new opportunity will influence your career trajectory and how it will benefit the employer. Will you be able to acquire or utilize new skills, manage different populations of patients, or make yourself more marketable in the future? Can you tell a story of why you made this change? Or is it just a parallel move to a similar employer? This may be acceptable, but be up-front about the reasons for making a change and the expectations of the new job. Does the institution stand to benefit (i.e., a win-win) from your joining them? You'll need to articulate this to them, casting a vision for how they stand to benefit by choosing you over other candidates. Often, experienced radiation oncologists may be more marketable than a new graduate.

Equally important, how will this change impact your personal life and/or family? Changing jobs for any reason may cause initial financial, social, and psychological disruptions. Your salary may change, and you may have to uproot children from schools and friends. A spouse may have to find a new job. Frequently these decisions are complex and require input from multiple stakeholders to weigh all the pros and cons. Like any interpersonal relationship, compromise is needed; however, evaluating the short-term and long-term impacts on yourself and your loved ones is necessary to ensure whether a transition is successful professionally and personally. The importance of family and social networks cannot be understated.

Your career will have seasons and may not take the linear, well-ordered path you had envisioned when you started. This is acceptable, and in fact, you may end up in a better place as a result. Consider this quote from John Gardner:

> You wonder whether you climbed the wrong mountain. But the metaphor is all wrong. Life isn't a mountain that has a summit. Nor is it – as some suppose – a riddle that has an answer. Nor a game that has a final score. Life is an endless unfolding and – if we wish it to be – an endless process of self-discovery, an endless and unpredictable dialogue between our own potentialities and the life situations in which we find ourselves. By potentialities I mean not

just intellectual gifts but the full range of one's capacities for learning, sensing, wondering, understanding, loving and aspiring. Perhaps you think that by age 35 or 45 or even 55 you will have explored those potentialities pretty fully. Don't deceive yourself! The capacities you actually develop to the full come out as the result of an interplay between you and life's challenges – and the challenges keep coming.

What Type of Change?

Within your career, it is desirable to define "must-haves", "should haves," and "could haves." It helps to make a list. The "must-haves" are top priority that should not be forgotten (especially in the face of enticing incentives). Think about what you are passionate about and why. What are your unique skills and strengths that you can bring to an institution? What are your values professionally and personally? For example, you may desire a career with a large and diverse clinical component versus one with substantial research and/or teaching, and a super-selective, small clinical expertise. Does your current job align with your interests and values? It may be that your ideal job could be found in multiple settings (Table 1). For example, many radiation oncologists have highly impactful careers with a primary clinical focus whether in private practice, a hospital setting, or academia.

Table 1 Factors to consider when changing jobs[a]

Factor	Consideration
Type of practice	Academic vs. private vs. community Full-time vs. part-time vs. shared practice Urban vs. rural Primary site vs. satellite Teaching Industry Hybrid or combination of the above (e.g., mixed industry/academic)
Patient contact	Peer review platform, multidisciplinary rounds, incident-reporting system, etc. Coverage/on call/expected patient numbers/courses Mentorship available Support from others
Compensation	Salary, benefits, insurance, paid leave, vacation leave[a]
Academic	Research, teaching, administration expectations Potential for leadership, promotion, and other advancement Support for lab clinical scientists (MD-PhD) Support for other types of research or education career paths
Lifestyle	Geography, vacation, support for personal leave (parental, childcare, family, sick leave, other)
Reputation	Local/national/international Culture Work ethic and satisfaction of existing staff

[a]It is best to review any contract with a lawyer, administrator, and/or mentor before accepting a position

When one is a new staff, flexibility to advocate for yourself will be at its nadir within that organization. It may also be the time in your life when you need the most flexibility (e.g., starting a family). Leadership and colleagues may change, so it is important to try to ensure that the organization is well suited to you culturally, and that the role is one that matches both your personal and professional priorities.

How to Make a Change?

In those circumstances where one is forced to find new opportunities in new geographies, it helps to leverage connections. Although radiation oncology is a small field, there are opportunities at conferences, such as ASTRO, to seek the advice of others. Additionally, does your training program have alumni in the geographic area of interest? Often these individuals are helpful for informational interviews and connections locally. They may even be aware of opportunities that frequently aren't advertised. If you don't know anyone, looking through other alumni registries (college, medical school) or organizations you belong to might be another option. This process is easier in a way if the new location is in a different town or city (or state or country) from your current employer, since concerns about your current employer learning of your inquiries to change jobs are lower. Wherever possible, ask people you speak with for discretion, and if you provide any information about where you work, ask for them to let you know before they contact anyone at your current position. Most employers understand this sensitivity.

In demonstrating interest for a new geography, a visit to the area is highly recommended, especially in a different geographic region to where your present job is (more important with different country or culture). This allows one to set up some meetings at various groups in an area while allowing you to demonstrate your commitment to and knowledge of an area. Employers are often curious to confirm whether an applicant will really like living in a new location and being able to provide information on this from visits will increase their confidence. Engaging in your own geographic market, especially if small, can be more challenging and requires greater tact and sensitivity. Contact can be made by a mentor/sponsor via email or telephone to other institutions to notify them that you are looking and open for an opportunity. Unlike other fields of medicine, radiation oncology is small and therefore jobs may be competitive. Therefore, patience may be required, and this sort of conversation may occur over years rather than months or weeks.

Engaging Mentors and Connections

Having a network of mentors who know your interests and accomplishments, as well as life goals and circumstances, can be invaluable. Such individuals may help clarify your thinking, provide a sounding board, make calls/connections, and serve as resources. Try to cultivate mentorship at each level of training and in your professional life. Keep these people updated as you progress. Use some of the questions at the end of this chapter to have discussions that will help you learn more about where you want to head. Coaches and headhunters can also serve as valuable sources of information and guidance. There are multiple types of coaches that can assist with success at work, job hunting, career advancement, personal and/or athletic goals, and the like. Headhunters can help assess the job market and provide ideas and connections. LinkedIn, Twitter, and other social media can be yet another avenue for information, recruitment, and making connections.

When to Make a Change?

Give yourself as much lead time as you can to do your background research, cultivate leads/connections, and approach the job market from a position of strength and confidence rather than desperation. External circumstances may interfere, for example, if spouse needs to move right away or your hospital is closing in 6 months. If necessary, consider some short-term periods in locum tenens or with your current employer (if possible) until your new search has been completed to your satisfaction. Of course, you should never use current employer resources (e.g., email, phone, work time) to perform your search. Use your personal email, cell phone, vacation days, and own time for these pursuits. Making a timeline may be helpful, and ensure you give your present employer enough (but not too much) notice about your upcoming change. There is often a specified minimum time to give notice (e.g., 3 months). It is always best to leave on the best of terms as possible, and to be as gracious as possible to present employer. Radiation oncology is a small world.

Interacting with a Potential New Employer

Messaging the reasons for your transition is likely to be one of the more common, yet complex, questions you will have to answer. You are likely to be asked about why you are leaving your current employer. Reflect upon your true reasons and be honest and professional. Focus on what the new opportunity provides and look ahead rather than focus on what did not go right in your prior job. You will also have other difficult questions of your own, such as regarding salary expectations and work-life balance issues. Take care when asking these questions to be focused on the "right" reasons for pursuing the job and waiting until offers are in hand before asking these types of questions indirectly or directly.

Being Recruited/Approached

For those who are not actively looking for a job change, responding to career inquiries is an excellent way to make connections, learn about peers, and make yourself more marketable in your current role. This is all provided that you do not "lead on" a prospective employer into thinking you are very likely to take the job if you have no desire to take on a new job. It is acceptable to approach these situations with curiosity and openness. Ultimately a job offer may allow you to approach your current employer to help improve your situation. Or, you might end up taking the new job because it really is a better fit. Staying open, being honest, and reflecting on your priorities are critical.

Switching Between Academics and Private Practice

Studies have been performed within radiation oncology evaluating factors associated with entering academia versus private practice. The top three factors predicting an academic career straight out of residency were baseline interest pre-residency, academic role models, and research opportunities, whereas factors predicting private practice were baseline interest pre-residency, academic role models, and academic pressures/obligations [4]. Another study assessed radiation oncology residents' career decision variables. The top five variables associated with an academic career path were colleagues, clinical research, teaching, geography, and support staff, whereas the top five variables for those seeking private practice were lifestyle, practice environment, patient care, geography, and colleagues [5]. Interestingly, financial incentives were not among the top factors.

Do not underestimate the challenges of a job transition. Many radiation oncologists who have been in academia may (falsely) believe private practice to be "easier" and more lucrative. The private practice landscape has gotten tighter, and private practitioners often place high value on different character traits compared to academics (e.g., the three A's, affability, availability, and ability, in that order). Sometimes CVs can be considered too "academic" (i.e., too many papers and not enough clinical experience) by private practices. Additionally, some may worry that the clinical volumes may be too high for those used to practicing in an academic "protected" environment. Site visits can be critical in assessing the potential fit of the job, staff, and you.

The best advice is to approach a potential change with integrity, humility, and curiosity, learning what priorities a new practice has and how you might be able to contribute. Have a friend who is in private practice (if that is where you are transitioning to) review your CV and cover letter before submission. During interviews, speak about specific expertise you may have and connections you can offer. If possible, learn more about the market dynamics in that market and some basic business terminology that may be relevant to practice. Many hospital groups operate similarly to private practices in the sorts of skills they are looking for, so these types of exercises can be useful in both scenarios.

Switching Between Academic Centers

It is not unusual for radiation oncologists to change academic jobs over the course of a career. This may be to obtain some independence from the prior center (which may help in developing an international reputation and for possible future promotions), and/or to advance your career, e.g., due to a new opportunity or path for development and leadership. Within academics, you may consider a job transition if a position opens up advertising a prerequisite that you are uniquely qualified for. For example, if you have interest and expertise in medical education and a center is searching for a new residency program director, then your qualifications will stand out. Likewise, if someone who is renowned for brachytherapy retires and you have a brachytherapy fellowship with several publications and/or grants, you may be viewed as competitive for the position. Physicians typically change jobs within academia if they feel they have something valuable to bring to the new position, for example, a specialized skill or international reputation. Their experience and training may help them to be desirable as recruits to develop a new program (e.g., an oligo-metastatic program or a palliative medicine program). Furthermore, similar to any job transition, personal, family, and geography factors need to be considered.

Alternatively, one may be recruited to become a chair of a department, the head of a cancer center, or a CEO of a hospital or professional society. These types of career changes require more thought, as they require different skills than those needed to be an excellent clinician, such as management, business, and leadership skills. These positions are likely to lead to a substantial change in day-to-day activities, often with reduced clinical duties, but more administrative and financial responsibilities.

Leaving or Returning to Clinical Practice

Leaving clinical practice (permanently) is a particularly significant decision, and one that should be approached even more cautiously as returning even after only a couple of years away can be challenging (due to licensing/certification issues, need to take SPEX/demonstrate competency, and lack of experience and loss of modern radiation therapy skills, etc.). A study of US resident physicians reported that 45% of respondents reported symptoms of burnout and 14% reported career choice regret. Within this study, radiation oncology was included within radiology, and symptoms of burnout were reported in 35% and career choice regret in almost 17% [6]. This could motivate institutions to consider alternative practice models, such as part-time practice, job sharing, modifications to family leave, etc., to help to improve job satisfaction and in retention of diverse faculty. It is always desirable to not leave clinical practice for extended times, if there is a possibility of returning in the future. An alternative may be transitioning to part-time position or locum tenens or taking a temporary personal leave. The decision to leave clinical practice permanently is different than more temporary personal leaves, which are expected during a lifetime and covered in the Family Medical Leave Act.

Even more substantive informational interviews are needed, especially when considering nonclinical paths such as working in industry, consulting, or others. If possible, short-term or part-time work may allow one to gain greater exposure and increase marketability simultaneously. Some short-term assignments (e.g., government service or sabbatical with industry) may enable you to return in the future, so when possible, try to get information from others who have done things similarly.

If you have made the decision to move, it is always best to maintain connections with current employers as much as possible. Maintain graciousness and kindness as you never know if your paths will intersect again in the future.

Dealing with Current Employer/References

As discussed above, sensitivity is required with current employment, both in terms of remaining committed to your job and its responsibilities and in keeping discussions with other potential employers separate.

If you are leaving, be gracious and kind, and remember that while you don't have an obligation (other than contractual) to your current employer, our field is small and one should always do the right thing. This may mean staying a little longer until a replacement can be identified, making sure your patients are appropriately transferred to another radiation oncologist with letters sent to patients in advance to notify them of their future plans, and taking on less desirable responsibilities immediately before you leave (as you will not be the go-to person for future opportunities once it is known that you are leaving).

Staying in the same market and moving to a competitor is likely the most complicated transition and not desirable in general. It will be addressed more below.

Medicolegal, Insurance, and Logistical Considerations

As with all contracts, it is important to have a trained lawyer review contracts before you sign. If your current employment contract has ramifications for your transition (e.g., noncompete, non-solicitation) mechanics, it is important to involve a lawyer early in the process as this will impact how your negotiations with a new employer will unfold. Buying into or out of partnerships even if the relocation is outside of a competition territory can be thorny, both legally and financially. Also, of import is tail or nose insurance (a policy that will cover you for work at the prior employer even after you have left). While your malpractice insurance covered you while you were at your previous employer, once you leave you can still be sued if you do not have tail (or nose coverage). These policies can be expensive, so it is important to clarify if your future or prior employer will pay for this, if not already contractually stipulated.

Be sure to allot plenty of time to change addresses, obtain licenses, and complete paperwork, in addition to the personal aspects of the transition. Whether across town or the country, it will take longer than you think.

Special Considerations: Layoffs/Downsizing, Termination, and Lawsuits

Sometimes the decision to leave an employer is made for you, by circumstances beyond your control (such as downsizing/integration), termination, or lawsuits. Such circumstances will make the process of looking for a new position more complicated and less orderly than an elective job search, but with appropriate advice and assistance, it can be managed. Engage an attorney who is responsible to your interests alone for advice and assistance in each of these circumstances. During a layoff, you are likely to have at least a little time to find a new job, and messaging the circumstances with a new employer will be easier. A termination (for cause or not) will be more challenging, and a capable attorney may be able to help you negotiate this sort of exit with an eye toward future questions in interviews, job/credentialing applications, and the like. As with all things, honesty is important at every stage, and engaging your mentors for advice and assistance is critical.

Stay Positive

Finding a new physician job is a challenging endeavor, no matter your background. It is best to practice self-awareness and self-reflection; you will learn something about yourself in this process and probably refine your goals. In the end, taking sufficient time to reflect on the why, what, and how to make a job change, always considering professional and personal factors, is likely to be beneficial in the long run. In radiation oncology, we are tremendously lucky to provide such effective treatments for our patients, and we are fortunate to have so many possible types of career paths. Making a job change is challenging, but when the time is right and a new career opportunity is aligned with one's values, goals, and priorities, such a change may be a fruitful way to reinvigorate one's career, increasing job satisfaction, which should also lead to better patient care.

Summary

- Changing jobs, whether by necessity or electively, can be a mechanism for crafting an interesting and exciting career.
- Be open to unplanned opportunities and make the most of wherever you are.
- Reflect and think carefully about reasons for wanting to change jobs, engaging mentors and colleagues frequently.
- Define your values and priorities and match to prospective opportunities.
- Recognize that you'll always know more about your current role than your future one.
- Engage outside professionals (attorney, tax advisor) where needed to understand the various considerations impacting your transition.

For Discussion with a Mentor or Colleague

- What are my priorities? What are my career priorities and personal priorities? How do they align?
- What do I envision as my career trajectory? What sorts of skills or experiences do I need to acquire? Where do I want to be in 5 years? In 10+ years?
- Do you know individuals in a specific career or location who would be willing to speak with me?
- Do you know individuals with similar life/personal considerations to me, either at my career stage or slightly ahead, who could give me advice on how to approach my career?

References

1. Kahn J, Goodman CR, Albert A, et al. Top concerns of radiation oncology trainees in 2019: job market, board examinations, and residency expansion. Int J Radiat Oncol Biol Phys. 2020;106:19–25.
2. Fung CY, Chen E, Vapiwala N, et al. The American Society for Radiation Oncology 2017 radiation oncologist workforce study. Int J Radiat Oncol Biol Phys. 2019;103:547–56.
3. Sambunjak D, Straus S, Marusic A. The impact of mentorship: systematic review. JAMA. 2006;296:1103–15.
4. Chang DT, Shaffer JL, Haffty BG, et al. Factors that determine academic versus private practice career interest in radiation oncology residents in the United States: results of a nationwide survey. Int J Radiat Oncol Biol Phys. 2013;87:464–70.
5. Wilson LD, Flynn DF, Haffty BG. Radiation oncology career decision variables for graduating trainees seeking positions in 2003-2004. Int J Radiat Oncol Biol Phys. 2005;62:519–25.
6. Dyrbye LN, Burke SE, Hardeman RR, et al. Association of clinical specialty with symptoms of burnout and career choice regret among US resident physicians. JAMA. 2018;320:1114–30.

Part III
Early Career Development

Identifying and Utilizing Mentors

Anna Lee, Lauren Colbert, and Clifton David Fuller

Introduction

The term "mentorship" is derived from Homer's "Odyssey" when the King of Ithaca, Odysseus, went to fight in the Trojan War. During this time, he entrusted the care of his son, Telemachus, to Mentor who provided guidance, counsel, and support [4]. While the concept of mentorship has existed for a long time, there are many definitions which reflect the varied ways it manifests depending on the context. In medicine, it can be generalized to a two-way relationship in which an individual invests personal knowledge, energy, and time in order to help another individual grow and develop [22].

The benefits of mentorship in academic medicine have been well described with respect to job satisfaction, career success, personal development, reflection, and self-direction of learning [8, 11, 35, 43, 49]. Furthermore, mentorship has shown to help alleviate stress and prevent burnout [55], which is particularly salient in radiation oncology where a nationwide survey reported approximately one-third of residents in the field reporting high levels of burnout symptoms [41]. Given an increasingly competitive job market [10], access to mentorship is important for both professional development and to promote wellness through the high-pressure years of training and the early-career period. Still, half of radiation oncology junior faculty and residents report not having a mentor, while females report more difficulty in finding mentors compared to their male counterparts [5, 17, 26]. Here, we offer a practical guide to mentorship with insights and studied frameworks that may maximize the mentorship experience.

A. Lee · L. Colbert · C. D. Fuller (✉)
The Department of Radiation Oncology, The University of Texas MD Anderson Cancer Center, Houston, TX, USA
e-mail: CDFuller@mdanderson.org

© Springer Nature Switzerland AG 2021
R. A. Chandra et al. (eds.), *Career Development in Academic Radiation Oncology*, https://doi.org/10.1007/978-3-030-71855-8_8

Identifying a Mentor or Mentor Team

Development of mentoring relationships can be challenging depending on one's interests and availability of opportunities in one's environment. However, mentorship can take place in different forms, and even when it does, it may not seem obvious or formalized. During the process of identifying a mentor, it is important to be open to formal, informal, spot, and peer mentoring opportunities, which can take place both inside and outside one's institution or practice. The best mentors may not necessarily be people who look and think like you and, above all, should embody ideal characteristics that will set up the mentee for success. A study by Cho et al. found words or phrases that mentees used to describe an ideal mentor included generosity, selflessness, patience, and understanding. Furthermore, they were honest, particularly about their own failures and real-life stories, and had exceptional communication skills, namely, active listening [9]. Other more practical considerations include being available and approachable [20] as well as being able to assess the strengths and weaknesses of the mentee without judgment. The interpersonal skill of providing constructive feedback in a supportive manner is also helpful in helping the mentee progress in achieving their goal. An efficient way to ascertain whether a mentor may embody these attributes is to see the long-term impact of the trainees that have worked with them in the past or even speaking to current/former protégés about their mentorship experience.

The process of identifying a mentor or principal investigator (PI) for the physician-scientists in our field can be more involved as the process also involves selecting a research laboratory. In an inductive, qualitative study, 42 early-stage doctoral students in biological science programs were asked about their decisions in finding the right fit with a PI and within a lab [31]. The most important factor was finding a PI with whom they felt had potential for a relationship to remain productive and positive over time, which included attributes such as authenticity, comfort, communication, respect, and interest. Eighty-eight percent of students indicated that mentoring style ("hands-on" versus a more "hands-off" approach) was a factor in their selection. Finally, a substantial amount of students (67%) felt the fit with lab mates and fit (75%) with the research conducted were important key criteria. With regard to finding an environment that was amenable to their working styles and interests, students noted that "choosing a permanent lab home…is probably one of the most important decisions you make for the rest of your life, besides what graduate school you go to and what spouse you decide to marry. It very much impacts future career opportunities, people you may postdoc with, what field you choose to pursue after your research, what field you land in and specialize in." Among students who left their first lab, lack of funding was the largest concern, which is integral to long-term stability. In sum, this study highlights the need for residency programs to provide opportunity for candid discussions between physician-scientists and PIs in the lab selection process.

Formal Versus Informal Channels

Mentorship can occur through both formal and informal channels. Informal mentoring is more likely to occur spontaneously, by choice, and is typically developed when protégés and mentors readily identify with each other. An informal mentorship may be initiated by a colleague introducing you to a faculty member at a conference or by meeting a resident during an away rotation with whom you maintained contact. One study found informal is more beneficial than formal mentorship in that informal mentors were more likely to engage in positive psychosocial activities such as counseling, facilitating social interactions, role modeling, and providing friendship [38]. Protégés were also more satisfied with their informal mentors than with formal mentors. This may be because the mentor sees oneself in the protégé and the protégé may be trying to emulate the mentor's qualities. Interestingly, an informal mentorship questionnaire conducted among medical professionals found older age and a longer mentoring relationship contributed to positive perceptions of interpersonal aspects of informal mentoring [32]. Older age as a surrogate of experience supports the notion that informal mentorship is typically initiated by the more seasoned or extroverted mentee; thus, the drawback may be that it could lead to social exclusion where it may indirectly leave out introverted or marginalized groups.

In radiation oncology, recent efforts to develop formal mentorship programs and evaluate them have been emerging since the publication of the Radiation Oncology Academic Development and Mentorship Assessment Project showing faculty who report having a mentor had higher objective measures of academic productivity [23] and another report revealing only half of residents in the field reported having a mentor [17]. A survey study of female residents in radiation oncology found 41% stated they did not feel they had adequate mentorship in residency and over half (51%) reported lack of mentorship affected career ambitions [34].

Formalizing mentorship provides a mechanism whereby residents feel comfortable seeking guidance from faculty, especially since many individuals do not have the opportunity to develop a mentoring relationship in an informal way. There can be drawbacks to formal mentoring such as the sense of a binding commitment from both the mentor and mentee via signing of formal agreements as well as a strict selection and training process, which may not always meet the expectations of the parties involved. However, studies addressing the impact of structured mentorship curriculums in radiation oncology showed very high rates of satisfaction. A survey of 126 residents in the Northeast found 90% of those involved in a formal mentorship program were satisfied with their experience [45]. Another study found 74% of residents reported a desire to participate in a formal mentorship program and 85% felt mentorship plays a critical role in residency training and career development [17]. One residency examined a formal program for trainees to regularly assess career goals with their mentors through an individual development plan, which significantly increased residents' confidence in achieving career goals and bolstered the mentor-mentee relationship [25]. Given the importance of mentorship in terms of resident satisfaction and future success, national programs in the field have developed these formal opportunities as outlined in Table 2 at all stages of one's career.

Intramural Versus Extramural Channels

Identifying the right mentor may require a search in many places—inside and outside the department and institution. A study of mentorship experiences of early-career academic radiation oncologists found women reported lower rates of mentor relationships with specialties outside the field, which may be particularly important to facilitate success in basic science research [26]. The importance of extramural mentorship particularly for physician-scientists is highlighted by National Institutes of Health (NIH)-sponsored training programs which have mentored career ("K") awards under the guidance of an experienced mentor or mentoring team, which often include involved parties from outside one's field and institution.

Extramural channels are important for career advancement in academic medicine as promotion at certain institutions may be tied to recommendations from respected peers and mentors outside the institution. Rush University recently evaluated their research mentoring program as part of their faculty development in academic medicine and found that mentees reported a strength of the program being the interprofessional collaboration and mentoring outside of one's college and that even more informal connections outside their college/department could be pursued. Their mentoring approach has resulted in high faculty retention, promotion, satisfaction, and scholarly productivity of mentees [44].

Working with a Mentor or Mentor Team

There are several approaches to mentorship. They can take place in dyadic, multiple, apprenticeship, and team forms and can be delivered in different methods such as peer, senior, distance, and virtual, which are outlined in Table 1 [22]. The most traditional form is the dyadic model that is delivered via the senior mentoring approach where the mentor who is more knowledgeable and seasoned is paired with a less experienced protégé. Although this is the most common, there is growing evidence for improved mentorship experiences that challenge the hierarchical and dyadic form. Williams et al. have described multilevel mentoring for junior faculty where peers, senior faculty, and private-practice physicians are involved [51]. Another study examined peer-group mentoring and found participants had more opportunities to learn and expand their knowledge and endorsed a greater sense of empowerment [37]. One study utilizing telephone interviews with 100 former recipients of NIH-mentored career development awards and their mentors found several themes that were consistent such as the improbability of finding a single person who

Table 1 Mentoring models and method of delivery [22]

Form of mentorship	Definition
Dyadic	Dyadic mentoring is the traditional mentoring model in which there is a one-to-one relationship between mentor and mentee, and it has been the most common mentoring model and has influenced the progress of mentorship [9]
Multiple	Multiple mentoring is very reminiscent of dyadic; however, in this model the mentee is mentored by several mentors simultaneously and noting that each mentor is facilitating the development of a particular area [2]
Apprenticeship	While this form is not a significant form of mentorship in itself, it may fall under that of dyadic mentoring—it is when the mentee observes and emulates the skills of the mentor [7]. The difference between this model of mentoring and that of the dyadic is that in this model, the mentor may facilitate educational knowledge but may not be involved in helping the mentee in developing their careers or providing holistic support [7]
Team	Resembling the multiple mentoring models is the team-mentoring model that standardizes the concept of several mentors into a formal committee, just as in multiple mentoring. Each mentor brings a different knowledge, but that also has interaction and communication between the several mentors whereby facilitating more efficient and effective mentoring [2]
Method of delivery	**Definition**
Peer mentoring	Very collaborative and mutually beneficial as the relationship is formed among the mentors, peers, or colleagues. In this situation, the mentee may be more inclined to share their difficulties and questions with peers, who are at an equal or similar level of knowledge and seniority, as opposed to senior faculty [2]
Senior mentoring	The most common form of delivery [7] in which there is a senior faculty taking the role of the mentor and a junior mentee
Distance and virtual mentoring	Distance mentoring and virtual mentoring may be considered under the same category as distance mentoring is when the mentor and mentee are in different locations [5]. It may be related to virtual mentoring wherein social media could be used as a tool to achieve goals, particularly with respect to biomedical research faculty, but which could be further researched in other fields

can fulfill the diverse mentoring needs of an individual and the importance and composition of mentor networks. The key insight was the importance of building mentoring networks tailored to each faculty member's unique career trajectory and needs [14].

Educational Aspect

The holistic model of mentoring has been described in the context of general medical practice, which is a three-pronged framework starting with the educational component of mentorship [19], which entails helping acquire and integrate new knowledge. Typically, this may be most pronounced in radiation oncology for physician-scientists where the principal investigator may be guiding experimental design and methodology for testing hypotheses. In the clinical setting, this is most visible in fellowship where trainees have been found to primarily pursue additional training to specialize in a technique (i.e., brachytherapy, proton therapy) or a clinical subsite (i.e., pediatrics) [18]. This may manifest as an apprenticeship-style mentorship where education often includes pearls from experience beyond what a textbook can offer.

Professional Aspect

Perhaps the most well-identified component of mentoring is the professional piece where the goal is to help maximize potential of a mentee to become a fulfilled and achieving practitioner [42]. Success in radiation oncology requires hard work and talent, but often achievements alone do not guarantee promotion or appointment to high-profile leadership positions. Thus, the concept of sponsorship has emerged where the focus is on enhancing the visibility, credibility, and professional networks of talented individuals [21]. A semi-structured interview study at Johns Hopkins looking at sponsorship found that (1) sponsorship is episodic and focused on specific opportunities; (2) effective sponsors are career-established and well-connected; (3) effective protégés rise to the task and remain loyal; (4) trust, respect, and weighing risks are key to successful sponsorship relationships; and (5) sponsorship is critical to career advancement [3]. The benefits of sponsorship are two-way—for the protégé, sponsorship has shown to improve job satisfaction, higher likelihood of being promoted, increased salary, and inclusion on major projects. For sponsors, they may be perceived by others as having exceptional ability to discover unrecognized talent, which then improves the reputation of the sponsor [36].

Some concrete actions a budding sponsor can take as recommended by Dr. Reed A. Omary, a radiologist at Vanderbilt University Medical Center, are the following:

1. Schedule time on your calendars to formally sponsor one or more of your colleagues such as nominating them for an award, asking a colleague at another institution to invite them as a visiting professor, or presenting them with an opportunity for a new leadership position.
2. Amplify your impact by sponsoring someone anonymously, which can sometimes be more effective for the recipient.

He also recommends the following for those who aim to be sponsored: (1) Ask someone directly for his or her assistance to sponsor you. For instance, if someone you know is enrolled in a leadership development program, ask that person to help nominate you for next year's program. (2) Develop as many professional relationships as possible with leaders from outside fields. These are potential first steps in using sponsorship as a deliberate career-advancement strategy as we understand its distinction from mentorship [15].

Personal Aspect

The third aspect of the holistic model of mentoring is the personal one where the mentor helps manage transitional states through counseling and listening. A questionnaire administered to internal medicine residents specifically explored personal aspects of the mentoring relationship and found 57% felt their mentor was important to personal development while 52% felt they had a meaningful personal relationship with their mentor [40]. This is especially important for trainees and early-career faculty where burnout is a topic of ongoing discussion. A qualitative analysis of the characteristics of outstanding mentors found support of a personal/professional balance to be one of the five themes as mentees looked to their mentors as role models for work-life integration. In addition, mentors who offered support to mentees during periods of stress or personal struggle were found to be more impactful [9]. For example, a mentor shares with a mentee her struggles with balancing children and key early-career decisions, which helped the mentee relates to her mentor and creates a safe space where they could open up about personal issues, particularly as they affect one's professional life. This underscores that mentees seek guidance not only academically but personally and sharing one's life experiences, whether good or bad, can leave a lasting impression on mentees.

Special Considerations

Mentorship and Gender

There are now numerous studies published on mentorship and its benefit to women in medicine as females in academic medicine face unique challenges with significant gender disparities in medical leadership [22]. It has been suggested that women pursue career-advancement opportunities differently than men in which men tend to make more informal network connections and be more self-promoting, whereas women may feel more hesitant to advance into a new role or negotiate for higher salary [3, 21, 48]. Thus, as the potential value of sponsorship for underrepresented groups is better understood, formal sponsorship programs are being developed in academic medicine so that women have access to the type of beneficial relationships that will advance one's career. Opportunities to find mentors through organized medical groups for women can be found in Table 2.

Interestingly, effective mentorship does not require same-gender pairings [13, 24], and there are studies supporting the contribution of gender diversity to collective intelligence [52]. A study of abstracts selected for presentation at the American Society for Radiation Oncology annual meeting found cross-gender mentorship pairings of the primary and senior author were more likely than same-gender pairings to obtain journal publication in higher-impact journals, suggesting a possible independent benefit to gender diversity in research mentorship [27].

Table 2 Formal mentorship opportunities in radiation oncology

Organization	Target group	Website for sign-up
American Association of Physicists in Medicine (AAPM) Science Council Associates Mentorship Program	PhD candidates Med phys junior faculty	http://gaf.aapm.org/
American College of Radiation Oncology (ACRO) Mentorship Program	Medical students Residents Attendings	https://www.acro.org/residents/resident-mentor-program/
American Society for Radiation Oncology (ASTRO) Grant Review Mentorship Program	Junior faculty	https://www.astro.org/Patient-Care-and-Research/Research/Mentoring
Association of Residents in Radiation Oncology (ARRO) Global Health Subcommittee Mutual Mentorship Program	Residents	https://www.astro.org/Affiliate/ARRO/Global-Health/Mutual-Mentorship-Program
American Association for Women in Radiology (AAWR) Mentorship Program	Residents Fellows Attendings	https://www.aawr.org/Events/AAWR-Mentoring-Program
Society for Women in Radiation Oncology (SWRO) Mentorship Program	Medical students Residents Attendings	https://www.societywomenradiationoncology.com/mentorship

Mentorship and Underrepresented Minorities

The field of radiation oncology has made efforts to increase diversity; however, there is still much work to be done in this regard as underrepresented minorities (URM) only comprise 9% of radiation oncology trainees even though they make up 15% of medical school graduates [16]. A diverse workforce can better understand the diverse patient population which the field serves as cancer affects all ethnicities, sexual orientations, religions, and socioeconomic statuses in the USA. Four themes have been identified that are associated with a dearth of URM in radiation oncology, namely, exposure, interest, preparation/mentorship, and unconscious bias [29]. In a survey of program directors in 2018, the top three factors in selecting applicants to interview were USMLE Step 1 scores, letters of recommendation, and research [33], the latter two likely requiring some level of mentorship. Boston University has developed the formalized radiation oncology mentorship initiative (ROMI) since 2003 where medical students are paired with faculty and have reported long-term success with match rates and practice in academic settings [7]. This model could be improved by focusing exposure of the field to medical schools with larger number of URM and encouraging application for national-level specialty-specific programs to help foster mentorship relationships and research opportunities. Fortunately, a compilation of programs to increase exposure early on is available [2].

Tips for Mentors (From OHSU Mentoring Website)

- Evaluate your skills and time.
- Say no, if you want to say no.
- Be available.
- Be curious.
- Be courteous.
- Be in touch.
- Be honest about the relationship.
- Play a role in career advancement.
- Help establish goals.
- Give feedback.
- Listen.
- Uphold professional standards.
- Get your own personal "coaching staff" in place to support you.
- Additional tips can be found in "Nature's Guide for Mentors" [28].

Tips for Mentees (From OHSU Mentoring Website)

- Have realistic expectations.
- Ask for specific advice and be receptive to input.
- Evaluate feedback and advice.
- Evaluate the relationship.
- Take responsibility for the relationship.
- Keep in touch.
- Be considerate.
- Be prepared.
- Establish the nature of the relationship.
- Realize that relationships are dynamic.
- Don't discount the value of peers.
- Maintain confidentiality.
- Express appreciation.
- Additional tips can be found in "Making the Most of Mentors: A Guide for Mentees" [54].

Challenges and Pitfalls in Mentorship

Distance Mentoring

Long-distance mentoring has shown to be one solution to multiple scenarios including but not limited to a scarcity of local mentors, establishing relationships outside one's institution or field and maintaining relationships during a pandemic where social distancing is the rule (COVID-19). They are becoming more common as both mentees and mentors move institutions or as a mentee seeks specific expertise [30]. Some ways to make long-distance mentoring more successful include establishing the relationship in a face-to-face meeting and then continuing it at a distance with occasional face time at conferences. Furthermore, setting clear expectations at the beginning can help define roles and goals. There are plenty of platforms beyond the phone call, e-mail, and text that can help facilitate mentorship in a virtual way including social media and online video platforms.

Mentee Missteps

Upon entering a mentorship relationship, the mentee may feel his/her role is daunting and that they have to be perfect from the outset; however, the beauty of cultivating a mentee's career is in the development and learning process. Vaughn et al. describe six phenotypes of missteps that most commonly occur with shared behaviors or traits such as conflict avoidance (the overcommitter, the ghost, the doormat), lack of confidence (the vampire, the lone wolf, the backstabber), and failure to understand the expectations of menteeship [50]. To avoid such missteps, mentees should begin by delineating personal and career goals and explicitly stating them so as to minimize conflict and maximize benefit for both parties. Furthermore, stating that the misstep has occurred candidly can strengthen the relationship and help for future success.

How to Break Up with Your Mentor

Sometimes a relationship can be established within a formal mentoring program, but this may not necessarily mean a true mentorship relationship has been established [42]. A formal mentorship program with a predefined time interval may allow a natural separation if goals do not align or there is simply not enough "chemistry" between the mentor and mentee. Dysfunctional mentoring relationships can have a negative impact on the professional development of protégés; namely, difficulties with self-esteem and low satisfaction of the workplace institution are potential consequences [46]. When one is in the middle of a mentor-mentee relationship and the quality of the relationship is low enough, there is little guidance as to how to navigate a mismatched or unsuccessful relationship. A few tips have been outlined in a post published by the American Society of Clinical Oncology (ASCO) Connection that posit the breakup in a stepwise, thoughtful process [1].

Assessment of Mentorship

Studies examining predictors for successful mentoring relationships found satisfaction with the mentoring relationship to the most reliable predictor [39, 53]. Thus, it's important to use validated tools to assess satisfaction and quality of mentoring and to do interval assessments to evaluate the weighted satisfaction of mentoring relationships.

Munich-Evaluation-of-Mentoring-Questionnaire (MEMeQ)

The MEMeQ is a validated questionnaire that was originally designed to evaluate mentorship programs in undergraduate medical education [47]. It weighs satisfaction based on importance of seven areas of interest and provides a descriptive profile of each protégé's areas of interest regarding their mentoring relationships. A survey study of radiation oncology mentorship among residents utilized the MEMeQ and found those in formal programs reported higher rates of satisfaction over those who were not in formal programs (90% vs. 9%, $p < 0.001$) [45].

Mentorship Profile Questionnaire and Mentorship Effectiveness Scale (Johns Hopkins University)

As formal and informal mentorship programs in medicine have been put in place across the nation, criteria for evaluating the effectiveness of these programs are needed. Within this context, the Ad Hoc Faculty Mentoring Committee at Johns Hopkins University School of Nursing developed generic instruments to measure the effectiveness of a faculty mentoring relationship [6]. The first is the Mentorship Profile Questionnaire, which describes the characteristics and outcome measures from the perspective of the mentee, and the Mentorship Effectiveness Scale, a 12-item 6-point agree-disagree-format Likert-type rating scale, which evaluates 12 behavioral characteristics of the mentor.

Conclusion

The field of radiation oncology is small and evidence-based with a high emphasis on research, characteristics that highlight the importance of mentorship. This relationship can exist in multiple forms to fulfill the needs of the mentee educationally, professionally, and personally. Mentorship helps maintain positive associations in the field, and more effort is needed to formalize sponsorship programs to help advance the careers of trainees and early-career faculty.

Summary

1. Mentorship exists in several models—dyadic, multiple, apprenticeship, and team—that can be delivered in various means, formal, informal, peer, senior, distance, and virtual.
2. Mentorship and, in particular, sponsorship are proven to be important components of career advancement. Women and underrepresented minorities can particularly benefit from sponsorship.
3. Mentors and mentor teams for physician-scientists in the field are the mainstay—relationships outside the institution and field are especially important for success.

For Discussion with a Mentor or Colleague [12]

- What does the term mentor mean to you?
- What are your previous experiences being a mentor and/or a mentee?
- What characteristics should the ideal mentor and mentee have?
- How do you foresee your needs regarding mentorship changing throughout your training and career?
- How is sponsorship different than mentorship?

Additional Reading/Resources

1. Oregon Health Sciences University Mentorship Website: https://www.ohsu.edu/school-of-medicine/mentoring/getting-started
2. University of Minnesota Online Mentorship Course: https://www.ctsi.umn.edu/education-and-training/mentoring/mentor-training
3. Stanford Radiation Oncology Mentorship Website: https://radonc.stanford.edu/about/mentorship.html

References

1. Abuali I. How to break up with your mentor. 2020. Retrieved 7 May 2020, from https://connection.asco.org/tec/career/how-break-your-mentor.
2. Agarwal A, DeNunzio NJ, Ahuja D, Hirsch AE. Beyond the standard curriculum: a review of available opportunities for medical students to prepare for a career in radiation oncology. Int J Radiat Oncol Biol Phys. 2014;88(1):39–44.
3. Ayyala MS, Skarupski K, Bodurtha JN, Gonzalez-Fernandez M, Ishii LE, Fivush B, Levine RB. Mentorship is not enough: exploring sponsorship and its role in career advancement in academic medicine. Acad Med. 2019;94(1):94–100.
4. Barondess JA. A brief history of mentoring. Trans Am Clin Climatol Assoc. 1995;106:1–24.
5. Barry PN, Miller KH, Ziegler C, Hertz R, Hanna N, Dragun AE. Factors affecting gender-based experiences for residents in radiation oncology. Int J Radiat Oncol Biol Phys. 2016;95(3):1009–16.
6. Berk RA, Berg J, Mortimer R, Walton-Moss B, Yeo TP. Measuring the effectiveness of faculty mentoring relationships. Acad Med. 2005;80(1):66–71.
7. Boyd GH, Rand AE, DeNunzio NJ, Agarwal A, Hirsch AE. The radiation oncology mentorship initiative: analysis of a formal mentoring initiative for medical students interested in radiation oncology. J Cancer Educ. 2019;35(7) https://doi.org/10.1007/s13187-019-01539-w.
8. Buddeberg-Fischer B, Herta KD. Formal mentoring programmes for medical students and doctors--a review of the Medline literature. Med Teach. 2006;28(3):248–57.
9. Cho CS, Ramanan RA, Feldman MD. Defining the ideal qualities of mentorship: a qualitative analysis of the characteristics of outstanding mentors. Am J Med. 2011;124(5):453–8.
10. Chowdhary M, Chhabra AM, Switchenko JM, Jhaveri J, Sen N, Patel PR, Curran WJ Jr, Abrams RA, Patel KR, Marwaha G. Domestic job shortage or job maldistribution? A geographic analysis of the current radiation oncology job market. Int J Radiat Oncol Biol Phys. 2017;99(1):9–15.
11. Connor MP, Bynoe AG, Redfern N, Pokora J, Clarke J. Developing senior doctors as mentors: a form of continuing professional development. Report of an initiative to develop a network of senior doctors as mentors: 1994-99. Med Educ. 2000;34(9):747–53.
12. Croke J, Milne E, Bezjak A, Millar BA, Giuliani M, Heeneman S. Mentorship needs for radiation oncology residents: implications for programme design. Clin Oncol (R Coll Radiol). 2020;32(4):e119–25.
13. DeCastro R, Griffith KA, Ubel PA, Stewart A, Jagsi R. Mentoring and the career satisfaction of male and female academic medical faculty. Acad Med. 2014;89(2):301–11.
14. DeCastro R, Sambuco D, Ubel PA, Stewart A, Jagsi R. Mentor networks in academic medicine: moving beyond a dyadic conception of mentoring for junior faculty researchers. Acad Med. 2013;88(4):488–96.
15. Deitte LA, McGinty GB, Canon CL, Omary RA, Johnson PT, Slanetz PJ. Shifting from mentorship to sponsorship-a game changer! J Am Coll Radiol. 2019;16(4 Pt A):498–500.
16. Deville C, Hwang WT, Burgos R, Chapman CH, Both S, Thomas CR Jr. Diversity in graduate medical education in the United States by race, ethnicity, and sex, 2012. JAMA Intern Med. 2015;175(10):1706–8.
17. Dhami G, Gao W, Gensheimer MF, Trister AD, Kane G, Zeng J. Mentorship programs in radiation oncology residency training programs: a critical unmet need. Int J Radiat Oncol Biol Phys. 2016;94(1):27–30.
18. Doke K, Mohamad O, Royce TJ, Meyer J, Chen AM. Fellowship training programs in radiation oncology: a snapshot from 2005 to 2017. Int J Radiat Oncol Biol Phys. 2019;104(4):765–72.
19. Freeman R. Towards effective mentoring in general practice. Br J Gen Pract. 1997;47(420):457–60.
20. Garmel GM. Mentoring medical students in academic emergency medicine. Acad Emerg Med. 2004;11(12):1351–7.

21. Gottlieb AS, Travis EL. Rationale and models for career advancement sponsorship in academic medicine: the time is Here; the time is now. Acad Med. 2018;93(11):1620–3.
22. Henry-Noel N, Bishop M, Gwede CK, Petkova E, Szumacher E. Mentorship in medicine and other health professions. J Cancer Educ. 2019;34(4):629–37.
23. Holliday EB, Jagsi R, Thomas CR Jr, Wilson LD, Fuller CD. Standing on the shoulders of giants: results from the radiation oncology academic development and mentorship assessment project (ROADMAP). Int J Radiat Oncol Biol Phys. 2014;88(1):18–24.
24. Jackson VA, Palepu A, Szalacha L, Caswell C, Carr PL, Inui T. "Having the right chemistry": a qualitative study of mentoring in academic medicine. Acad Med. 2003;78(3):328–34.
25. Ko HC, Kimple RJ. The resident individual development plan as a guide for radiation oncology mentorship. Int J Radiat Oncol Biol Phys. 2018;101(4):786–8.
26. Lalani N, Griffith KA, Jones RD, Spratt DE, Croke J, Jagsi R. Mentorship experiences of early-career academic radiation oncologists in North America. Int J Radiat Oncol Biol Phys. 2018;101(3):732–40.
27. Lee A, Albert A, Griffith K, Evans S, Rahimy E, Park HS, Cervino LI, Moran JM, Jagsi R. Mentorship in radiation oncology: role of gender diversity in abstract presenting and senior author dyads on subsequent high-impact publications. Adv Radiat Oncol. 2020;5(2):292–6.
28. Lee A, Dennis C, Campbell P. Nature's guide for mentors. Nature. 2007;447(7146):791–7.
29. Lightfoote JB, Fielding JR, Deville C, Gunderman RB, Morgan GN, Pandharipande PV, Duerinckx AJ, Wynn RB, Macura KJ. Improving diversity, inclusion, and representation in radiology and radiation oncology part 1: why these matter. J Am Coll Radiol. 2014;11(7):673–80.
30. Luckhaupt SE, Chin MH, Mangione CM, Phillips RS, Bell D, Leonard AC, Tsevat J. Mentorship in academic general internal medicine. Results of a survey of mentors. J Gen Intern Med. 2005;20(11):1014–8.
31. Maher MA, Wofford AM, Roksa J, Feldon DF. Finding a fit: biological science doctoral students' selection of a principal infestivator and research laboratory. CBE Life Sci Educ. 2020;19(3):1–15.
32. Mohtady HA, Konings KD, Al-Eraky MM, Muijtjens AMM, van Merrienboer JJG. High enthusiasm about long lasting mentoring relationships and older mentors. BMC Med Educ. 2019;19(1):364.
33. NRMP. Results of the 2018 NRMP Program Director Survey. 2018. Retrieved 5 May 2020, from   https://www.nrmp.org/wp-content/uploads/2018/07/NRMP-2018-Program-Director-Survey-for-WWW.pdf.
34. Osborn VW, Doke K, Griffith KA, Jones R, Lee A, Maquilan G, Masters AH, Albert AA, Dover LL, Puckett LL, Hentz C, Kahn JM, Colbert LE, Barry PN, Jagsi R. A survey study of female radiation oncology residents' experiences to inform change. Int J Radiat Oncol Biol Phys. 2019;104(5):999–1008.
35. Overeem K, Driessen EW, Arah OA, Lombarts KM, Wollersheim HC, Grol RP. Peer mentoring in doctor performance assessment: strategies, obstacles and benefits. Med Educ. 2010;44(2):140–7.
36. Perry RE, Parikh JR. Sponsorship: a proven strategy for promoting career advancement and diversity in radiology. J Am Coll Radiol. 2019;16(8):1102–7.
37. Pololi L, Knight S. Mentoring faculty in academic medicine. A new paradigm? J Gen Intern Med. 2005;20(9):866–70.
38. Ragins BR, Cotton JL. Mentor functions and outcomes: a comparison of men and women in formal and informal mentoring relationships. J Appl Psychol. 1999;84(4):529–50.
39. Ragins BR, Cotton JL, Miller JS. Marginal mentoring: the effects of type of mentor, quality of relationship, and program design on work and career attitudes. Acad Manag J. 2000;6:1177–94.
40. Ramanan RA, Taylor WC, Davis RB, Phillips RS. Mentoring matters. Mentoring and career preparation in internal medicine residency training. J Gen Intern Med. 2006;21(4):340–5.
41. Ramey SJ, Ahmed AA, Takita C, Wilson LD, Thomas CR Jr, Yechieli R. Burnout evaluation of radiation residents nationwide: results of a survey of United States residents. Int J Radiat Oncol Biol Phys. 2017;99(3):530–8.

42. Sambunjak D, Marusic A. Mentoring: what's in a name? JAMA. 2009;302(23):2591–2.
43. Sambunjak D, Straus SE, Marusic A. Mentoring in academic medicine: a systematic review. JAMA. 2006;296(9):1103–15.
44. Sandi G, Chubinskaya S. A faculty development model that promotes success of early career faculty in academic medicine. J Contin Educ Heal Prof. 2020;40(1):69–72.
45. Sayan M, Ohri N, Lee A, Abou Yehia Z, Gupta A, Byun J, Jabbour SK, Wagman R, Haffty BG, Weiner J, Kim S. The impact of formal mentorship experience among radiation oncology residents from the northeast. Front Oncol. 2019;9:1369.
46. Scandura TA. Dysfunctional mentoring relationships and outcomes. J Manag. 1998;24:449–67.
47. Schafer M, Pander T, Pinilla S, Fischer MR, von der Borch P, Dimitriadis K. The Munich-Evaluation-of-Mentoring-Questionnaire (MEMeQ)--a novel instrument for evaluating proteges' satisfaction with mentoring relationships in medical education. BMC Med Educ. 2015;15:201.
48. Shakil S, Redberg RF. Gender disparities in sponsorship-how they perpetuate the glass ceiling. JAMA Intern Med. 2017;177(4):582.
49. van Schaik S, Plant J, O'Sullivan P. Promoting self-directed learning through portfolios in undergraduate medical education: the mentors' perspective. Med Teach. 2013;35(2):139–44.
50. Vaughn V, Saint S, Chopra V. Mentee missteps: Tales from the academic trenches. JAMA. 2017;317(5):475–6.
51. Williams LL, Levine JB, Malhotra S, Holtzheimer P. The good-enough mentoring relationship. Acad Psychiatry. 2004;28(2):111–5.
52. Woolley AW, Chabris CF, Pentland A, Hashmi N, Malone TW. Evidence for a collective intelligence factor in the performance of human groups. Science. 2010;330(6004):686–8.
53. Xu X, Payne SC. Quantiy, quality, and satisfaction with mentoring: what matters most? J Career Dev. 2014;41:507–25.
54. Zerzan JT, Hess R, Schur E, Phillips RS, Rigotti N. Making the Most of mentors: a guide for mentees. Acad Med. 2009;84(1):140–4.
55. Zhang H, Isaac A, Wright ED, Alrajhi Y, Seikaly H. Formal mentorship in a surgical residency training program: a prospective interventional study. J Otolaryngol Head Neck Surg. 2017;46(1):13.

Conflict Resolution and Interpersonal Strategies

Eric M. Chang, Ritchell van Dams, and Michael L. Steinberg

Modern healthcare is complex, requiring the collaboration of specialized multidisciplinary teams [1]. Though unified in the common goal of delivering high-quality patient care, providers often have differing priorities and are working in stressful environments—as such, the potential for conflict is inevitable [1]. This may be intensified in the academic setting, where the inherent hierarchical structure may compel behavior that would otherwise be inconsistent with one's beliefs and values [2]. Importantly, this conflict may not be benign. While unresolved conflict may result in poor staff morale, communication, and productivity in the business setting, this can translate into poor patient outcomes in a clinical care setting [1, 3, 4]. Given these critical consequences, there is growing awareness of the need for dedicated training in conflict resolution in undergraduate and graduate medical education. The Accreditation Council for Graduate Medical Education (ACGME) mandates that residents achieve competency in "communicating effectively with physicians, other health professionals, and health-related agencies" as well as in "working effectively as a member or leader of a healthcare team" [5]. However, with few validated tools available to teach these skills, interpersonal education in practice may often occur primarily through the hidden curriculum of on-the-job training [1, 4]. Furthermore, upon graduation or completion of residency training, many young physicians may avoid conflict for fear of "rocking the boat" [6]. They are often promoted based on their clinical skills, academic productivity, or other aspects of their individual

E. M. Chang
Department of Radiation Oncology, University of California Los Angeles,
Los Angeles, CA, USA

Department of Radiation Medicine, Oregon Health & Science University, Portland, OR, USA

R. van Dams · M. L. Steinberg (✉)
Department of Radiation Oncology, University of California Los Angeles,
Los Angeles, CA, USA
e-mail: RVanDams@mednet.ucla.edu; MSteinberg@mednet.ucla.edu

© Springer Nature Switzerland AG 2021   107
R. A. Chandra et al. (eds.), *Career Development in Academic Radiation Oncology*, https://doi.org/10.1007/978-3-030-71855-8_9

performance, and may be unprepared for the leadership roles they may assume as their career advances [3]. Radiation oncologists, in particular, must become adept at leading teams with diverse training backgrounds while managing, at times, challenging relationships with providers from other disciplines. In this chapter, we will provide an overview of conflict and how it arises in the healthcare setting, emphasizing practical tips for conflict resolution. As radiation oncologists are charged with leadership roles, we will also review strategies for conflict management, with a view that conflict is not necessarily a hindrance but rather a driver of change, crucial to the performance of high-functioning healthcare teams.

What Is Conflict?

Conflict can be defined as a disagreement with one's self or with others that causes harm or has the potential to harm [1]. An important distinction in this definition is that while disagreement may be a precursor to conflict, the expression of differing opinions does not always lead to a situation in which damage can occur [1, 6]. Disagreement can be a reflection of diversity, encouraging productive discussion and creativity; conflict, in contrast, is associated with negative emotions, such as frustration and bitterness [3, 6]. One may experience conflict over a situation without ever outwardly expressing disagreement to the offending party [6]. A related misconception is that conflict is abnormal, the result of insurmountable personality problems [1]. Given the widely different values, perspectives, priorities, and preferences held in society, conflict may be more productively viewed as a natural occurrence, with the establishment of healthy approaches to conflict resolution an expectation of every workplace [7].

Sources of Conflict

An important component of conflict resolution is reflecting on the driving forces that caused a conflict to occur. In healthcare, sources of conflict can arise at multiple levels of interaction [8]. To adapt terminology from the social sciences, these can be conceptualized to occur at the micro- (between individuals in their social settings), meso- (at the level of groups or institutions), and macro- (due to large-scale forces, such as legislative or economic) levels [8]. Examples of micro-level conflicts are differences in personality or contradictory views regarding scope of practice. Examples of meso-level conflicts may be issues of patient volume or with financial compensation; examples of macro-level conflicts may be changes in governmental reimbursement policies [8].

At the level of the healthcare team, conflict has been categorized as substantive—dealing with aspects of the group's work, such as differing views on adequate quality of care or the roles and responsibilities of team members—versus affective, dealing with the interpersonal relationships between group members, such as conflicting personalities or communication styles [3, 9]. Having a grasp of this distinction may help guide the most appropriate conflict resolution strategy, as often affective conflicts can be inappropriately reframed as substantive conflicts, hindering productive communication. However, these types of conflict are also often interrelated. For example, a physician may disagree with a colleague regarding the proper treatment fractionation scheme for a patient. Should the physician begin to view the colleague's preference for longer fractionation schemes as solely driven by personal financial incentive rather than patient tolerance or efficacy, a potentially substantive conflict could drive a persistent emotional mistrust.

The Progression of Conflict

Having a framework for how conflict naturally progresses may help both in anticipating when conflict is likely to occur and in deciding the most effective time to intervene. In his well-known model of group development, psychologist Bruce Tuckman described that conflict characterizes the "storming" phase of team development [10]. This phase occurs toward the beginning of the formation of a team, when members are gaining enough trust in each other to begin expressing disagreement and interpersonal differences start to arise [4, 10]. Unresolved conflict at this time can hinder a team's performance until goals, processes, and roles become solidified—the goal of conflict resolution in this case should be to shorten the duration of this period and prevent a team from reentering this phase as new challenges occur [4]. Throughout medical training, this phase may have become a familiar experience, felt at each new clinical rotation after the initial excitement of team formation has worn off but before the team has had a chance to coalesce.

When conflict arises, it can be described as progressing through four phases [1]. In the first phase, the stimulus occurs, causing the parties involved to experience frustration. In the second phase, the parties attempt to rationalize their frustration, to conceptualize a cause for why it arose. In the third phase, the parties enact behaviors targeted at addressing the cause. In the final phase, these behaviors result in destructive outcomes, establishing the conflict. Importantly, the rationalization that occurs in the second phase may be rapid and inaccurate, resulting in behaviors in the third phase that are misguided. While the stimulus and rationalization may be unavoidable, with greater awareness of this process, the subsequent behaviors may be modified—as such, the best time to intervene may be between the second and third phases.

Conflict Resolution

Though a relatively new area of research in medicine, the negative and positive effects of conflict have been studied for decades in other disciplines, from developmental psychology to organizational management [3]. Conflict resolution, in particular, has been studied extensively in the world of business management, in an effort to avoid its negative impact on productivity [4]. While undoubtedly a physician will have to develop a personalized approach to conflict resolution over the course of his or her career, in this section we will review the principles for effective conflict management to assist in this process.

Conflict Management Styles

A well-regarded instrument for describing conflict management styles was put forth by Kenneth Thomas and Ralph Kilmann in 1974 [11]. In this framework, individuals are recognized to have inherent differences in their personalities and values, which drives their style for approaching interpersonal conflict. While the instrument acknowledges that one's response may vary based on the situation and stakes at hand, it attempts to describe one's default nature when facing conflict. In this manner, it can serve as a springboard for assessing one's strengths and weaknesses when honing conflict resolution skills.

The Thomas-Kilmann conflict mode instrument is based on the managerial grid model defined by Robert Blake and Jane Mouton and describes conflict resolution styles on two dimensions of behavior: assertiveness, or the degree to which one attempts to satisfy his or her own concerns in a conflict, and cooperativeness, the degree to which one attempts to satisfy other's concerns [11, 12]. Considering these two dimensions on axes, five styles of conflict resolution are defined (Fig. 1) [3]:

1. *Competing*: Competing maximizes assertiveness while minimizing cooperativeness. It exemplifies the "win-lose" style of negotiation, in which one focuses on his or her priorities at the expense of those of others, sometimes at all cost.
2. *Accommodating*: The opposite of competing, accommodating maximizes cooperativeness while minimizing assertiveness. The focus is on building and maintaining relationships, accommodating other parties' concerns at times at the expense of one's own.
3. *Avoiding*: Avoiding minimizes both assertiveness and cooperativeness. Exemplifying the "take whatever you can get" attitude, avoiding neglects both one's own concerns and those of others in an effort to not address the conflict.
4. *Collaborating*: The opposite of avoiding, collaborating attempts to maximize assertiveness and cooperativeness. It exemplifies the "win-win" style of negotiation, in which one attempts to work with others to understand their interests and find a solution that fully satisfies the needs of both parties.

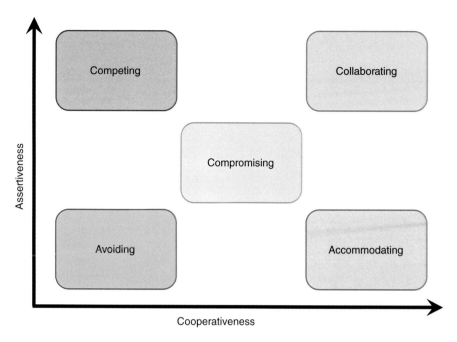

Fig. 1 The Thomas-Kilmann conflict modes

5. *Compromising*: Compromising is balanced in both assertiveness and cooperativeness. Compromising attempts to find a middle-ground position and is distinct
   from collaborating in that concessions are made on both sides. It is in effect a
   "lose-lose" negotiation, in that both parties are only partially satisfied.

In addition to evaluating one's style at baseline, it can be useful to assess how
one's approach to conflict changes based on the people involved; for instance, one's
style may vary in conflicts with peers, supervisors, and patients, or in personal relationships [4]. It may also be beneficial to learn how others approach conflict so that
one's style can be tailored to the other party's in order to be most effective [3]. In
healthcare, studies applying the Thomas-Kilmann instrument have suggested that
different conflict styles may be favored based on physician specialty [13]. Although
it may appear that certain conflict management styles are inherently "better" than
others, styles may be adaptive based on the situation [3]. Collaborating, while ideal
in that both parties are fully satisfied, requires time and trust; compromising may
allow for resolution when time is limited. Competing can harm team unity but may
be appropriate when the stakes are high, such as when conflicts occur over patient
safety. Though avoiding conflict may not be the most productive approach, it may
be reasonable when the conflict is not of vital importance or might be better
addressed at a later time. As differences in opinion are never elucidated, accommodating may not be successful in the long term but may be useful when maintaining
team harmony is critical.

Striving for Collaboration

By fully satisfying the needs of all parties involved, the collaborating style of conflict management may serve as the ideal for achieving long-term resolution. In a small study applying the Thomas-Kilmann instrument in medical residents, residents who successfully executed administrative duties were more likely to exhibit a collaborative management style, with positive correlations seen between residents' collaborating scores and faculty evaluations [14]. Collaboration is time-intensive, requiring a thorough exploration of each party's perspectives, priorities, and goals; even after undergoing this painstaking process, collaboration may not be possible. However, strategies have been described to increase the chances of successful collaboration. In his popular book *The 7 Habits of Highly Effective People*, Stephen Covey discusses that achieving true collaboration often requires a change in mindset, such that the needs of the opposing party become viewed as integral to meeting one's own [15]. Adopting the mentality that resources are not scarce but rather can become increasingly plentiful with cooperation may repress the desire to compete during conflict resolution. Both parties may need to demonstrate an internal commitment to collaboration so that other strategies are not accepted as less demanding alternatives.

Covey further details that collaboration can be facilitated by taking time outside of the conflict setting to invest in long-term relationships [15]. If there is already an established level of trust between both parties prior to a conflict, even when anger or frustration arises, there will likely remain good faith that the conflict can be resolved and that relationship will return to its positive baseline. In contrast, without trust, parties may be quick to misinterpret each other's actions or compete for fear of being taken advantage of [3]. Behaviors for establishing trust described by Covey include taking the time to learn about an individual's background, engaging in small acts of kindness or courtesy, keeping faithful to commitments, explicitly clarifying expectations when making requests, treating everyone by the same set of principles, and apologizing sincerely after wronging others [15]. Conversely, trust can be easily eroded through discourtesy, disrespect, or lack of empathy.

The Importance of Communication Skills

In many ways, communication can be viewed as the medium through which conflict resolution must occur, and thus honing one's communication skills is crucial for effective conflict management. Tactless communication can lead to a breakdown in discussions; imprecise communication is often the source of medical errors. In an analysis of near-miss and adverse events in radiation oncology, communication and human behaviors were the most common errors affecting all types of events [16]. Furthermore, in a separate study focusing on communication errors, the radiation oncology physician was the most common source of error [17]. In the setting of conflict, presuming both parties are committed to resolution, communication allows for the voicing of priorities and acknowledgment of needs [3]. Notably, while to the untrained eye effective communication in a conflict can appear to be innate to the speaker, these skills are learnable and practicable [6].

When communicating during a conflict, it may be helpful to have guiding principles to ensure the conversation is productive. In their book *Getting to Yes*, negotiation experts Roger Fisher and William Ury describe a principle-based approach to conflict resolution [18]. The first principle, "Separate the people from the problem," acknowledges that both parties bring their own emotions into a conflict and that these often get entangled within the discussion of the objective problem. As parties become more and more resolute in their positions, the discussion can become more of a "battle of wills" aimed at ego preservation and "winning" the argument rather than at active listening and productive communication [19]. While maintaining objectivity and focusing on data can combat this tendency, the authors note that glossing over or assuming the other party's intentions may only amplify the chances of misunderstanding. Being willing to explore each side's perceptions and name emotions can help keep communication open. This may be particularly important in healthcare, where certain conflicts may call for more focus on relationship building to achieve resolution: for instance, in a study comparing the conflict management styles of intensivists and palliative care specialists in the critical care setting, palliative care specialists were observed to use fewer task-based statements (e.g., discussing the prognosis or clinical situation) and more relationship-building statements (e.g., asking about the patient's interests or values), which was perceived to be potentially more effective [20]. Fisher and Ury's second principle, "Focus on interests, not positions," recognizes that parties often begin negotiations by stating positions (e.g., "I am stuck with more inpatient consults than the other physicians") rather than underlying interests (e.g., "weekend clinical work is limiting my time to work on research and be with family"). Positions are often much less flexible, and thus limiting communication to positions can lead to an impasse. In contrast, there may be many positions to satisfy a single interest. Parties may also have multiple interests, leaving greater opportunity for finding commonality.

At a more granular level, choosing words intentionally can help communicate ideas without conveying criticism or stimulating emotion (Table 1). For example, management consultant Stanley Wachs discourages making absolute statements or using superlatives; in their extremism these may encourage quick disagreement and protest [6]. Likewise, one should refrain from labeling or categorizing people in discussions. These stereotypes can feel disrespectful and belittling and may even internally create negative expectations of others. The use of the word "but" in a conflict can signal a sense of criticism; replacing this with "and" may be more constructive without provoking defensiveness. Beginning statements with "I" rather than "you" is a way to state a problem without assigning blame. Nonviolent communication, a tool developed by psychologist Marshall Rosenberg, suggests that a fundamental component of effective communication is expressing clear observations and requests without mixing in evaluations or being critical of others [21].

Table 1 Tips for effective communication during a conflict

Tip	Example
Avoid absolute statements	"You are always late to clinic" becomes "You have been late to clinic a few times this week"
Avoid superlatives	"Dr. Smith is the worst doctor" "Todd is the laziest resident"
Avoid labels or categorizing others	"Stacy is such a complainer" "Justin is a know-it-all"
Replace "but" with "and"	"Our meetings are productive but they are not efficient" becomes "Our meetings are productive and I hope we can think about ways to make them more efficient"
Use "I" statements	"You don't respect my opinion" becomes "I sometimes feel unheard"

Lastly, it should be recognized that communication is not only what is said—a great deal of what is expressed is nonverbal. Thus, in addition to engaging in active listening by outwardly acknowledging and paraphrasing the other party's opinions and feelings, one should play close attention to what he or she is communicating through nonverbal cues [13]. Elements of nonverbal communication include sounds, ways of talking, posture, appearance, head movements, closeness, body contact, facial expression, and eye movements [4]. Taking the time to make certain one's nonverbal cues communicate a sense of engagement and are consistent with what is said out loud may ensure the other party feels acknowledged and remains receptive.

Preparing for a Conflict

If a discussion about a conflict is anticipated, taking certain steps ahead of time to prepare can increase the chances of positive outcomes. Envisioning best- and worst-case scenarios as well as the outcome one is willing to accept may help during discussions of priorities [1]. Self-reflecting on one's own role in the conflict in particular can ensure the conversation does not become excessively critical [6]. The nature of a discussion can change dramatically depending on the timing and setting as well as who is in attendance and their relationships with each other [1]. Planning to hold the discussion in a safe and neutral environment may be beneficial; inviting a third party to mediate can be useful though escalating to a supervisor without first addressing the issue directly can breed resentment [22]. Opening the conflict directly by saying "I need to talk with you about a difficult issue" rather than by minimizing ("I'd like to chat") or with a critique ("You've been slacking off lately") can appropriately set the tone without making the other party feel ambushed or provoking defensiveness [6]. Rehearsing with a colleague may help alleviate anxiety over the discussion [1]. Lastly, envisioning a common goal ahead of time may be useful as an anchor to return to when guiding the conversation. Often in the clinical setting, this is patient care or patient safety [22].

It can be helpful to have a framework to guide the discussion. In the surgical literature, Liz Lee and colleagues provided a model for conflict resolution based on the history and physical format familiar to all physicians (Table 2) [19]. In the history, each party describes their view of the conflict and how it occurred. Similar to a patient interview, there is a focus on listening empathetically. During the physical, objective data pertaining to each party's position is discussed; if presented without judgment or critique, objective data, such as the number of consults seen by a physician, can help bring a party to see the other's perspective. In the assessment/plan, the parties formulate possible reasons for the conflict and outline a plan for resolution. During the informed consent, the parties review the proposed plan to identify possible problems that may arise. The time-out is a reminder that there needs to be constant communication between the conflicting parties when enacting the plan to ensure expectations are met and further conflicts are avoided. In the Operation, the plan is enacted following the steps outlined in the assessment/plan. Finally, during postoperative care, the outcomes of the plan are assessed. Similar to after a procedure, regular follow-up and re-evaluation are stressed to ensure both parties remain feeling validated and involved.

Table 2 The history and physical model of conflict resolution [19]

History	Each party describes their perspective of the conflict, including its causes and outcomes Emphasis on active listening and empathizing with the other party without defensiveness
Physical exam	Each party presents objective data pertinent to their position Data should be presented without judgment or critique; the goal is to foster collaboration rather than prove the other side "wrong"
Differential diagnosis and assessment/plan	The parties formulate possible underlying reasons for the conflict The parties outline a plan for conflict resolution
Preoperative preparation/ informed consent	The parties review the proposed plan to identify possible problems that may arise Emphasis on ensuring each party felt validated and respected during development of the plan
Time-out	Serves as a reminder that constant communication between the conflicting parties is needed as the plan is enacted Regular communication may ensure expectations are met and further conflicts are anticipated and avoided
Operation	The plan is enacted following the steps outlined in the assessment/ plan
Postoperative care	The outcomes of the plan are assessed, with regular re-evaluation to ensure both parties remain feeling validated and involved Flexibility may be required should a party feel its needs are no longer being met as the plan is enacted

Assessing the Outcomes of a Conflict

In Fisher and Ury's *Getting to Yes*, the fourth principle for successful negotiation is "Insist on using objective criteria" [18]. If possible, the authors recommend both parties should agree upon a set of objective criteria by which to assess the outcome of the negotiation. Ideally, these criteria should be independent of each party's will as well as legitimate and practical. To achieve this, it can be useful to rely on accepted fair standards: for instance, one might research the number of inpatient consults seen on average at similarly sized academic centers to determine what is fair for a physician to see. In addition to these objective measures, it is also important following a conflict to reflect on its subjective outcomes. After a constructive conflict, group unity improves, productivity rises, and commitment increases. In contrast, after a destructive conflict, negativism results, groups divide, and satisfaction decreases [1]. It may be that a conflict cannot be resolved in one discussion—in these instances, having set start and end times can be useful to ensure a conversation does not drag on unproductively [1]. Regardless of the outcome, taking time for self-reflection after a conflict can provide a deeper understanding of one's own values and assumptions, which may assist when revisiting the conflict or in resolving new conflicts moving forward [23].

Emotional Intelligence

In the history of medical training, physicians have traditionally been taught to exhibit a "detached concern" in practice, engaging empathetically with patients but without becoming emotionally involved [13]. However, in recent years, there has been growing awareness that vital capabilities of the twenty-first-century physician—effectively leading teams and engendering behavior change in patients and colleagues—require high emotional intelligence [24]. Emotional intelligence recognizes that humans are both rational and emotional beings, and that complete focus on logic and objective data ignores a critical driver of human behavior [24, 25]. Proponents argue that emotions underlie powerful forces, such as energy, commitment, and motivation, and as such cannot be "left at home" when entering the workplace [25]. Emotions may be of particular importance in the setting of a conflict, where influential sentiments—feeling valued and respected—are crucial in achieving long-lasting resolution.

Importantly, exhibiting emotional intelligence does not mean uncontrollably expressing one's emotions. Rather, the first steps to cultivating emotional intelligence involve a rigorous process of introspection and self-governance, so that one can learn to identify and understand the drivers of his or her emotions, managing the internal response prior to enacting destructive behaviors [25]. While a complete discussion of this process is beyond the scope of this chapter, experts at the Emotional Intelligence and Diversity Institute recommend starting by asking one's

Fig. 2 Initial questions
during a conflict for
developing emotional
intelligence[25]

Questions for developing emotional intelligence

- What emotions are operating in this conflict for both myself and others?
- What are both the rational and emotional elements of this conflict?
- What does my emotional reaction to this conflict tell me about what matters to me?
- How does my body show its emotions? What signs are visible in others?
- How are my emotions influencing my behavior?

self a series of initial questions (Fig. 2) [25]. Once a fluency in emotions is achieved, one can begin turning these skills outward, communicating feelings and needs effectively as well as learning to acknowledge the diversity of emotional responses in colleagues [25]. In this manner, emotions can be used to shape a workplace environment that both is engaging for co-workers and benefits from differences in perspective [25].

Conflict in Organizational Development: A Primer

Radiation oncologists are charged to lead a multidisciplinary team, relying extensively on the specialized knowledge of nurses, medical physicists, dosimetrists, radiation therapists, and administrative staff in the safe and effective delivery of radiation therapy and the ongoing medical management of their patients. As a team leader, it is important to recognize that high-performing work environments do not happen by accident but are rather consciously and purposefully guided to create a climate of energy and productivity [25]. The destructive outcomes of conflict—pessimism, poor morale, and selfishness—may be especially damaging to workplace culture. Furthermore, conflict is in essence rooted in the differences between people [7]. Thus, learning to harness conflict effectively can allow diverse opinion to become a source of innovation at the organizational level, with successful resolution an important driver of team unity.

Health consultant Tim Porter-O'Grady describes that an organization's culture surrounding conflict is heavily influenced by the leader's disposition toward conflict resolution [7]. Thus, making an active effort to improve one's personal response to conflict via the methods discussed above is an important first step in shaping how others respond. For example, if a leader exhibits discomfort when approaching conflict, this may cause others to be unwilling to speak up when it occurs, leading to prolonged discordance. Avoiding assigning blame in discussions of conflict can help reframe it as an opportunity for change rather than discipline. In a study of employees from multiple countries, researchers Jeanine Prime and Elizabeth Salib identified humility as a key leadership trait for making workers of varying demographic backgrounds feel included [26]. This feeling of inclusion was further associated with more innovation, more engagement in selfless behavior, and greater feelings of belongingness and uniqueness. Strategies to embrace a selfless leadership style include openly discussing one's mistakes and being willing to support and learn from others when they voice concerns. The experts at the Emotional Intelligence and Diversity Institute further recommend taking the time to meet individually with co-workers to learn about their needs and personal drivers of behavior [25]. Humility may be of particular importance in the academic setting, where the hierarchical structure can serve as a barrier to open communication [3].

When serving in an administrative role, creating a formal mechanism for conflict resolution can help frame conflict as an ordinary occurrence in the functioning of the workplace [7]. In addition to staff mediation programs, in radiation oncology this may involve participation in formal systems to learn from patient safety-related events, such as the Radiation Oncology Incident Learning System (RO-ILS) co-sponsored by the American Society for Radiation Oncology (ASTRO) and American Association of Physicists in Medicine (AAPM) [27]. Beyond commitment from leadership, dedicated training in conflict resolution skills should be available for workers at all levels, with conflict resolution program and mediation activities reviewed regularly to ensure their continued effectiveness and applicability [7].

Conclusions

Effectively collaborating with colleagues can be a greater undertaking at times than the task itself [22]. In medicine, where individuals of diverse training backgrounds must come together to perform highly complex tasks, conflict is a given. As a physician, one should learn that effective resolution does not mean the complete elimination of conflict [22]. Rather, by taking an active approach to practicing conflict resolution skills, one can develop a level of comfort with conflict when it arises, embracing it as a source of productivity and unity necessary in the delivery of high-quality patient care.

Summary

- Conflict can be defined as a disagreement with one's self or with others that causes harm or has the potential to harm.
- Assessing one's default conflict management style can serve as a starting point when honing conflict resolution skills.
- Developing communication skills and emotional intelligence are crucial for effective conflict resolution.

- Taking time for preparation prior to and self-reflection following the discussion of a conflict may increase the chances of positive outcomes.
- Embracing conflict as normative can allow it to become a source of productivity and innovation for the healthcare team.

For Discussion with a Mentor or Colleague

- What is your conflict management style as described in the Thomas-Kilmann model (competing/accommodating/avoiding/collaborating/compromising)? How does your style change in conflicts with peers, supervisors, patients, or in personal relationships?
- Can you recall specific instances in which a conflict has resulted in positive or negative outcomes? What were the similarities and differences in your approaches to these conflicts?
- What leadership qualities are important in establishing a workplace culture that embraces conflict and the differences between colleagues?

References

1. Saltman DC. Conflict management: a primer for doctors in training. Postgrad Med J. 2006;82(963):9–12.
2. Rosenbaum JR, Bradley EH, Holmboe ES, Farrell MH, Krumholz HM. Sources of ethical conflict in medical housestaff training: a qualitative study. Am J Med. 2004;116(6):402–7.
3. Quinn JF, White BAA. Cultivating leadership in medicine. Dubuque: Kendall Hunt Publishing Company; 2019.
4. Wolfe AD, Hoang KB, Denniston SF. Teaching conflict resolution in medicine: lessons from business, diplomacy, and theatre. MedEdPORTAL. 2018;14:10672.
5. ACGME. Common program requirements (residency): Accreditation Council for Graduate Medical Education; 2019. https://www.acgme.org/Portals/0/PFAssets/ProgramRequirements/CPRResidency2019.pdf. Accessed 10 Apr 2020.
6. Wachs SR. Put conflict resolution skills to work. J Oncol Pract. 2008;4(1):37–40.
7. Porter-O'Grady T. Embracing conflict: building a healthy community. Health Care Manag Rev. 2004;29(3):181–7.
8. Brown J, Lewis L, Ellis K, Stewart M, Freeman TR, Kasperski MJ. Conflict on interprofessional primary health care teams – can it be resolved? J Interprof Care. 2011;25(1):4–10.
9. Payne M. Teamwork in multiprofessional care. Chicago: Lyceum Books; 2000.
10. Tuckman BW. Developmental sequence in small groups. Psychol Bull. 1965;63(6):384–99.
11. Thomas K, Kilmann R. The Thomas-Kilmann conflict mode instrument. XICOM: Tuxedo; 1974.
12. Blake R, Mouton J. The managerial grid: the key to leadership excellence. Houston: Gulf Publishing Company; 1964.
13. Sinskey JL, Chang JM, Shibata GS, Infosino AJ, Rouine-Rapp K. Applying conflict management strategies to the pediatric operating room. Anesth Analg. 2019;129(4):1109–17.
14. Ogunyemi D, Fong S, Elmore G, Korwin D, Azziz R. The associations between residents' behavior and the Thomas-Kilmann Conflict MODE Instrument. J Grad Med Educ. 2010;2(1):118–25.

15. Covey SR. The seven habits of highly effective people: powerful lessons in personal change. London: Simon & Schuster; 2004.

16. Spraker MB, Fain R, Gopan O, Zeng J, Nyflot M, Jordan L, et al. Evaluation of near-miss and adverse events in radiation oncology using a comprehensive causal factor taxonomy. Pract Radiat Oncol. 2017 Oct;7(5):346–53.

17. Blakaj A, Wootton L, Zeng J, Nyflot M, Ford EC, Spraker MB. Let's talk: communication errors in radiation oncology. Int J Radiat Oncol Biol Phys. 2017;99(2):E547.

18. Fisher R, Ury W. Getting to yes: negotiating agreement without giving in. Boston: Houghton Mifflin; 1981.

19. Lee L, Berger DH, Awad SS, Brandt ML, Martinez G, Brunicardi FC. Conflict resolution: practical principles for surgeons. World J Surg. 2008;32(11):2331–5.

20. Chiarchiaro J, White DB, Ernecoff NC, Buddadhumaruk P, Schuster RA, Arnold RM. Conflict management strategies in the ICU differ between palliative care specialists and intensivists. Crit Care Med. 2016;44(5):934–42.

21. Rosenberg M, Molho P. Nonviolent (empathic) communication for health care providers. Haemophilia. 1998;4(4):335–40.

22. Mallidi J, Frye RL. How to handle conflict with poise?: a fellow's perspective. J Am Coll Cardiol. 2015;65(1):98–100.

23. Hocking BA. Using reflection to resolve conflict. AORN J. 2006;84(2):249–50, 253–9.

24. Emanuel EJ, Gudbranson E. Does medicine overemphasize IQ? JAMA. 2018;319(7):651.

25. Gardenswartz L, Cherbosque J, Rowe A. Emotional intelligence for managing results in a diverse world: the hard truth about soft skills in the workplace. Davies-Black Pub: Mountain View; 2008.

26. Prime J, Salib E. Inclusive leadership: the view from six countries. Catalyst. 2014. https://www.catalyst.org/research/inclusive-leadership-the-view-from-six-countries. Accessed 17 Apr 2020.

27. Radiation Oncology Incident Learning System (RO-ILS). American Society for Radiation Oncology. 2020. https://www.astro.org/Patient-Care-and-Research/Patient-Safety/RO-ILS. Accessed 17 Apr 2020.

Aligning Your Goals with Your Colleagues, Department, and Institution

Nadia N. Laack

Introduction

To be successful in any field, professionals must identify, set, evaluate, and often reevaluate their personal career goals. Yet, true success in a professional setting involves more than simply achieving one's personal goals. Each individual, be they clinician, researcher, or educator, academic faculty or industry consultant, resident or emeritus, is part of a broad, interwoven fabric that ties together the radiation oncology field as a whole. In today's vibrant nexus of healthcare organizations, academic institutions, private technology companies, and governmental funding agencies, it is crucial for individuals to ensure that their career goals are not only personally meaningful, but that they also align with the priorities of other parts of the field.

Healthcare institutions are facing enormous challenges and are often under pressure to generate new revenue sources. These can include everything from clinical initiatives to innovative industry partnerships to seeking highly competitive grant funding from governmental or private foundations. At a time when there is less and less money to go around, professionals and institutions alike must work together to ensure that the goals they pursue are aligned to continue improving the field of radiation oncology. In this chapter, we will discuss how to identify your career goals, how to ensure that they align with your colleagues, department, and institution, how to achieve these goals – and how to reevaluate and adapt when previous goals are no longer attainable.

N. N. Laack (✉)
Department of Radiation Oncology, Mayo Clinic, Rochester, MN, USA
e-mail: Laack.Nadia@mayo.edu

121
R. A. Chandra et al. (eds.), *Career Development in Academic Radiation Oncology*, https://doi.org/10.1007/978-3-030-71855-8_10

Identifying Your Career Goals

The type of radiation oncology career that you aspire to will often determine the types of goals you should set for you career. The types of careers available can broadly be categorized as private practice, clinician-educator, translational scientist, and basic scientist [1]. However, the training to become an oncologist is grueling, and the workload and patient stresses often lead to high levels of burnout, depression, and dissatisfaction both at work and at home. It is now more important than ever to ensure that your professional aspirations align, first and foremost, with your personal passions.

A recent study of 1367 medical faculty who had received National Institutes of Health (NIH) career development awards identified several common career motivators that respondents placed high importance on. These included publishing high-quality research, conducting patient care, teaching, publishing prolifically, work–life balance, salary, reputation, and leadership positions [2]. As Shanafelt et al. noted, "Once the ideal job type is identified, it becomes easier to evaluate and compare specific job opportunities" [1]. They further identified a list of insightful questions to help guide the process of professional goal setting:

- Why did I choose to become a physician?
- Why did I choose to become an oncologist?
- What do I like most about my job?
- What motivates me professionally?
- By the end of my career, what three things do I hope to have accomplished?

While identifying and setting career goals that align with personal preferences is essential to maintaining a healthier work–life balance, it is also important to keep in mind that your interests and priorities will likely change over time. What is intriguing to you during your residency training may not be interesting 10 years from now. The above questions can be utilized at both at the outset of identifying your career goals and during ongoing reevaluations.

As radiation oncologists, we begin setting goals even before selecting a residency. Because it is difficult to transition from a small, community-focused program and compete for academic positions at large institutions, medical students who believe they want to pursue an academic career will attempt to match at larger academic programs. In addition, medical students interested in a translational lab or clinical scientist track will attempt to match at residencies with strong basic science programs. During residency, our goals may evolve and focus as we learn more about the roles and responsibilities of the different academic positions. In addition, other factors, such as geography and proximity to support can also become increasingly important as many residents prepare to grow their families.

As with many specialties, academic radiation oncology is a small field with relatively few available positions each year. Understanding your priorities is important in your choice of an academic position. For example, if you are passionate about pediatric radiation oncology and that is your most important career goal, you may need to be more flexible in the size, geographic location, and research and leadership of the practice. If you are more flexible in your disease site of interest, you may be able to prioritize location or salary and promotion structure.

Once you've identified what's important to you in your work and home lives, and have established what motivates you and what you aspire to achieve, it's time to lay out simple, realistic, and measurable goals. Imagine if you were to set a vague goal to "publish more and better papers." How would you know if and when you had achieved this goal? The goal in this example has no clear definitions of the start or end, and no plan for how to succeed.

One well-known and popular goal-setting framework is known as the SMART method [3, 4], which is an acronym that stands for

- **S**pecific
- **M**easurable
- **A**chievable
- **R**elevant
- **T**ime bound

The SMART framework helps define what exactly you want to achieve, which specific steps you will take to work toward this goal, how and when you will measure success, and most importantly – it keeps the focus on setting goals that are realistic, meaningful, and attainable.

Table 1 is a sample worksheet demonstrating how to use the SMART model to set and meet both career and personal goals. The goal example above is used in this worksheet to show specific actions that could be taken, problems that can be anticipated ahead of time, and realistic evaluation strategies.

Table 1 SMART goal worksheet

Name:					Date Prepared: 1/1/2020	
	S Specific	**M** Measurable	**A** Attainable	**R** Results-Based	**T** Time-Bound	**Date Achieved**
Goal	List specific actions you can take to work toward this goal	How will you measure whether your actions are helping you make progress?	Be sure that goals are not too easy to reach and not impossible to meet	How will you know that your goal is on-track and has been achieved?	Assign a timeframe for when you want to achieve this goal.	
Publish more and better papers	• Read three journal articles each week • Attend workshop to improve writing skills • Schedule weekly meeting with co-authors • Block time on calendar for writing • Start writing support group with colleagues	• Monthly report on ratio of writing meetings actually held to meetings cancelled • Monthly review of spreadsheet tracking progress on papers and submissions	I will increase my publication rate by 50% each year, and will publish in at least one high-impact journal each year, within the next three years.	*I published two articles in 2019.* Goals: 2020 = 3 papers 2021 = 4.5 (5) papers 2022 = 6.75 papers At least 1 annually will be in a journal with an IF ≥5.	• Writing progress will be tracking spreadsheet • Meeting attendance will be reviewed monthly • Overall success will be evaluated 12/31/2022	

As we move through this chapter, we will consider how to ensure that your goals are not only personally fulfilling, but are also realistically achievable in your department, institution, and broader community.

Aligning Your Goals with Your Colleagues

Developing an attitude of partnership and cooperation is vital in a field like radiation oncology, a practice which is inherently multidisciplinary. Patients with cancer often undergo multimodality therapy involving surgery, chemotherapy, radiation, and immunotherapy at various timepoints. Even more broadly, the average radiation oncologist on any given day can consult with colleagues in neurology, pulmonology, orthopedics, pediatrics, radiology, and cardiology – sometimes before noon.

Far too often, the personal and professional goals of individuals lead to intense competition, rather than supportive collaboration. In fact, there is almost no discussion in the scholarly literature or organizational blogosphere about how to align one's own goals with their colleagues' goals. There are occasional references to coworkers coming together to accomplish "shared goals" for an organization. Yet the concept of aligning goals between colleagues for mutual benefit is sorely lacking.

Yet, it is not enough to merely engage in successful communication and patient care with colleagues from other departments. The importance of aligning your own goals with the work of your colleagues is deeply connected to building a fulfilling, and successful, career as well as truly improving the outcomes for our patients. Despite perverse and competitive reward systems that exist in some academic institutions, it is important to remain true to the priorities and passions that drove you to an academic career.

The primary benefit of involving a diverse team of colleagues in your efforts is to improve the quality of your work which will in turn have the highest likelihood of benefitting your patients. Just as we know that companies and boardrooms function more effectively and are more successful, including experienced colleagues as well as junior colleagues and other collaborators from a diverse background will help identify blind spots in your projects and goals. An inclusive policy of collaboration is also a method to ensure areas of alignment with your colleagues both within and outside the department. If you are struggling to get others involved, it may be a sign that your project isn't well aligned. In addition, multidisciplinary collaborations increase your visibility in your institution. Finally, successfully completing a multidisciplinary project helps you establish credibility and broadens your network of collaborators, as your colleagues will be more likely to recommend others in their network collaborate with you.

Aligning Your Goals with Your Department's Priorities

One of the key factors in job satisfaction is how closely aligned your professional interests and goals are with the areas prioritized by your department. While the overall mission of your department may be shared with you at some point during the interview and hiring process, you may be too nervous or focused on other areas to pay close attention. Yet once you become an active member of the department, it is vital that you develop and maintain an understanding of its guiding vision to ensure your work will be valued and supported [5].

Department priorities are generally set out by groups of individuals on committees, and may be more or less clearly communicated depending on the department's culture. As with personal preferences and goals, a department's goals are likely to change over time and in response to situational factors, so it's vital to ensure you have ways to keep in touch with what's happening in the department.

There are generally two types of organizational engagement methods to help keep you informed about departmental plans: Formal structures (committees, boards, workshops, etc.) and informal networks (department picnics, holiday parties, hallway chats, etc.) [6, 7]. Involvement in departmental committees is important to developing a sense of engagement and ownership in the departmental priorities. Depending on your career area of interest, you may request to join departmental research, education, or clinical practice–related committees. As time for scholarly pursuits is critically important in the early years for faculty, it is important to balance stewardship and citizenship with personal goals and responsibilities.

Informal networks are also important both to developing joy and well-being in the workplace, as well as connecting to sources of information for departmental and institutional plans and goals. Although the extent and depth to which people engage in their informal networks may depend somewhat on personality types, attending departmental functions can help build important social and professional bonds and maintains connection to what's happening in the department. Being curious and making an effort to learn something about your colleagues on a daily basis will help establish trust and break down barriers that may develop when a new staff member joins, especially in departmental cultures that lean more competitive. Finally, everyone appreciates being recognized for what they do and are more likely to help and mentor you if you take the time to genuinely express appreciation for your colleagues' support, example, leadership, or scholarly ability. Asking colleagues for advice and expressing sincere interest in their suggestions for success will not only build important relationships for networking, but help you learn the "insider" tricks for navigating in the department and institution.

As was mentioned earlier in this chapter, most academic and healthcare centers have been experiencing increasing financial strain in recent years. Because of this unfortunate reality, many department priorities are now becoming aligned with areas that can provide reliable sources of funding. For example, most radiation oncology faculty are able to pursue some type of federal grant funding for projects. Your department may also have an established relationship with one or more personal benefactors who are interested in supporting work with a specific focus. There may also be internal department or institutional funding opportunities that are offered on a recurring cycle, or for specialized projects with high importance.

Although historically more common in medical oncology, industry is an increasingly important source of funding in radiation oncology. Both pharma and technology vendors are engaging with academic radiation oncology departments to support clinical trials of new drug–radiation combinations or novel treatment delivery devices or techniques. Determining the industries with which your department already has relationships can provide opportunities for aligning your goals with successful partnerships.

While aligning your interests and skills with these myriad funding opportunities and the priorities of your department can be a fulfilling way to achieve your goals, it can also be confusing and overwhelming at times. Many departments have mentoring processes to help connect young faculty to senior faculty, and the process of mentorship has continually been shown to be successful even across institutions [8]. Establishing a trusting, professional, and oftentimes personal relationship with more experienced department leaders has been shown to lead to increased career satisfaction, promotions, and psychosocial benefits [9].

Aligning Your Goals with Institutional Priorities

Most well-established organizations have developed a mission statement or central values that are used as a touchstone to guide decisions that need to be made as new challenges and opportunities arise. These can usually be found on the department or institution's webpages and are important to become familiar with.

To help guide the evaluation of an institution's mission, Girod suggests reviewing them by asking the following questions [10]:

- What are the institutional goals and strategic initiatives by school/hospital/ department?
- What parts of these goals and plans are relevant to my position in this institution?
- Do the goals of my department/division align with the school's/hospital's mission and therefore will my work be supported? If not, which areas of work are likely to be supported that are related to my area of expertise?
- What are the strengths and the areas of excellence of the institutional/departmental/divisional performance, programmatic criteria, and leadership in the academic missions related to my position?

Regardless of the career path and type of institution you choose, all institutional missions should be to serve their end user and all goals should keep the end user at the forefront. For example, a private practice clinic or medical center should have the goal of providing the best care possible to patients who require treatment. A research organization should strive to develop the best diagnostic, imaging, and therapeutic interventions for patients. An academic institution's goal should be to train the most competent and engaged professionals using the most cutting-edge educational methods available. Evaluating your institution's priorities by asking questions such as those above will help you to better understand what your institution will expect from you in your role. That knowledge can then guide you in outlining your professional career goals.

As you consider how your goals align with your institution, identifying high-functioning multidisciplinary teams can help clarify areas of possible alignment, as well as serve as an aspirational model if the team in your area of interest and expertise is still developing. Connecting with others in successful multidisciplinary teams for guidance and advice will not only assist you toward your goals, but increase your network within your institution.

As you establish a network within your department and institution of those who can provide guidance and support for your goals, you also will be able to influence the direction of the department and institution. Junior staff members often have unique perspectives on the rapidly changing science, technology, and overall landscape of our field. Your perspective is valuable to your department and institution. By demonstrating that your goals are aligned with the institution, leaders in the institution will trust your perspective and suggestions are shared with the intent of benefiting the institutional mission, not just your own career.

How to Achieve and Evolve Your Goals

Once you have identified your motivations and priorities and aligned them at various levels, the next step is to establish how, and when, you will measure your progress. Looking at the SMART goal model once again, this is the "M" (Measurement) column. In our original example of someone who "wants to publish more and better papers," this could be "measured" by performing monthly reviews of a tracking spreadsheet to concretely visualize progress. Defining clear, measurable goal markers can also help motivate you to reach smaller, more easily achievable milestones alone the way – which also provides a boost in self-confidence.

Working through an organized strategy such as the SMART model can provide a framework to help you methodically work toward achieving concrete goals. Yet over the course of your career, there will inevitably be changes that throw a wrench into even the most clearly defined goals. Identifying, aligning, and measuring goals over time may help you successfully achieve the goals you originally set – but only if those goals are still relevant and applicable in the current environment. Colleagues or collaborators with new or different expertise may join or leave the practice, changes in department chair or institutional leadership can result in a change in the department/institutional priorities. Regular review of the SMART goals, and annually at the least, is advisable to pivot and realign as needed.

Technology in the radiation oncology field and the world at-large continues to evolve so rapidly it can be hard to keep up at times. The broad field of healthcare is directly affected by new technological advancements, but also experiences additional challenges resulting from shifting societal values, new state and federal laws, local administrative issues, and global health crises. While prior research showed that faculty commonly endorsed publishing, reputation, and leadership positions as professional goals, the future of radiation oncology may see faculty prioritizing the development of computer algorithms, meeting the needs of underserved populations, and sharing knowledge and technology from developed countries with providers and patients in low- and middle-income countries.

There will also almost certainly be times throughout your career when you develop new interests, want a change of pace or direction, or are presented with an exciting new opportunity. In a study of NIH career grant recipients, the researchers noted that, "Goals appear to evolve in response to challenges over time" [2].The experience of confronting an unexpected challenge may be an ideal time to reassess your previously set goals. Furthermore, it may be inspiring to view the new challenge as an obstacle to overcome, and develop problem-specific goals to creatively turn the challenge into an opportunity. Clearly it is just as important to take time to periodically reevaluate your goals in light of your current interests, situation, skills, and broader institutional priorities as it is to set those goals in the first place.

Conclusion

- Identifying your personal and professional goals is important to your fulfillment and career satisfaction.
- Multidisciplinary collaboration, both within and outside the department, is a central tenet of successful clinical and academic radiation oncology practice.
- Alignment with departmental and institutional goals will often provide more opportunities for funding and support, both financial and expertise.
- Demonstrating successful completion of multidisciplinary, department/institutionally aligned projects builds credibility and trust, increases your network, and can increase your influence to shape future goals.

For Discussion with a Mentor or Colleague

- What are the institutional goals and strategic initiatives for our school/hospital/department?
- What are the strengths and the areas of excellence of the institutional/departmental/divisional performance, programmatic criteria, and leadership in the academic missions related to my position?
- Which departmental initiatives align closely with institutional strategies?
- Do you see my work/interests being aligned with any of the departmental/institutional initiatives?
- Who are the colleagues and coworkers that are leading efforts most closely aligned to my interests and departmental/institutional priorities?

References

1. Shanafelt T, Chung H, White H, Lyckholm LJ. Shaping your career to maximize personal satisfaction in the practice of oncology. J Clin Oncol. 2006;24(24):4020–6.
2. Jones RD, Griffith KA, Ubel PA, Stewart A, Jagsi R. A mixed-methods investigation of the motivations, goals, and aspirations of male and female academic medical faculty. Acad Med. 2016;91(8):1089–97.
3. Drucker PF. The practice of management. New York: HarperCollins Publishers, Inc.; 1954.
4. Team MTC. SMART goals: how to make your goals achievable 2019. Available from: https://www.mindtools.com/pages/article/smart-goals.htm
5. Hilty DMH, Robert E. Aligning your goals with those of colleagues, the department, and the institution. In: LWH R, Donald M, editors. Handbook of career development in academic psychiatry and behavioral sciences. 2nd ed. Arlington: American Psychiatric Association Publishing; 2017. p. 127–40.
6. Leaders If. How informal and formal networks hurt and help performance 2020. Available from: https://www.ideasforleaders.com/ideas/how-informal-and-formal-networks-hurt-and-help-performance.
7. Soda GZ. Akbar. A network perspective on organizational architecture: performance effects of the interplay of formal and informal organization. Strateg Manag J. 2012;33(6):751–71.
8. Esbenshade AJ, Kahalley LS, Baertschiger R, Dasgupta R, Goldsmith KC, Nathan PC, et al. Mentors' perspectives on the successes and challenges of mentoring in the COG Young Investigator mentorship program: a report from the Children's Oncology Group. Pediatr Blood Cancer. 2019;66(10):e27920.
9. Allen TD, Eby LT, Poteet ML, Lentz E, Lima L. Career benefits associated with mentoring for protegee: a meta-analysis. J Appl Psychol. 2004;89(1):127–36.
10. Girod SC. How to align individual goals with institutional goals. In: Roberts LW, editor. The academic medicine handbook: a guide to achievement and fulfillment for academic faculty. New York: Springer Science+Business Media; 2013. p. 27–31.

Working with Colleagues and Staff

Wendy A. Woodward

Introduction

Working with staff and colleagues is arguably the most critical aspect of career development and success in every field. Several unique aspects of radiation oncology warrant consideration when addressing the challenges and opportunities in working with others. First, radiation oncology is a relatively small field. Many future radiation oncologists will meet other residency candidates on the interview trail whom they will ultimately know their whole career. Senior physicians are connected to one another across the country – and, indeed, around the world – and can often obtain a first-hand reference on any new faculty applicant with one phone call. For better or worse, narratives of both negative and positive interactions are often widely available. Second, radiation oncology brings together many interdisciplinary specialists; physicists, multi-disciplinary clinical teams, therapists, dosimetrists, diagnostic imagers, radiologists, and administrators are all critical to the progress and function of radiation oncology departments, and in academics, biologists, statisticians, and other research disciplines add to this intersection of disciplines. Without a doubt, different disciplines bring different skills and communication styles. Together, these issues make it paramount to engage in professional interactions that contribute positively to one's reputation, which happens in great part through the investment of substantial commitment to understanding how to communicate across demographics and how to increase the effectiveness of the many teams that are critical to your career goals. As such, this chapter provides an overview of data regarding teams and team communication, and specifically delves into some of the differences in communicating with clinical, research, leadership, and external teams in radiation oncology.

W. A. Woodward (✉)
The University of Texas MD Anderson Cancer Center, Houston, TX, USA
e-mail: wwoodward@mdanderson.org

© Springer Nature Switzerland AG 2021
R. A. Chandra et al. (eds.), *Career Development in Academic Radiation Oncology*, https://doi.org/10.1007/978-3-030-71855-8_11

Being a Part of an Effective Team

On the road to a fulfilling career in radiation oncology, most will wear numerous hats and in doing so will work with many teams, and it is useful to consider working with colleagues as synonymous with working in teams. These are all opportunities to build relationships, and these relationships, whether strong or weak, positive or negative, have a dramatic impact on your career in a small field like radiation oncology. In subsequent sections of this chapter, practical advice regarding succeeding with the typical teams encountered in a radiation oncology career will be considered. The first and most important of these teams is the nuclear clinical team taking care of patients and the related, extended team working to plan radiotherapy and treat patients and provide multi-disciplinary care. For some, the second significant team in their career development will be the research team, which often includes technicians, analysts, trainees, collaborators, grant coordinators, and others. The administrative staff and leadership team represent another important team radiation oncologists interact with. External teams in national societies or cooperative groups are to be considered as well. Of course, each of these groups of colleagues brings its own hierarchy (or lack of it), function, and engagement, and each requires different roles from a radiation oncologist to contribute as effectively as possible. Across all such groups, optimal, deliberate communication skills including managing conflict and setting boundaries will enhance the probability of productivity. Being a part of effective teams across all of these realms provides the groundwork for a reputation of effectiveness, collegiality, and respect and will aid in shaping a desirable and joyful career.

Independent of the type of team, let's first consider what is known broadly about effective teams. No doubt most radiation oncology faculty will have had an experience working with an ineffective team – a study group in medical school, an academic or sporting team, a work-related committee, or something else. The most common misconception about team success is that it is related to the intelligence of the members. Two recent studies highlight three aspects of more successful teams that counter the simple assumption that the intelligence quotient of the members is a safe recipe for success [1–3]. In one study of more than 700 people organized into teams that assessed collective intelligence, teams with higher average IQs were not clearly superior. Similarly, results were no better for teams with members who reported being more engaged in the task, or teams with more extroverts. The three significant predictors for more successful teams were having no clear leader, i.e., no single predominant speaker; having more members with high scores on a test of reading others' emotions; and having more women. Interestingly, although the test for reading others emotions involves visual cues, these factors hold in online groups where visual tools are not available [1].

What can you do with this information? First, recognize the importance of understanding the emotions and drivers of yourself and your team members. Get to know your colleagues in every job position and take the time to solicit and listen to the challenges they face in meeting the expectations of them (which are undoubtedly different from the expectations of physicians). Follow-up by creating an open space to communicate when you perceive a team member is worried or concerned to address issues head-on. Next, actively hire or advocate to build diverse teams. Make a mental list of colleagues who bring a unique perspective or background and volunteer their names when teams are being developed. Ask to be involved in hiring the staff you work with and be a leader in conquering implicit bias. Notably, Iris Bohnet notes in her book describing measures that work to reduce gender inequity that token diversity is worse than no representation [4]. The broad benefits of building and sustaining a substantially diverse team cannot be over-emphasized [5, 6]. Lastly, be a part of fostering an environment in which each member feels empowered to speak freely and contribute. Although physicians are in some ways de facto leaders of their nuclear, clinical, and other teams, be careful not to be the only voice. Key to this are recognizing the experience and expertise of your team members and never speaking for them when they can offer their input directly or when they have more knowledge about the problem than you do. In a group, when someone else does this, invite the colleague or staff member who knows this topic to contribute. If silence makes you uncomfortable, get over it. For those for whom mental answers form before a speaker has finished a comment or question (including some extroverts), suppress the temptation to interrupt, so that those who wait for others to speak will have a chance to share their insights and will not judge you as a poor listener. Be self-critical of the words you share without being so restrictive that you never contribute. Does what you want to say add value? Does the whole group need to know this now? If not, your words are competing for time from others who value colleagues and listen and feel critical of those who don't. A separate key aspect of self-review is to critically evaluate how you respond when others speak. Does it increase or decrease the chance of them trying again? Importantly, create situations for introverts to contribute on their terms. The Meyers-Briggs Personality Inventory loosely defines introverts as people who recharge best on their own or by creating space as opposed to drawing energy from interpersonal interactions to recharge [7]. Much has been written about the inherent and unique talents of introverts [8, 9]. Since introverts are typically less likely to volunteer their opinion in a group and may favor thinking critically about a response over being put on the spot, deliberate efforts to engage the whole team include sending out an agenda so all can consider their input ahead of time, inviting written input, and personally talking one on one with team members who don't always speak up in a group.

Of course, much of this is easy when we are at our best and harder when emotion or fatigue comes into play. There is no question that emotion is natural in all human beings and will at times be on display at work. It is similarly true that developing the skills to manage your own emotions is crucial to building the most productive and successful team possible. Managing your own emotions ensures that you are never a part of making someone who feels they have less power than yourself feel vulnerable at work is crucial to building the most productive and successful team possible. Indeed, studies of clinicians who are reported by staff for bad behavior show that these doctors have worse patient outcomes [10–12]. These studies also demonstrate that most clinicians will evoke no further reporting after a single low-pressure, direct conversation from a peer about their behavior [13]. Take it upon yourself to politely but directly call out disruptive behavior when you see it. Incivility reduces providers' ability to respond to stress [14], and calling it out has a strong positive ripple effect on all who observe it [14, 15].

Finally, on a broader scope, it is worth considering that what drives effective communication can differ in person and online, although as above the predictors of effective teams remain the same online and in person [1]. Certainly massive amounts of communication occur via email. More recently, communication via online communities such as Twitter or Facebook groups has become commonplace in radiation oncology and since the COVID19 pandemic, Zoom, Web-ex, and other virtual meeting platforms are the new norm. Rachel Happe, founder of the Community Roundtable, provides a strong set of recommendations for enhancing online engagement. Most importantly, she notes that this requires stepping back from the style of delivering declarative, well-thought-out complete thoughts that are common when we communicate to demonstrate expertise in a clinic or academic setting. The more complete a thought is, the less engagement it requires. She writes that people who get the most engagement online have a writing style that is "modest, imperfect, inquisitive, solicitous and often vulnerable" [16]. This may seem incongruous when you are hoping to convey that you have transitioned from a trainee to an attending, or when you are overcoming imposter syndrome in an academic setting. Indeed, it is a fine balance to ensure that you are not underestimated, yet create space for all to contribute; but this is certainly a skill that can be fine-tuned with proper attention to truly optimize your engagement with colleagues near and far.

Real-World Example (1)

The issue Dr. Brogan is a physician with outstanding Press Ganey patient satisfaction scores who is regarded as highly competent by her peers. She is engaged in ensuring that her clinic runs on time and instructs her nursing team when to put each patient in a room. She expects perfection of herself and others and routinely offers instructions to her nurse practitioner and nursing team to optimize efficiency. She often manages details herself to avoid doing work twice.

When the nurses on-board a new staff member, a senior nurse simplifies "best practices" for working with this doctor by saying, "Say yes to everything Dr. Brogan says. Just do what she asks and don't talk." Not surprisingly, Dr. Brogan is disappointed to learn that this is how her practice is perceived.

In fact, her faculty leader recognizes that this team has several causes for underperforming. The staff has low morale because they view themselves as caring, competent members of the oncology team at a top hospital who are functioning below their licenses as technicians; they are given instructions at each step. Turnover is high, resulting in time and money spent on recruiting and training. The team can't make on-the-ground improvements to the patient experience because the details of how problems arise will not be brought up in this team when there is a perceived risk in speaking up. Finally, the clinic grinds to a halt if the physician is pulled away because all direction comes from the physician.

The intervention Although it was critical that a peer or leader had multiple direct conversations with this faculty member, real change came from leadership training and introspection by this physician. The conversations with leadership didn't reveal the problem to the doctor; she was self-aware, but was failing to solve the issue with willpower, as is commonly the case. The conversation highlighted the need to address the issues by learning new skills. Eventually with Dr. Brogan committing to trust the team and let go of control; morale and flow improved.

The moral Know your weaknesses. Ask for feedback and believe it when you get it. Strive to understand effective teams and seek out support and skills to be the best team member you can be.

What is the challenge in the above example if you are Dr. Brogan? The Challenge is overcoming the beleife that the crux of the problem is something that is lacking on the part of other team members. Brene Brown, a renowned research expert in shame and empathy, suggests an exercise whereby you list employees or colleagues that fill you with frustration and then assume they are absolutely doing the best they can do in that moment [17]. She contends that by doing so it is easier to move on from reiterating the same issues without progress, to teaching the team, re-assessing skill gaps, and reassigning or letting go if needed. This represents a commitment to stop respecting and evaluating people based solely on what we think they should accomplish and start respecting them for who they are and holding them accountable for what they are actually doing and possibly by doing so have greater clarity about your own gaps. Although clinicians are not typically direct managers of their team members, they are instrumental in conversations with the team and team supervisors, and approaching team management from a position of leadership can be transformative. The more joy in work your team experiences, the more effective they will be and the more joy clinic will bring to you.

Communicating with Clinical Colleagues

In the current medical climate, the focus on quality often translates into metrics achieved by increasing the number of electronic health record (EHR) tasks completed for each patient. The clinical team is under significant pressure from sources beyond the physician to document metrics during clinic in addition to the standard work of greeting and registering patients, taking vitals, educating, and performing assessments. Nothing creates more frustration at work than opposing expectations, i.e., nursing leadership requiring perfect documentation but clinicians expecting faster throughput than can be achieved. Critical to optimizing these potentially competing issues is regular, even daily, huddles with the clinic team to review the schedule and have overview discussions with an eye toward ensuring that the first patients are scheduled when everyone is present and ready to start; that the flow of patients on the template allows all of the work that needs to be done by the whole team; that the time it takes patients to check in is accounted for, considering all clinics running at the same time; and that the staffing required to manage the clinics is available. Communicating with the "boots-on-the-ground" team members to understand the issues the clinic team faces makes it easier to avoid frustration in the clinic and to focus instead on finding solutions and working together. Notably, when change is needed and the team isn't used to change, preferring to respond "that's not how we do it," it is helpful to first understand from peers if barriers to change exist that aren't immediately obvious. Change can then be approached by presenting the case for it, with process and follow-up plans to the stakeholders, moving forward one the team is engaged. In general, this approach – getting input and buy-in from the team – will bring greater cohesiveness and build trust. Although some cases may require asking leadership to mandate change, this approach sometimes creates more problems to be managed in the future or leads to increased turnover.

Real-World Example (2)

The issue Clinicians note that the nursing notes and information gathered at the start of the patient visit are not relevant to the work the physician does during the consult and that this information is not stored in a place where it can be reviewed or used in the final documentation. Nurses are doing the work they have been expected to do for years, plus documenting new metrics, and are leery both of being criticized and of being asked to take on more unspecified work. Nursing leadership balked at new expectations, citing lack of bandwidth.

The intervention Face-to-face discussions between the clinicians and nurses reinforced to all that the clinicians well understand that the nurses are strongly committed to their patients and to doing work that matters. With a better understanding of how the proposed change could help patients, nurses met with their supervisor to proactively say that they could see value and feasibility in the proposal.

The outcome Nurses agreed to create a new assessment form, working with a clinician to ensure that the form includes the most relevant information for the practice – that is, is this patient ready for radiation, are they interested in having it here, and what is the timing for radiation planning? – and participated in creating an education timeline led by the clinicians to get up to speed on the oncology issues that influence these answers. With ongoing check-in, this approach replaced the prior less-relevant assessment, the nurses learned more about the oncologic specifics of the patients they care for, and the physicians increased the number of patients they saw without a trainee or advanced practice provider, thus improving throughput in clinic.

A unique aspect of radiation oncology clinical teams is the absolute reliance on clinical physicists and the dosimetry team typically led by physics. Personality inventory testing in physicists suggests they are often introverted and cautious [18]. Wilson and Jackson report common traits including particularly careful, controlled, and inhibited [18]. The advantage of careful and controlled personality traits in the professionals who ensure that the linear accelerators are correctly commissioned and review dose and planning parameters for patient care is obvious. For physicians who often deal in less quantifiable uncertainties than physicists accept in their discipline (the so-called "art" of medicine), than physicists accept in their discipline, it is critical to take time to understand the parameters medical physics are monitoring in plans and machine quality assurance, and to create an environment where physics can easily bring up any concerns. Given the possibility for baseline communication style to differ between physicists and physicians, time spent building a relationship and mutual understanding is critical in radiation oncology. Empowering physicists to "stop the line" for patient safety requires a culture that values physicists' input and never overrides physicists' concerns. From the beginning of training, radiation oncology residents should be trained to look to physics for input regarding robustness of any treatment and to include them proactively in the treatment team.

Running a Productive and Creative Research Team

In some ways, the challenges related to interacting with a research team are very different than those in a clinic team because the variation in staff roles is greater than in the clinic. Clinic staff who are beyond the onboarding stage and therefore well established in their role at the institution are doing a job for which they are fully trained. They have a clear understanding of what is needed each day and whether they are meeting their goals. A research team often includes trainees with various stages of expertise about the specific project, collaborators with their own priorities about being involved and varied expertise for the project, senior investigators (if you are not leading the project), and staff who are critical to the project, such as grant submission or statistical analysis teams, who must complete their tasks in advance of "hard" deadlines. Such teams require a highly varied amount of "situational leadership." The fundamental principle of the situational leadership model is that there is no single "best" style of leadership. Effective leadership is task-relevant, and the most successful leaders are those who adapt their leadership style to the *performance readiness* (ability and willingness) of the individual or group they are attempting to lead or influence.

Real-World Example (3)

The issue When a faculty primary investigator leaves the institution, a research scientist from that investigator's group, one who will continue to be funded by a persisting funding mechanism for the program and who has been doing good work, is retained and transitioned to Dr. Black's research team. Dr. Black is a member of the broader science team of the departing faculty, so the work is at some level synergistic. Dr. Black was delighted to have this senior, capable staff scientist without finding a new funding stream. Dr. Black incorporated the staff scientist into lab meetings and offered her various assignments, including data analysis on several stale projects, assisting with lab coordination efforts, and collaborative studies with another lab. In lab meetings, updates were vague and inquiries repeated over time led to assurances that tasks would be done. In the absence of receiving direct results, Dr. Black set up biweekly meetings with the staff scientist at which goals were discussed and deadlines set. Ultimately, the staff scientist reported that tasks were done, but follow-up demonstrated that they had not been completed. In short, the reports of success were not substantiated.

The intervention Dr. Black met with the staff scientist and presented the issues. When confronted, the scientist reported that she had never known how to do any of the tasks she'd been asked to do and was embarrassed to be judged as incapable after strong recommendations. She had already interviewed for another job, which she ultimately took. She was reportedly as effective in her next job as she had been previously.

The moral Dr. Black never knew that this staff scientist, who had been competent in the scope of her previous duties, was not competent in her new scope. Dr. Black had not planned an objective way to evaluate progress, and thus was never able to provide training or realign this employee with work that was in scope. The employee handled this badly, but better situational leadership by Dr. Black may have avoided this job transition.

Communication between faculty team members can also be unique in research teams. If you are doing research where you are not the senior researcher on a project, it is important to remember that every communication you have reflects on the person leading your efforts, so communicate with them before you communicate with collaborators or program officers on mentored grants. Don't surprise them. The senior author will feel protective of their relationships with the team involved, so look to them for guidance when you are first working in that team. Alternatively, in research where you are functioning as the independent, lead, or senior investigator in a space where you are fully up to speed, you can improve your team's effectiveness by communicating about this to the junior members. Make sure that they know, explicitly, what to present to you for approval prior to distribution. Know your deadlines and send reminders that you need to see the abstract or poster with time to finalize it for collaborator review that isn't done at the last minute. Grant coordinators and statisticians understand that their jobs are similar to staff at tax preparation agencies, that is, that things are busier around grant deadlines. That is a part of the job, but there is a limit to what you can expect, and it is important to understand the workload of those team members to set expectations realistically and plan to meet them. You may be able to "sweet talk" the staff into overriding the deadlines they need and push the limits, but you are not doing yourself or them any favors when this happens. Creating last-minute emergencies through failure to plan or through procrastination will create ill will and increase burnout and turnover in your staff. This decreases knowledge and competence, and the overall net effect on your research is negative.

Communicating with Leadership

One of the most delicate challenges in communicating with colleagues is in communicating with your leadership team. The leadership team needs your honest input to identify issues and solve them, but leaders are not uniformly accepting of criticism and rightfully expect maturity and professionalism in communication. Noting that the entire faculty likely brings their concerns or challenges to the same leader, it makes sense that that leader will run out of good will if they are barraged with a litany of complaints and emotion each day. So how do you provide input in a productive way that ensures that your leadership has the impression that you are the competent, problem-solving, game, smart, faculty member that you are?

Without question, the first and last principle in communication with your leadership is be professional; other principles are to be authentic and to focus on obvious shared values such as patient care, staff care, junior faculty care, self-care, and so on. Seek to understand. Have questions before you have answers, but have answers. You may know more about "the weeds" of the issues that you are challenged by, and in some cases offering a solution or offering to lead a team to find a solution is an easy win for the leadership. However, you may learn that your solution doesn't take some less obvious issues into account, or isn't something your leadership supports. It is still an act of good faith and a seed from which to start a positive conversation to think through the solutions before you talk. What about change that you don't have time to lead or that you could lead but at the cost of the work you should be focused on? In those cases, highlight the benefits of finding a solution, ask what work is ongoing (as this shows your leader you trust there is work ongoing), and ask explicitly for the change you are hoping for.

Real-World Example (4)

The issue Dr. Monroe has complained to her one-up, Dr. Walters, on several occasions that the process by which shared research nursing resources are allocated across the group isn't fair. Dr. Monroe has many funded trials but notes that she was never allowed to start a trial without funding, unlike Dr. Feld, who had been there forever and has never gotten a grant. Several other frustrations often appear in these conversations. Dr. Walters has made some statements about closing unfunded trials to create resources for other trials, but Dr. Monroe remains frustrated and continues to write grants to fund trials. Dr. Walters has typically empathized with the frustrations but has never explicitly addressed what can or will be done to resolve this. Dr. Monroe ultimately complains more broadly to other leaders looking for change and, more explicitly, expressing frustration that Dr. Walters has failed to address these issues.

The intervention Learning that Dr. Monroe has taken these issues to others, Dr. Walters understands the complaint differently. Dr. Walters had not recognized these complaints as a request for change; rather, he had heard them as venting about frustrations that had reasonable origins from a faculty who was very successful and had never brought an unfunded concept to the table. He thought that providing a sounding board for venting and recognizing Dr. Monroe's success had addressed the concern. Dr. Walters initiated a conversation with an apology for failing to understand the "ask" and to request more information. He explained the details and divisional priorities that led to the support of Dr. Feld's study. He also expressed his wish that Dr. Monroe had brought an unfunded concept for discussion to push the need to realign the resources. Dr. Walters committed to explicitly creating an opportunity for Dr. Monroe and other faculty to use the shared resources.

The moral Dr. Monroe might have had an earlier resolution with a more direct ask, "Can I start this study using shared resources like Dr. Feld has?" Presumably, Dr. Monroe didn't see this as a viable option, which is a failing by Dr. Walters to create an open environment, but the direct ask may have prompted action.

Lastly, it is important to note that most people, and as such most leaders, have an "in group" owing to a well-studied phenomenon called in-group bias [19–21]. Research suggests that the most common factor predicting association with an in-group is how similar a person is to that leader. In some ways, this makes sense; we believe that we understand people who seem similar to us or whom we believe share culture, and we may have to work harder to connect with people who are different. The best leaders recognize this unconscious bias and actively work to bridge it. When they don't, there is very little an individual can do to overcome this bias and be integrated into the in-group, which leaves the individual faculty member with a difficult decision: Does your happiness and desired career progression rely on the support and advocacy of the direct leadership? Can you get that support in other places in the organization or within the society? Are you happy keeping your head down and focusing on the challenges available to you? If the answer to any of these questions is no, then critical thought is needed on looking for an opportunity that brings greater satisfaction. Take emotion and ego out of this equation. Be open to changes where you are, and take your time to make decisions that offer you the best balance of the values that bring you joy in work.

External Professional Relationships

Work on society committees such as the American Society for Radiation Oncology, American Radium Society, or Radiation Research Society are fulfilling opportunities to build relationships nationally and to get involved in moving the field forward. Work in cooperative groups can lead to developing trials or eventually being involved in changing the standard of care. These are relationships that are often fostered by facilitators, a senior colleague who makes introductions or recommends you. That doesn't mean you can't make progress in this space without a local contact to help; it is possible to reach out to faculty involved in the work you are interested in joining and simply ask them to advise you on getting involved. You can volunteer for society committees, and you can attend any public cooperative group meetings. Most importantly, for committee work, you are one name on a roster of people who likely don't know everyone and who largely communicate by conference calls. You can make an impression by engaging or not engaging. A few tips can have substantial impact. Respond to all emails sent to the group requesting feedback, even if it is just to formally agree or thank the team for including you. On conference calls or at a microphone, identify yourself before offering input or asking a question. Prepare for the call so you can engage. The society staff on these calls often have input regarding membership, and if you are present and engaged they will remember you. The faculty chair will appreciate your input and in some cases may develop an availability bias in your favor when the need arises for someone who is engaged. The tips regarding teams noted above are even more important on a conference call. Don't fill the silence; lift up and attribute the comments of others when you agree with them, and be mindful to engage in ways that add value. If that proves difficult, formally discuss with the staff whether they feel you are adding value to the committee in a way you aren't appreciating. It is reasonable to leave a committee that isn't in your scope rather than be billed as a non-contributor, or to be explicit that you don't see a way to contribute but you are appreciating the experience and are glad to remain.

In conclusion, good communication is often about listening and soliciting the input of others to ensure that all relevant data and priorities are on the table. Establishing strong relationships makes it easier to be direct and avoid miscommunication. Nuances will vary according to your role, the expertise of the persons you interact with, time pressures, culture, and other factors, but with authentic respect as a guiding principle you will start with a strong foundation for all settings.

Bullets

- Be careful not to be the dominant voice on your teams. Foster an environment that solicits input from the entire group, offering your input when it adds value.

- Solicit and listen to the challenges your team members face to meet the expectations of them.
- Actively hire and/or advocate to build diverse teams.
- Recognize the experience and expertise of your team members by not speaking for them.
- Listen, actively.
- Address conflict professionally and directly without emotion.
- Ask leadership directly for the solutions you need.

For Discussion with a Mentor or Colleague

- What resources in your organization have helped you improve their communication skills?
- What national resources are of high value for communication?
- Which are the most effective clinic teams in the organization that I might learn from observing?

References

1. Engel D, et al. Reading the mind in the eyes or reading between the lines? Theory of mind predicts collective intelligence equally well online and face-to-face. PLoS One. 2014;9(12):e115212.
2. Woolley A, Malone T. What makes a team smarter? More women. Harv Bus Rev. 2011;89(6):32–3.
3. Woolley AW, et al. Evidence for a collective intelligence factor in the performance of human groups. Science. 2010;330(6004):686–8.
4. Bohnet I. What works: gender equality by design. Cambridge: The Belknap Press of Harvard University Press. xi; 2016. 385 pages.
5. Homan AC, et al. Leading diversity: towards a theory of functional leadership in diverse teams. J Appl Psychol. 2020;105(10):1101–28.
6. Parsons SK, et al. Promoting high-quality Cancer care and equity through disciplinary diversity in team composition. J Oncol Pract. 2016;12(11):1141–7.
7. Carlyn M. An assessment of the Myers-Briggs Type indicator. J Pers Assess. 1977;41(5):461–73.
8. Cain S. Quiet : the power of introverts in a world that can't stop talking. 1st ed. New York: Crown Publishers; 2012. x, 333 p.
9. Cain S, Mone G, Snider G. Quiet power: the secret strengths of introverts. New York: Dial Books for Young Readers; 2016. 270 pages.
10. Cooper WO, et al. Use of unsolicited patient observations to identify surgeons with increased risk for postoperative complications. JAMA Surg. 2017;152(6):522–9.
11. Martinez, W., et al., Qualitative content analysis of coworkers' safety reports of unprofessional behavior by physicians and advanced practice professionals. J Patient Saf, 2018.
12. Webb LE, et al. Using Coworker observations to promote accountability for disrespectful and unsafe behaviors by physicians and advanced practice professionals. Jt Comm J Qual Patient Saf. 2016;42(4):149–64.

13. Swiggart WH, et al. A plan for identification, treatment, and remediation of disruptive behaviors in physicians. Front Health Serv Manag. 2009;25(4):3–11.
14. Gilin Oore D, et al. When respect deteriorates: incivility as a moderator of the stressor-strain relationship among hospital workers. J Nurs Manag. 2010;18(8):878–88.
15. Sutton RI. The no asshole rule: building a civilized workplace and surviving one that isn't. 1st trade ed. New York: Business Plus; 2010. 238 p.
16. Happe R. The language of engagement. Available from: https://communityroundtable. com/grow/language-engagement/?fbclid=IwAR0Qtr3BbCRc_lUPmKZe2V9RSzEEz fgv8cX5Gx3U8xovOxmSTHAdGurYHy4.
17. Brown B. Assume others are doing the best they can. 2020 [cited 2020 5/23/2020]; Available from: https://www.thegrowthfaculty.com/blog/BrenBrowntoptipassumeothersaredoingthe besttheycan.
18. Wilson G, Jackson C. The personality of physicists. Personal Individ Differ. 1994;16(1):187–9.
19. Bass A, et al. In-group bias in residency selection. Med Teach. 2013;35(9):747–51.
20. Fischer R, Derham C. Is in-group bias culture-dependent? A meta-analysis across 18 societies. Springerplus. 2016;5:70.
21. Rudman LA, Goodwin SA. Gender differences in automatic in-group bias: why do women like women more than men like men? J Pers Soc Psychol. 2004;87(4):494–509.

Becoming a Clinician: Organization, Interprofessional Considerations, Documentation, Billing, and Insurance

Ritchell van Dams, Eric M. Chang, and Michael L. Steinberg

The scope of modern clinical medicine is vast, and the gap between the skills taught in medical school and residency and the skills needed to thrive as a clinician have never been wider. The expansion of evidence-based medicine has yielded a wealth of valuable data about the clinical efficacy and effectiveness of our interventions in radiation oncology and has led to dramatic breakthroughs that improve the quantity and quality of life for our patients. Hand in hand with this expansion of academic knowledge is a responsibility for the clinician to obtain, absorb, synthesize, and deploy advances in medical understanding in ways that are appropriate and timely for the individual patient. Coexistent with this deluge of new research knowledge is a complex and ever-changing regulatory landscape of various documentation, billing, and insurance considerations that are essential to delivering high-value care while maintaining the financial stability of a practice. As a field, radiation oncology sits at a unique nexus that combines high-technology treatment options, a culture of evidence-based practice, and the rich network of interprofessional relationships that are a necessary relational component of our tertiary referral specialty (i.e., radiation oncologists receive referrals mostly from secondary care specialists).

Due to this ever-changing practice environment, no fixed set of facts or rules can remain true and useful for more than a few years. As a result, this chapter is organized around four guiding principles that provide a framework for the clinical practice of radiation oncology. When followed, these principles will allow a radiation oncologist to be successful across a range of circumstances. Each section introduces

R. van Dams · M. L. Steinberg (✉)
Department of Radiation Oncology, University of California Los Angeles, Los Angeles, CA, USA
e-mail: RVanDams@mednet.ucla.edu; MSteinberg@mednet.ucla.edu

E. M. Chang
Department of Radiation Oncology, University of California Los Angeles, Los Angeles, CA, USA

Department of Radiation Medicine, Oregon Health & Science University, Portland, OR, USA

© Springer Nature Switzerland AG 2021
R. A. Chandra et al. (eds.), *Career Development in Academic Radiation Oncology*, https://doi.org/10.1007/978-3-030-71855-8_12

the principle, its rationale, and concrete examples of how it can be implemented or how it affects the practice of a radiation oncologist. Change is inevitable, but we believe that having a set of guiding principles can help the new and seasoned clinician alike make sense of change and allow for the adaptation necessary to thrive.

Principle 1: The Patient Comes First

The "value" in value-based care is not merely financial

> Every patient you see is a lesson in much more than the malady from which he suffers. – Sir William Osler

Our relationship with our patients and to society as a whole is unique and sacrosanct. No other profession is expected to poke, prod, and potentially cause harm with the aim of eventual cure or comfort. There has also been a shift in recent decades away from a paternalistic model of the physician-patient relationship to a shared decision-making model in which the physician considers not only the medically optimal treatment approach but also the broader biopsychosocial context of the patient's disease process. This imposes a duty to reflect on the practice of medicine and the set of values that we and our patients carry.

Some of these values are financially based and are becoming increasingly enmeshed with the formal structures that measure how we are evaluated and remunerated. In an effort to mitigate rising costs in a fee-for-service-based payment model, payers are increasingly moving toward a value-based system of repayment in an effort to shift the focus away from the volume of services to the quality of services. Although the standard formulation for value is the outcomes divided by the costs [1], a more complete accounting of value takes into consideration total quality as a function of health care structure, process, and outcomes such that a more accurate formulation is that value = quality/cost [2]. These value metrics stem from a goal to provide the most good for the least cost and are codified in quality measures assessed by the Centers for Medicare & Medicaid Services (CMS) and other payers. Casalino and Khullar [3] describe three contexts in which financial incentives can be used with an aim of improving value-based purchasing: (1) external payer (e.g., CMS) to a hospital or medical group, (2) external payer to individual physicians, and (3) internal incentives between hospitals or medical groups to its own physicians. In the first context, the size of the patient population seen in hospitals and medical groups allows for statistically meaningful outcomes data that can be subject to measurement incentives leveed by external payers. The second arrangement, however, between the same payers and individual practitioners is more fraught. The smaller scale of this context leads to higher variability in measured outcomes, and the administrative burden of measurement may be proportionally higher. As a result, there is a risk for unintended consequences such as physician avoidance of more complex patients or perverse incentives in a pay-for-performance structure. Among other things, the authors advocate for non-financial incentives that may achieve the desired outcome of value-based care more effectively. As an example, high-performing physicians or practices may earn exemption from certain reporting or prior authorization requirements for a period of time. They also advocate for broader use of the final context, in which organizations structure and measure incentives and metrics internally. This context provides individual physicians with more autonomy and representation to define meaningful metrics within their particular practice setting.

These outside payer quality measures can be thought of as the minimum requirements for delivering care but may not adequately measure actual patient-centered care. More often, more nuanced considerations of the individual patient's preferences will be required. These measures can measure patient experience. Addressing patient experience is rapidly becoming a critical component for health systems everywhere. Understanding patient preferences and aligning them with the best evidence-based practice are not always straightforward. Zulman et al. [4] used a Delphi process to develop five clinical practices to foster more meaningful connections during our patient encounters. The five practices, with examples of their relevance to a radiation oncology consultation, are described below:

1. *Prepare with intention*: This practice has two components: (1) personalized preparation for the encounter and (2) pausing and focusing before the encounter. The initial consultation in radiation oncology is often exemplary for the first component. Patients seen in initial consultation typically have an extensive oncologic history that requires careful review before any recommendation can be made. Furthermore, in many academic settings, the presence of a trainee (e.g., resident or fellow) provides a natural context for careful review of the patient's history prior to the encounter. The pause to focus is less embedded in the current culture of medicine, but is nevertheless a valuable habit in the context of modern radiation oncology clinical schedules that often involve over-booking consultations, follow-ups, and on-treatment visits simultaneously. The use of these mindfulness techniques has been shown to reduce clinician stress and anxiety, which can widen our psychological and emotional bandwidth during busy clinic days [5].

2. *Listen intently and completely*: This practice combines the importance of careful listening and avoidance of interruptions. Importantly, physicians should be attentive to how their body language conveys listening and receptiveness, and simple techniques such as sitting (as opposed to standing) and orienting one's body toward the patient even when typing in the health record can greatly improve the patient's sense of being heard [6]. Reducing interruptions, and staying silent during pauses, can provide a wealth of information that a patient may otherwise be reluctant to share.

3. *Agree on what matters most*: Our patients are often faced with a variety of potential treatment options. The treatment of intermediate-risk prostate cancer, for instance, can encompass a wide range of options including surgery and multiple modalities and fractionation schema for radiation. In helping our patients navigate these wide range of options, it can be helpful to proactively elicit the

patient's goals for the encounter and the priorities that contribute most to their sense of high quality of life. In affirming these priorities and values, the patient not only feels heard but is also more likely to feel their eventual treatment plan is in the best interest of their goals.

4. *Connect with the patient's story*: This practice element emphasizes the importance of being empathetic toward our patients' sociocultural backgrounds and circumstances as well as the benefits of positive framing and celebration of successes. Radiation therapy is not only resource-intensive to deliver, but it is also resource-intensive to undergo. Being attuned to a patient's circumstances, including financial hardship or travel distance, can help to inform decisions around treatment modalities or fractionation schema when multiple treatment options are appropriate. Our treatments can also be physically and emotionally taxing, and frequent small praises can go a long way to boosting patient morale and maximizing patient compliance with recommended therapy [7].

5. *Explore emotional cues*: This final practice is the most nuanced but potentially the most useful. By taking careful inventory of a patient's verbal and nonverbal emotional cues and actively inquiring about their emotional state, we can not only improve patient satisfaction and comprehension but also potentially reduce symptom burden [8]. While broader emotional intelligence can be taught in self-administered or small group seminar sessions, the best approach may be through direct observation. To this end, residents would do well to reflect on their attending physicians' approaches to decoding nonverbal emotional cues and those physicians should strive to model this behavior when working with trainees.

Consistent application of these five practices will not only improve patient's understanding of their treatment recommendations, but also bring a higher sense of purpose and alignment within the physician. The intrinsic desire to provide the best care possible for our patients serves as a powerful motivator for the remaining three principles. The primacy and centrality of the principle of keeping the patient first can provide context and meaning for engaging in literature searches when facing a challenging case, can help establish your reputation among your colleagues as a patient-centered physician, and can provide clarity in your justification of a treatment plan in your documentation and correspondence.

Principle 2: Train and Retrain

Organizing your time, developing your practice, and committing to lifelong learning

> The education upon which [we are] engaged is not a college course, not a medical course, but a life course, for which the work of a few years under teachers is but a preparation. – Sir William Osler

Clinicians emerge from residency as if from a period of delayed adolescence. The modern residency is set within a framework of strict medicolegal, regulatory, and educational guardrails developed and enforced by the Accreditation Council for

Graduate Medical Education (ACGME) that ensure broad oversight and account-ability for every document, prescription, and procedure. While this structured over-sight contributes significantly to improved patient safety and educational quality, the transition to independent practice has become steeper as residents are given full autonomy and accountability on their first day of attending practice and are expected to be able to jump right in. It becomes crucial, then, for junior clinicians to organize and shelter their time. The urgent and important work of day-to-day practice can seem all-consuming and if given the opportunity can replace the time needed for the equally important but less urgent needs of developing your practice, meeting aca-demic goals, and committing to lifelong learning.

On a day-to-day level, decisions around how to structure one's time and attention can be aided by the classic Eisenhower matrix (Fig. 1). The Eisenhower matrix is derived from an observation Dwight D. Eisenhower made about his work: "I have two kinds of problems, the urgent and the important. The urgent are not important, and the important are never urgent." Using the Eisenhower matrix, tasks are evalu-ated using the criteria of urgency and importance. Important, time-sensitive tasks that need your immediate attention should always be addressed personally, includ-ing issues that arise at the treatment machine or processes of care that require timely review such as simulation setup. Many tasks, however, appear important by virtue of their urgency but in reality can be delegated or delayed. Most emails and phone calls can be set aside for dedicated review periods each day, and many patient que-ries can be successfully delegated to nurses, nurse practitioners, or physician assis-tants. The less urgent – but no less important – tasks often require more careful

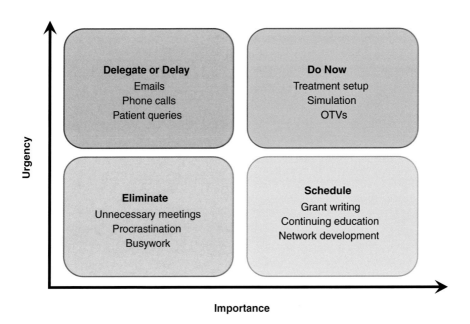

Fig. 1 Using the Eisenhower matrix to prioritize tasks in radiation oncology

attention as signs of neglect may not manifest until the damage is quite severe. These tasks often benefit from structural support in the form of scheduling and reminders.

Tasks in this quadrant include long-term research work such as grant writing, professional development including portfolio-building and network development, and perhaps most chiefly continuing education. Upon graduation from residency, the typical US-trained radiation oncologist will likely have completed no less than 13 years of post-secondary education and will have taken at least eight high-stakes examinations. After finally passing the oral boards, it can be tempting to feel a sense that one's education is "complete." If the examinations throughout college, medical school, and residency have a unifying trend, it is that the information tested becomes more dynamic and relevant over time. The physics and chemistry seen on the Medical College Admissions Test (MCAT) have not changed significantly in decades. The American Board of Radiology (ABR) written and oral exams, on the other hand, must adapt to annual changes in research findings and clinical guidelines. In prior years, the ABR has used a traditional decennial examination as part of its Maintenance of Certification (MOC) process. In 2016, they announced a shift to an Online Longitudinal Assessment (OLA) model in which practicing physicians are presented with a continuous but manageable stream of questions designed to assess "walking-around knowledge" that the typical radiation oncologist is expected to know. This format may be advantageous for many reasons. It distributes the energy and efforts of the examinee over a broad swath of time rather than forcing a once-per-decade rush of exam preparation. It also reinforces learning rather than simply testing learning by reintroducing questions in deficient topic areas. Finally, it is more responsive and adaptive, with constant feedback from examinees regarding the appropriateness of questions and the ability to quickly incorporate important, new clinical developments in the testing base.

The constant stream of new research articles can be overwhelming, but certain routines or behaviors may prove helpful for identifying and making sense of the highest impact findings. In her excellent compilation of tips for success as an academic clinical investigator, Lee [9] notes that early and precise specialization allows for more efficient maintenance of your area of expertise and offers the advice that your research focus should synergize with your clinical practice. Most journals offer an option to receive an email of the latest issue's table of contents, allowing for rapid scanning of topics that may be relevant to one's area of practice. There are also dedicated radiation-oncology-specific newsletters that send daily or weekly updates about the most important recent journal articles. Even these condensed and abbreviated information streams can be overwhelming when received daily or multiple times per day, so it may help to set up electronic rules within the email platform to automatically route these emails to a special folder that is reviewed at a set time each week. One task that should not be put off too long is keeping your CV up to date, as dates of invited talks can disappear in the clutter of a busy calendar and participation on committees can fade out of memory [9].

Another intervention that may be surprisingly easy is a special attention during departmental chart rounds or interdepartmental tumor boards for any non-standard treatment approaches. These cases provide a unique opportunity to engage with a colleague on a potentially difficult case and learn the set of treatment principles that guided them to their plan. Interactions with colleagues from different disciplines in particular may help you keep up to date on the most relevant developments outside of radiation oncology. The ever-advancing nature of radiation oncology practice offers both an opportunity to improve our treatment approaches and the responsibility to provide our patients with the best care as supported by the latest high-level evidence.

Principle 3: Friend to Everyone, Enemy of No One

Interprofessional considerations and building a professional portfolio

Showing up is 80 percent of life. – W. Allen

Radiation oncology exists as a tertiary referral specialty, and as a result we often do not have direct access to newly diagnosed patients who need treatment. In addition, our colleagues often have an incomplete understanding of the work we do. This necessitates the cultivation of relationships at several levels to ensure both a healthy practice and a working relationship that serves our patients best. Within the department, we must maintain productive relationships with our administrative and research staff, nurses, therapists, dosimetrists, physicists, and fellow radiation oncologists. Outside of our department, we often need to develop and nurture relationships with surgeons, medical oncologists, and primary care physicians both within and beyond the walls of our institution. These efforts addressing relationship development take years to establish a baseline and will never cease as long as you practice medicine.

There is no secret to building these relationships. It is a truism, though no less true, that to be depended upon you must be dependable, and to be seen you must show up. To the extent that your schedule allows, take on clinical responsibilities and leadership roles that mesh with your professional interests. These may be aligned with your desired anatomic sub-site for treatment or may be grouped by academic domain, such as quality improvement, health systems care, or education. At regional and national conferences, attend the sessions germane to your areas of passion, ask questions, and volunteer when committee opportunities arise. Fully commit to the projects you take on and pay careful attention to meeting external deadlines – if you cannot, learn to decline graciously [9].

The same applies when developing relationships with referring providers. This task may seem daunting at first, but the *Journal of Oncology Practice* [10] offers some clear and concrete guidance on the topic (Table 1). A senior physician in your area of specialization may offer key introductions to fellow surgeons and medical oncologists, allowing you to leverage their established trust to start building your relationships with them. Attend tumor boards and engage with the interdisciplinary team on complex patients. Consistently demonstrate the value of your treatment

Table 1 Tips for building and maintaining a referral base [10]

Tip	Example
Let them know who you are	Seek introductions from senior physicians and mentors When on call, capitalize on the opportunity to form a relationship with the consulting team
Involve the referrer	See the patient quickly, within a day if possible Communicate your thoughts clearly and in the preferred medium of your referrer (e.g., telephone)
Clarify your role	If you cover more than one disease subsite, make it known Be proactive about introducing radiotherapeutic treatment options at tumor board if it appears the group is unaware
Teach	Let your referring primary care physicians know what you do and how you do it Participate in cross-specialty medical conferences or grand rounds
Don't avoid the awkward	Provide direct and honest feedback when receiving an inappropriate referral or if the prior treatment plan was inadequate Importantly, be open and receptive to criticism that your referring providers have for you

modality, which may include guest lectures at their regional or national conferences or tumor boards. Being available to take your colleagues' calls is the surest way to building trust and rapport that improved referrals. Once a referral is obtained, maintain those lines of communication at the level and in the mode that the physician prefers. Some physicians find email to be a substandard alternative to the phone. Respect that preference. This work can be initially thankless and seemingly stagnant. A determined and consistent effort is important, however, as a single shared case may be enough to "win over" a colleague and kick start a productive career-long working relationship.

Principle 4: You Are Responsible for Everything You Do

Documentation, billing, and insurance

The best preparation for tomorrow is to do today's work superbly well. – Sir William Osler

Documentation, billing, and insurance are often seen as necessary evils in the practice of a modern physician. With the right perspective and approach, however, all three may be used as tools for better understanding how we practice and for quality improvement. As a field, radiation oncology has a long history of innovation with the seemingly mundane task of documentation. Among the first electronic health record (EHR) systems in medicine were the record-and-verify systems used for planning and treatment in our specialty of radiation oncology. One of the earliest uses of documentation review was in the seminal Patterns of Clinical Care [11] study that examined individual patient records at a national level across 10 disease sites and hundreds of facilities to identify patterns in treatment processes and assess the quality of treatment at different facility types. Our documentation can also provide benefit on an individual level. Patients who are given access to their oncologist's notes report a higher level of understanding of their diagnosis, potential side effects, and reassurance about their treatment plan; a small minority of patients – under 5 percent – report regret regarding reading their oncologist's note [12]. Building good documentation practices is critical as it clarifies your thinking to yourself, to your colleagues, and in an emerging world of "open notes," to your patients. Medical care is increasingly complex and fragmented, and thorough documentation allows us to communicate the care plan with physicians between clinics and across months and years.

An understanding of how we bill and how insurance pays is fundamental to understanding the business of medicine at the physician level [13]. Although some health systems and practices rely on dedicated staff to assign billing codes, we recommend taking the initiative to seek advice and training from your faculty practice group regarding the documentation and recordkeeping standards that support your evaluation and management (E&M) and other codes used in the radiation oncology process of care. Ultimately, it is the physician's responsibility to ensure coding is performed correctly, and often the physician is the only party that truly knows what happened with a patient. Correct billing is critical; overbilling is intuitively understood and can be fraud, while underbilling not only harms the bottom line but also inadequately documents the process of care. Lastly, a detailed understanding of the documentation required to support your billing can ultimately save time by facilitating requests for authorization from insurance providers. Guidance for proper E&M documentation is regularly revised and provided by CMS, and multiple medical societies including the American Society for Radiation Oncology (ASTRO) provide conferences and online resources for up-to-date training in radiation oncology coding [14, 15].

Besides being a necessary component of a healthy practice, billing and insurance processes can provide valuable data for understanding how patients are cared for across the country. The Current Procedural Terminology (CPT) codes were defined by the American Medical Association (AMA) in effort to standardize the reporting of medical, surgical, and diagnostic services and procedures [16]. Correct use of CPT codes not only ensures accurate documentation of services rendered and allows for appropriate reimbursement for those services but also serves to document the process of care for the radiation oncology care. The codes can also be used at the national level to assess geographic and temporal trends to specific technologies or treatment techniques.

Our field is on the cusp of a generational change in our billing and insurance practices. The radiation oncology alternative payment model (RO APM) proposed by CMS in 2019 marks a sudden and dramatic shift in the way radiation oncology services will be reimbursed [17]. In the currently proposed RO APM, facilities and physicians will receive a single bundled payment per episode of care per patient, with the precise rate dependent upon the disease site, geographic location of the facility, historical reimbursement rate for the facility, and a number of other adjustment factors. Importantly, the need to understand billing and coding is not obviated by these episodes of care, as the proposed RO APM includes continued collection of this data for measurement of intensity of services and quality outcomes.

Ultimately, all of the financial risk is placed on the facility to reduce costs below the bundled payment for each episode or else each episode of care would incur a loss to the facility. While these kinds of transitions in reimbursement paradigms can be great opportunities for innovation and progress, attention must be paid that perverse incentives are not inadvertently generated. One common criticism of a bundled payment model is that it fosters a race to the bottom in terms of quality, in which providers seek the treatment approach with the lowest facility cost in order to maximize the revenue from the single episodic payment. Nevertheless, this payment paradigm also has the potential to spur innovation in new practices that provide isoeffective treatment at a lower cost – the definition of high-value care.

Conclusion

The process of becoming a clinician starts in medical school, continues throughout a career, and is never truly complete. Although the landscape of clinical radiation oncology will undoubtedly continue to change in the years and decades to come, certain core principles can guide the new and seasoned clinician alike through periods of turbulence and calm. By always prioritizing the patient, committing to ongoing learning, fostering meaningful interprofessional relationships, and diligently documenting our process of care, we can provide the best care possible for our patients regardless of the environment.

Summary

- The clinical environment of academic radiation oncology is ever-changing, requiring adaptability to new circumstances. Despite this, some core principles remain useful.
- The patient always comes first, and it behooves us to take careful inventory of each patient's preferences and values when determining how to best care for them.
- The knowledge landscape of radiation oncology is vast and requires constant attention to maintain excellence in the care we provide. The Online Longitudinal Assessment can be a useful tool for self-assessment of one's knowledge base.
- Building and maintaining a referral base require diligence and time but can offer lasting and fruitful working relationships.
- Documentation, billing, and insurance are a necessary part of a healthy practice and can provide valuable data and insight into improving the outcomes that our patients experience.

For Discussion with a Mentor or Colleague

- Given the multiple duties of varying importance and ease of completion facing the physician (e.g., grant writing, research projects, clinical care, email correspondence), what strategies do you use to prioritize tasks on a daily, monthly, and yearly basis? How have you learned to balance your clinical and academic responsibilities?
- What routines have you developed to stay on top of the latest developments in research and clinical care? What resources have you have found most useful?
- Can you tell me about a time you "won over" a colleague and earned his or her trust? Can you tell me about a challenging relationship you have had with a colleague and what strategies you used to improve the relationship?
- Given that coding and billing are not routine aspects of medical training, how did you familiarize yourself with financial management when starting out as a junior physician? How do you refresh your knowledge in an ever-changing financial landscape?

References

1. Porter ME. What is value in health care? N Engl J Med. 2010;363(26):2477–81.
2. Teckie S, McCloskey SA, Steinberg ML. Value: a framework for radiation oncology. J Clin Oncol. Am Soc Clin Oncol. 2014;32:2864–70.
3. Casalino LP, Khullar D. Value-based purchasing and physician professionalism. JAMA. 2019;322(17):1647.
4. Zulman DM, Haverfield MC, Shaw JG, Brown-Johnson CG, Schwartz R, Tierney AA, et al. Practices to Foster physician presence and connection with patients in the clinical encounter. JAMA. 2020;323(1):70.
5. Lomas T, Medina JC, Ivtzan I, Rupprecht S, Eiroa-Orosa FJ. A systematic review of the impact of mindfulness on the well-being of healthcare professionals. J Clin Psychol. 2018;74(3):319–55.
6. Merel SE, McKinney CM, Ufkes P, Kwan AC, White AA. Sitting at patients' bedsides may improve patients' perceptions of physician communication skills. J Hosp Med. 2016;11(12):865–8.
7. Ramfelt E, Lützén K. Patients with cancer: their approaches to participation in treatment plan decisions. Nurs Ethics. 2005;12(2):143–55.
8. Rakel D, Barrett B, Zhang Z, Hoeft T, Chewning B, Marchand L, et al. Perception of empathy in the therapeutic encounter: effects on the common cold. Patient Educ Couns. 2011;85(3):390–7.
9. Lee SJ. Tips for success as an academic clinical investigator. J Clin Oncol. 2013;31(6):811–3.
10. Building and maintaining a referral base. J Oncol Pract. 2007;3(4):227–30.
11. Kramer S, Hanks GE, Diamond JJ, MacLean CJ. The study of the patterns of clinical care in radiation therapy in the United States. CA Cancer J Clin. 1984;34(2):75–85.
12. Shaverdian N, Chang EM, Chu FI, Morasso EG, Pfeffer MA, Cheng EM, et al. Impact of open access to physician notes on radiation oncology patients: results from an exploratory survey. Pract Radiat Oncol. 2019;9(2):102–7.
13. Financial management in oncology practice, part 2: billing and collections. J Oncol Pract. 2008;4(4):195–9.

14. Evaluation & Management Visits | CMS [Internet]. [cited 2020 Apr 29]. Available from: https://www.cms.gov/Medicare/Medicare-Fee-for-Service-Payment/PhysicianFeeSched/Evaluation-and-Management-Visits.
15. Coding - American Society for Radiation Oncology (ASTRO) - American Society for Radiation Oncology (ASTRO) [Internet]. [cited 2020 Apr 29]. Available from: https://www.astro.org/Daily-Practice/Coding.
16. CPT® overview and code approval | American Medical Association [Internet]. [cited 2020 Apr 29]. Available from: https://www.ama-assn.org/practice-management/cpt/cpt-overview-and-code-approval.
17. Proposed Radiation Oncology (RO) Model | CMS [Internet]. [cited 2020 Apr 29]. Available from: https://www.cms.gov/newsroom/fact-sheets/proposed-radiation-oncology-ro-model.

Becoming an Educator: Giving Feedback, Supervising Trainees, Formal Didactics

Daniel W. Golden and Ravi A. Chandra

The Educator as a Career Path

Academic medicine has three pillars – clinical care, research, and education. Academic institutions expect faculty members to contribute to all three of these academic missions, although individual faculty members may have different balances across these three domains. Often the analogy of "filling a bucket" is used to describe how to envision the amount of effort dedicated to these three academic roles. A busy academic clinical radiation oncologist may primarily focus their effort on building a regional, national, or international reputation in their specific disease site with a smaller percentage of their effort dedicated to research or education. Conversely, a radiation oncologist that is hired as a physician-scientist with significant protected time to secure extramural grant funding and run a laboratory may dedicate less time to clinical care and education. We are beginning to see the emergence of radiation oncology educators who focus significant effort on education as their primary scholarly focus [1]. When promotion committees assess a faculty member for reappointment or promotion, the combination of their effort in these three domains (clinical care, research, education) determine if the faculty member meets the criteria for advancement. Though all prospective and junior faculty are encouraged to learn the criteria their individual institution uses when evaluating these three domains, this is especially the case for those planning to pursue a career as an educator within radiation oncology.

D. W. Golden (✉)
Radiation and Cellular Oncology, Pritzker School of Medicine, The University of Chicago, Chicago, IL, USA
e-mail: dgolden@radonc.uchicago.edu

R. A. Chandra
Department of Radiation Medicine, Knight Cancer Institute, Oregon Health & Science University, Portland, OR, USA
e-mail: chandrav@ohsu.edu

© Springer Nature Switzerland AG 2021   157
R. A. Chandra et al. (eds.), *Career Development in Academic Radiation Oncology*, https://doi.org/10.1007/978-3-030-71855-8_13

With the above in mind, it is important to recognize that all faculty are expected to contribute at some level to all three pillars of the academic mission. Thus, it is imperative that all faculty view themselves as educators, even if the majority of their effort is directed elsewhere. Medical school and residency focus on development of clinical skills and learning research methods. However, all too often, when learning to be an educator, the trainee and, eventually, junior faculty member, is left to observation of their own teachers and clinical educators to learn best practices. The word "Doctor" comes from the Latin word, "Docere," which means "To teach." Thus, a primary role of a doctor is to function as an educator. This includes educating trainees and also educating patients. This chapter will focus on becoming an educator in the context of teaching trainees at the medical school/undergraduate medical education (UGME), and residency and fellowship/graduate medical education (GME) training levels.

The goal of an educator is to ensure their trainees are prepared to practice competently and independently at the end of their terminal training. However, an educator must consider the level of their trainee when deciding the goal and specific objectives of the particular learning experience the educator is responsible for. Common learning activities that a radiation oncology faculty member will be involved with include supervising residents during clinical rotations, interacting with rotating medical students, didactic lectures to residents and/or medical students, Socratic teaching of residents during clinical chart rounds, serving as a departmental examiner during objective structured case-based assessments (colloquially known as "mock orals"), and numerous other educational interactions with trainees. Other opportunities exist within this realm including formal and informal mentorship of trainees at all levels, including on research projects and in career development.

One area of internal tension that educators may experience is the conflicting goals of serving both as the learner's coach and the judge [2]. As the coach, the educator wants their trainee to be as successful as possible and can point out areas for improvement to the trainee, understanding that this is with the ultimate goal of the trainee succeeding. However, the educator is often asked at the end of an educational experience to assess, or judge, the trainee and provide a recommendation about level of competence. This can cause a tension between the trainee and educator. Therefore, an educator should explicitly state that their goal is to help the trainee succeed and any feedback is meant as constructive and formative, rather than critical or summative.

Circling back to the importance of education to reappointment and promotion, documentation of educational effort (hours, learners, frequency, outcomes) is critical for reappointment and promotion. Junior faculty should ensure their department is obtaining teaching evaluations from any residents or medical students that rotate on their clinical service. Additionally, the department should have a mechanism to obtain learner evaluations of other educational effort such as resident lectures, serving as an examiner for objective case-based skills assessments (mock orals), or other educational activities with direct learner contact. These evaluations will provide the educator with important insight into how they can improve their teaching effort and also are used by institutional committees when reviewing a faculty member for reappointment or promotion. Many institutions have educator's portfolios where effort in the domains of curricular development, direct and clinical teaching, and educational leadership can be documented separately from the curriculum vitae. This is especially important as many of the attributes and efforts of a committed educator may not fit the standard rubrics on a curriculum vitae.

Curriculum Models

An educator must carefully consider all components of the curriculum their learners are immersed in. There are three components of any curriculum – set, hidden, and null. The "set" curriculum represents what the learner is told they are going to learn. Examples include the goals and objectives provided at the start of a clinical rotation, a table of contents in a textbook, the syllabus provided at the outset of a radiation biology course, and the outline provided by the American Board of Radiology for written and oral boards. Learners are aware of the content in the set curriculum and expect to learn it during their training experience.

The second component of a curriculum is the "hidden" curriculum. This is often described as the socialization into medicine or a specific specialty (e.g., radiation oncology). The hidden curriculum provides both positive and negative learning experiences. An example of a positive experience is a resident observing their attending using high levels of compassion and empathy when discussing goals of care with a patient with metastatic pancreatic cancer requiring palliative radiotherapy for progressive local disease. Although the resident may not identify this as a specific learning experience, through observing the clinical interaction they are learning how to have these difficult discussions and will model compassion and empathy in future interactions. Unfortunately, the hidden curriculum also includes negative learning experiences. An example would be a medical student who observes an attending radiation oncologist belittling a dosimetrist for not achieving a requested dose constraint. Again, the medical student may not identify this as a learning experience, but as the medical student moves into residency and eventually independent practice they may have learned from observing this professional interaction that it is acceptable to belittle other staff in the radiation oncology clinic. Educators, and indeed all physicians, must therefore be conscious that they are modeling behavior for their learners at all times and are therefore "educating" learners at all times in the clinic.

The third component of a curriculum is the "null" curriculum. This represents the content that is excluded from the set and hidden components of a curriculum. Examples in radiation oncology include self-care and wellness, radiotherapy treatment plan evaluation, healthcare economics, and myriad other topics that are often excluded from a set curriculum due to time and resource constraints. Although it is impossible to teach learners everything, the astute educator should try to bring critical topics that they recognize have been relegated to the null curriculum into the set curriculum. This can be accomplished by providing a paper to a rotating resident that discusses wellness and burnout, ensuring medical students and residents are included in treatment plan evaluation activities, or volunteering to give an additional didactic lecture on healthcare economics.

These aspects of the curriculum can be leveraged in the education of trainees by holding sessions at the beginning and mid-point of rotations to achieve clarity on mutual goals and objectives. Targeted experiences may be envisaged to these ends. Reflection sessions on "questions that have arisen" and other lessons learned may provide fodder for discussion over more passively acquired elements of the curriculum. Though not a formal aspect of current rotations, future opportunities exist within the narrative space to encourage trainees to reflect on all they have learned in the course of their individual rotations.

Formal Didactics

There are multiple opportunities for direct teaching both within the radiation oncology department and the broader institution. Junior faculty should actively seek out opportunities at the UGME, GME, and continuing medical education (CME) levels. Additionally, there are opportunities to teach to other specialties and to patients.

At the UGME level, junior faculty can get involved with the medical student clerkship or in the preclinical medical student curriculum. Due to limited resources the medical student clerkship may not have a robust didactic curriculum. There are medical student clerkship curriculum materials available that can be introduced to provide all medical students with a strong foundation in radiation oncology [3]. Additionally, junior faculty can actively seek to include medical students on their clinical services and provide mentorship opportunities such as career development conversations and research opportunities. Small investments of time can yield tremendous dividends for individual students. Outside of the radiation oncology department junior faculty should evaluate if radiation oncology is integrated into the general medical school curriculum. Many institutions have no radiation oncology content in the general curriculum. Junior faculty can volunteer to provide a lecture during a clinical pathophysiology course to preclinical students, develop oncology modules, or can look to integrate a radiation oncology experience into a core clerkship such as medicine, surgery, or radiology.

At the GME level there are numerous opportunities for formal didactics. Most residency programs have a didactic seminar schedule which can be an excellent means for junior faculty to teach and develop connections with trainees. For example, if a junior faculty member has a specific clinical or research interest, they should approach the chief residents or program director about giving a talk on their topic of interest. Junior faculty can also develop and run hands-on workshops to teach fundamental skills such as contouring, plan evaluation, image verification, brachytherapy, and many other clinical skills. Residents enjoy interactive learning formats that are not the usual slide lecture format. These can include "chalk talks" or hands-on workshops. Many medical schools have simulation centers and educators are encouraged to devise creative means to incorporate such resources into their teaching. Faculty can also volunteer to give introductory seminars about radiation oncology to other department's residency or fellowship programs. Common learner groups for this kind of talk include an overview of radiation oncology for medical oncology fellows, surgical residents or surgical fellows, an overview of the role of radiotherapy and brachytherapy in the management gynecologic malignancies for gynecologic oncology fellows, and many other topics of interest.

At the CME level, faculty can volunteer to give a departmental seminar on a new clinical topic, research interest, or other topic of interest. Additionally, faculty can offer to give seminars to colleagues in other specialties such as before or after a tumor board to review new clinical guidelines or changes in standard of care. This can be a great mechanism to ensure their institution is providing cutting-edge care while also getting to know their colleagues in other specialties. Junior faculty can also look to give talks at national meetings (scientific or refresher) although these are more often invited talks rather than volunteer opportunities.

Lastly, there are numerous patient support groups that are always eager to invite physicians as speakers. This type of talk requires a different level of teaching with more of a focus on basic concepts and answering questions commonly asked by the lay public rather than focusing on data and high-level evidence. These talks can be quite rewarding for the physician and are a way to educate and contribute to the local community.

When giving lectures or running workshops, it is important to consider how to teach for retention. The educator needs to consider their learners' comfort with the material and how each individual learner responds to different levels of stress. The Yerkes–Dodson law [4] (Fig. 1) suggests that learners who are at low levels of stress (arousal) will not retain information due to lack of attention. An example is an early morning slide lecture with no interactive component that the learner sleeps through. On the other end of the spectrum, if the stress (arousal) level is too high the learner cannot concentrate on the learning experience and will not retain information. An example might be a learner who is uncomfortable being asked questions in front of a large group during departmental chart rounds. Different learners will respond

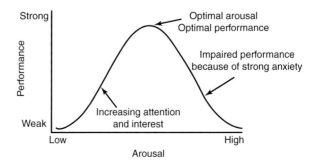

Fig. 1 Hebbian version of the Yerkes-Dodson law demonstrating an optimal level of arousal (stress) will maximize performance (learning)

differently to different levels of stress. The astute educator will determine, perhaps with input from the learner, what the appropriate level of stress is for the learner. One mechanism to prevent low levels of arousal is to keep the learners engaged through use of an audience response system and asking questions or discussing key points as a group throughout a lecture. There are numerous free audience response systems that can be easily integrated into a slide lecture.

Additionally, different learners have different preferred learning styles. There are numerous proposed models for learning styles. One common model is the Visual, Auditory, Reading, and Kinesthetic model. Any individual learner does not have one learning style, and most likely can, and needs to, learn with all of these teaching methods. However, individual learners may have learning "preferences." One learner may prefer slide lectures because they are most comfortable with auditory and reading as learning styles while another learner may prefer a hands-on workshop that is more visual and kinesthetic. Thus, an educator should develop teaching practices that allow different learners to learn using their learning preference. The takeaway here is not all learners are the same, and the educational strategy that works for one learner may not work for another. If a learner is struggling, rather than blame the learner, the educator should take a step back and consider how the educational strategy can be modified to play to the learner's preferred learning style and optimal level of stress. Excellent educators become facile in integrating these different mechanisms into their teaching and recognizing these attributes in learners with whom they interact.

One other concept that is key to ensuring long-term transfer of knowledge is spaced repetition. This is the idea that a particular fact or piece of knowledge can be reinforced through repetition. If an educator teaches a learner a key fact or skill, the educator should then ask the learner the next day, next week, or next month to recite the fact or demonstrate the skill again. This will optimize long-term retention. There is no harm in reinforcing key knowledge and skills to ensure your trainee will remember them years later when in independent practice.

The final point to make about formal structured didactics is how to appropriately utilize slide presentation software. Considering the Yerkes–Dodson curve, it is critical to ensure your audience remains engaged. Thus, as discussed previously, use of audience response systems is encouraged. Simpler methods such as interspersing multiple-choice questions about previously covered content or providing a fill-in-the-blank worksheet that can be completed during the presentation can increase learner engagement without inducing too much stress. Additionally, the slide set should include an initial overview of the lecture so the leaners know what to expect throughout the talk. Going back to this overview slide periodically during the talk can help remind learners what has been covered and what remains to be covered. Repeatedly including this overview slide throughout the talk can also be used by the speaker as a reminder to check for questions from the learners. Other recommendations for slide presentations include keeping the number of lines on a slide to seven or fewer; using high-quality images; and limiting use of extraneous graphics, backgrounds, transitions, and animations that distract from the content being presented. One common problem in radiation oncology is the "data dump" slide, which includes so much information it is impossible for the learners to distill key points of information. This should be avoided. Lastly, a common rule of thumb is to allow for at least 1 minute per slide. If the talk is scheduled for 60 minutes and the speaker has 90 slides, this is a set-up for failure. Either the speaker will cover the material too quickly, will not cover all the material, or will significantly run over their allotted time.

Teaching in Clinic

The other common teaching environment for junior faculty is the clinic. Residents and medical students will most likely rotate through the junior faculty's clinical service and it is important that they are provided with a structured clinical learning experience. As required by the Accreditation Council for Graduate Medical Education, all faculty should have clearly defined goals and objectives for their individual rotation. How to write goals and objectives is beyond the scope of this text, but can be found elsewhere [5].

The first point to consider when teaching in the clinic is the concept of "graduated responsibility." The training level of the resident and their individual competence should be carefully considered when deciding what level of supervision to provide. A junior resident will likely require direct supervision of clinical tasks such as counseling patients about adverse effects, contouring, and plan evaluation. A senior resident likely can be indirectly supervised by allowing them to independently enter target volumes, counsel patients about adverse effects, or evaluate treatment plans before the teaching physician gets involved. In these situations, the attending should put in extra effort to allow the senior resident to continue to learn and grow. Examples of how to do this include copying the resident's contours into a separate structure set before making revisions to the can compare their original contours to the teaching physician's final contours, observing the resident counseling a patient about adverse effects rather than assuming they are covering all necessary topics, and inviting the resident to review the treatment plan with the teaching physician before final plan approval and discussing why the teaching physician may have chosen something different than the resident. The teaching physician is encouraged to consider individual clinical activities as "entrustable professional activities" (EPAs) and then decide based on the resident's competency level whether direct or indirect supervision is required. A teaching physician that does not provide direct supervision of a trainee when it is needed misses the opportunity to teach best practices to the new trainee and prevent development of bad habits (e.g., not checking normal structures before contouring target volumes, not evaluating target volumes in three dimensions, etc.). Conversely, a teaching physician that provides too much direct supervision to an advanced trainee may stifle that trainee's ability to practice clinical skills independently in preparation for independent clinical practice.

A critical role of the teaching physician is to provide formative feedback during and at the end of clinical rotations. The teaching physician should not save feedback until the end of the clinical experience as it will not allow the trainee to respond to the feedback and demonstrate improvement. When providing feedback, it should be framed as such. One problem that is endemic in clinical medicine is teaching physicians often struggle to provide constructive feedback out of fear of offending the trainee or not knowing how to approach the trainee in a comfortable manner. One concept that can be used to explain feedback to a trainee is "radical candor" [6]. This is the idea that a supervisor should care personally and challenge directly. Thus, the teaching physician can frame a feedback session at the outset by stating "I *care personally* about you being as successful as possible, so I'm going to *challenge you directly* with areas for improvement that I've observed thus far during your clinical rotation with me." Of course, if the teaching physician hasn't demonstrated previously that they care personally about the trainee, this approach may not work. The teaching physician should schedule a time for feedback so the trainee is not taken by surprise. Prior to a feedback session, the teaching physician should write down the trainee's strengths and areas for improvement to ensure they are prepared for the discussion. Teaching physicians should provide both positive and constructive feedback. Acknowledging a trainee's strengths to reinforce positive behaviors is just as important as pointing out areas for improvement. Using this recommended approach can help teaching physicians broach the difficult subject of feedback and feel comfortable providing constructive feedback, not just positive feedback.

Diving Deeper: Acquiring Additional Educator's Skills

For those who wish to focus on education as their primary academic mission, being an excellent educator in the aforementioned areas common to all academicians is a necessary starting point. Other opportunities exist to develop as an educator, including attending conferences such as those run by the Association of American Medical Colleges (AAMC), American Medical Association (AMA), or the American Society for Radiation Oncology (ASTRO), participating in cooperative educational groups such as the Radiation Oncology Education Collaborative Study Group (ROECSG), and degree programs focused on medical education such as a Master of Health Professions Education. Conferences provide opportunities to connect with other like-minded individuals, share best practices and new ideas, and provide venues for collaboration. As educators, one should seek to be a resource to other faculty within a home department seeking to develop their skills. Numerous opportunities for service within an institution (e.g., UGME or GME curriculum committees) and national organizations (American Board of Radiology committees, ASTRO, etc.) exist in this space as well.

Medical Education Scholarship

A final topic to consider with regards to a faculty member's role as an educator is the potential for scholarship of teaching. Fincher and Work state, "Scholarship advances or transforms knowledge in a discipline through the application of the scholar's intellect in an informed, disciplined and creative manner. Scholarship is demonstrated by a peer-reviewed, publicly disseminated product" [7]. There are numerous opportunities for scholarship of teaching in radiation oncology. Needs assessments can be done to describe the current state of education with regards to a specific topic such as contouring, communications, or wellness. Subsequently, novel curriculum innovations can be developed, implemented, and evaluated which produces data that can be published and disseminated in peer-reviewed form. Methodology for the curriculum development is beyond the scope of this text and can be found elsewhere [8]. Scholarship of education can complement a clinical or research-focused career, or serve as a primary means of scholarship. For example, a clinician with an expertise in prostate brachytherapy can develop training innovations techniques to teach proper brachytherapy technique. With a little extra effort, data can be collected to demonstrate the effectiveness of an educational innovation and can be published in peer-reviewed literature. By publishing and disseminating the educational innovation, this now qualifies as scholarship. Lastly, scholarship of teaching can cut across disciplines and professions. There is ample opportunity to develop educational collaborations with other specialties (e.g., medical oncology, surgery, pathology, diagnostic radiology, etc.) or other professions (e.g., radiation physics, nursing, dosimetry, etc.). Writing and editing, including of textbooks and other enduring online materials (e.g., test preparation materials, podcasts, etc.) must not be overlooked in this area as well. Table 1 provides exemplary examples of scholarship of teaching in radiation oncology. Additional examples of education scholarship can be found elsewhere [5].

Table 1 Examples of radiation oncology scholarship of teaching

Study	Study design	Intervention	Outcome	Target learners
Neppala et al. [4]	Randomized trial	Interactive contouring module	Improved engagement and interest in radiation oncology	UGME
Golden et al. [3]	Cohort study	Structured clerkship curriculum	Improved objective knowledge	UGME
Ju et al. [9]	Feasibility	Objective structured clinical examination	Standardized patients can be used to teach radiation oncology residents	GME
Thaker et al. [10]	Feasibility	Prostate brachytherapy education using a phantom simulator	Simulation can be used to teach fundamental prostate brachytherapy skills	GME

UGME undergraduate medical education, *GME* graduate medical education

Conclusion

Education, as one of the three pillars of academic medicine, represents an opportunity for junior faculty to expand their presence in their department and institution. There are many formal teaching opportunities such as lectures and workshops along with the clinical preceptorship that must be provided to residents rotating on their service. It is imperative that teaching physicians consider their learner's training levels, strengths and weaknesses, and learning preferences when developing an educational program. Education is an often-overlooked opportunity for a faculty member to increase their scholarly output. Finally, for those interested in education as a primary scholarly focus, numerous opportunities exist for developing skills and creatively contributing within this space.

For Discussion with a Mentor or Colleague

- What aspects of medical education appeal to me most and in what areas do I want/need to enhance my skills?
- Are there specific medical education experiences (site visits, conferences/workshops, leadership/service opportunities) I should consider? Are there medical education needs within my department or institution? Are there medical education leaders within my department or institution with whom I should meet?
- Is scholarship of teaching considered a valid academic pursuit at my institution? What are the criteria for reappointment and promotion/advancement? Can scholarship of teaching be used to satisfy these requirements?

References

1. Fernandez C, Corbin KC, Golden DW. The radiation oncology 'medical educator' career path. Int J Radiat Oncol Biol Phys. 2020;106:50–1.
2. Cavalcanti RB, Detsky AS. The education and training of future physicians: why coaches can't be judges. JAMA. 2011;306:993–4.
3. Golden DW, et al. Objective evaluation of a didactic curriculum for the radiation oncology medical student clerkship. Int J Radiat Oncol Biol Phys. 2018;101:1039–45.
4. Diamond DM, Campbell AM, Park CR, Halonen J, Zoladz PR. The temporal dynamics model of emotional memory processing: a synthesis on the neurobiological basis of stress-induced amnesia, flashbulb and traumatic memories, and the Yerkes-Dodson law. Neural Plast. 2007;2007:60803. https://doi.org/10.1155/2007/60803. PMID: 17641736; PMCID: PMC1906714.
5. Golden DW, Ingledew PA. Radiation oncology education. In: Halperin EC, Wazer DE, Perez CA, Brady LW, editors. Perez and Brady's principles and practice of radiation oncology. 7th ed. Philadelphia: Wolters Kluwer Health/Lippincott Williams & Wilkins; 2018.

6. Scott K. Radical candor: fully revised & updated edition: be a kick-ass boss without losing your humanity: St. Martin's Press; 2019.
7. E Fincher R-M, Work JA. Perspectives on the scholarship of teaching. Med Educ. 2006;40:293–5.
8. Thomas PA. Curriculum development for medical education: a six-step approach. Baltimore: Johns Hopkins University Press; 2015.
9. Ju, Melody, Abigail T. Berman, Wei-Ting Hwang, Denise Lamarra, Cordelia Baffic, Gita Suneja, and Neha Vapiwala. 2014. "Assessing Interpersonal and Communication Skills in Radiation Oncology Residents: A Pilot Standardized Patient Program." International Journal of Radiation Oncology, Biology, Physics 88 (5): 1129–35. https://doi.org/10.1016/j.ijrobp.2014.01.007.
10. Thaker, Nikhil G., Rajat J. Kudchadker, David A. Swanson, Jeffrey M. Albert, Usama Mahmood, Thomas J. Pugh, Nicholas S. Boehling, et al. 2014. "Establishing High-Quality Prostate Brachytherapy Using a Phantom Simulator Training Program." International Journal of Radiation Oncology, Biology, Physics 90 (3): 579–86. https://doi.org/10.1016/j.ijrobp.2014.06.036.

Becoming a Researcher: Grants and Budgets, Reviewing and Writing Papers, and the Institutional Review Board (IRB)

Jennifer Yin Yee Kwan, Scott V. Bratman, and Fei-Fei Liu

Grants and Budgets

How to Write a Successful Grant

One of the basic tenets of academic medicine is original contribution of new knowledge, which will advance our field of Radiation Oncology, generated through research activities. This applies to the entire spectrum ranging from basic laboratory, translational, clinical trials, quality of life, health economics, imaging/technology, artificial intelligence, to education research activities. The conduct of research requires resources, such as supplies, personnel, and services, which need funding. Fortunately, our system has multiple sources for such funding, ranging from clinical departmental support, philanthropy, industry, to peer-reviewed agencies. Each source has slightly different criteria, but the basic principles to capture these funds successfully are fundamentally the same.

The essence of any successful request for funding is the compelling premise as to what new knowledge will be created by your proposal, and how will it impact our cancer patients? Then, as the hypothesis is being formulated and strengthened, the research proposal needs to be organized in a scientifically logical manner to address the overarching hypothesis. Commonly, there will be three major aims, each with sub-aims, which will either prove or refute the hypothesis, contribute insight into the process under investigation, and advance the state of knowledge in the chosen area of enquiry. The major aims need to be interrelated, but they cannot be

J. Y. Y. Kwan · S. V. Bratman · F.-F. Liu (✉)
Radiation Medicine Program, Princess Margaret Cancer Centre, University Health Network, Toronto, ON, Canada

Department of Radiation Oncology, University of Toronto, Toronto, ON, Canada
e-mail: Fei-Fei.Liu@rmp.uhn.ca

© Springer Nature Switzerland AG 2021
R. A. Chandra et al. (eds.), *Career Development in Academic Radiation Oncology*, https://doi.org/10.1007/978-3-030-71855-8_14

constructed to be interdependent, such that failure of one aim would lead to the collapse of the entire premise. As an example, if one were to examine the role of cyclins in altering radiosensitivity of human cancers, and one of the aims is too narrowly focused on a specific member of that pathway, and is proven to be irrelevant, then one might conclude cyclins play no role in affecting radiation response. Hence, it is important to design the aims thoughtfully to address the scientific hypothesis appropriately, but not so restrictive or dogmatic to lead to a dead end.

In order to convince the reviewers that the chosen area for investigation warrants further investigation, the provision of preliminary data is key and critical. Hence, during the preparation of a grant application, the investigator needs to plan carefully as to what pieces of evidence would be necessary to compel the reviewer (and the applicant him/herself) that the stated hypothesis is worthy of further enquiry. One way to think of this situation is from an investment perspective. Research dollars are precious; the reviewers need to decide that among the 10 grants they are currently reviewing, which one or two applications would they recommend investing, for the highest return on investment ("ROI")? The strength of the preliminary data is crucial in convincing reviewers to advocate for specific grants; these data need to be compelling and intriguing, hence the planning of experiments to generate the preliminary data is definitely worthy of significant time and energy expended by the applicant during this phase of grant writing.

Oftentimes, we are asked as to how much experimental details are necessary to include in a grant application. In general, young investigators would need to provide more details than a more experienced applicant [1]. The reviewer needs to be convinced that the applicant has the scientific know-how to successfully execute the proposed studies, particularly for complex and novel experiments (e.g., in 2020, it might be single-cell RNA sequencing). It is helpful to refer to previously published methodologies by the applicant to save space, or have a letter from a collaborator with expertise in the proposed methodology. On the topic of letters, as a new investigator, it is important to demonstrate independence from his/her previous mentor or supervisor. In fact, oftentimes, it would be prudent and valuable to have the previous supervisor provide such a letter specifying independence. This can be clarified by the previous supervisor indicating that a specific cell line or mouse model has now been gifted to the current applicant, or there is an agreement that the proposed area of enquiry will only be pursued by the younger investigator and no longer of interest to the senior supervisor.

One very important aspect of the design and construction of aims is to provide a section at the end of each aim, as "Anticipated Outcomes and Alternatives." This section refers to interpretation of the anticipated data, with an alternative plan briefly described, if the anticipated outcome were not observed. The value of providing this section is to first focus the reviewers' attention on the scientific objective of the proposed aim, and interpretation of the anticipated data. The second value of providing an "alternative" is to illustrate the scientific open-mindedness of the applicant; scientific roads are rarely linear, it is the pursuit of the unexpected, that often leads to the most exciting discoveries!

Finally, success comes to those who are best prepared, as summarized in publications on this topic [2, 3]. In addition to the planning and generation of preliminary data, it is critical to start writing drafts of these grants months ahead of the deadline. Not only does this allow editing the proposal as a function of newly generated data, but also allows feedback from mentors or colleagues prior to the final submission, particularly for young investigators. In some research-intensive institutions, there are internal grant review processes prior to submission, which are extremely valuable, and have been demonstrated to increase success rate of research grants, as one would expect. If such opportunities are available, they should definitely be capitalized, for obvious reasons. Persistence and passion are critical; if one is convinced of the value of a particular line of enquiry, even if not initially successful, persistence will pay off. Many of our scientific icons in oncology, such as Judah Folkman and John Dick, have both described personal difficulty in capturing external funding in their earlier years, since reviewers were averse to investing in untested hypotheses of tumor angiogenesis or cancer stem cells. It took them years to convince grant panels that these entities actually exist and are relevant – the rest is history!

Budgets

The easiest way to assemble a budget for any research proposal is to read a budget from a previous grant application of a similar nature, for the same funding agency. This is where networking and mentoring are key and critical since these mechanisms allow access to such previous applicants. The major elements of most research budgets include personnel, supplies, services, and "others." Each agency might have slightly different rules in terms of who can be funded, for what component of time, etc. It is critically important to read and follow the rules stated, and if they are unclear, contact the agency directly to ensure there is a clear understanding of the expectations in terms of documentations or other requirements.

For personnel requests, it is important to justify each individual's role in contributing to the research project. The justification does not need to be detailed to the minute or hour, but must make sense to the reviewer. For example, if there are very few mouse experiments proposed, yet there is a request for a full-time animal technician throughout the entire duration of the grant, reviewers will start to question that specific request; thereby risking reduction of that specific budgetary request. It is also helpful if specific individuals are identified (e.g., an actual name), which will strengthen the justification that such a person with appropriate skillsets has already been hired for that specific role (e.g., technician, graduate student, or postdoctoral fellow).

Similarly, requested supplies and reagents also need to be justified. For a first-time applicant, reading a previous budget would be critical to learn the appropriate amount of such requests, and strategy for justification. If a piece of equipment is requested, a quote from a vendor would need to be included; one needs to be thoughtful since some agencies mandate that once funded, that piece of equipment MUST be purchased from the original vendor, so it behooves the applicant to ensure that the best vendor has indeed been selected for that hardware.

If there are animal (e.g., mouse) experiments being proposed, the number of mice MUST be justified so statistical expertise would be required for such justifications. Clinical or translational studies would of course require biostatistical expertise to justify cohort size of groups of patients or number of samples. With any type of complex omics-data, bioinformatics expertise to assist in the design of such studies as well as their analyses are of paramount importance. Finally, with clinical studies, please remember to include underrepresented minority (URM) groups, and if such populations cannot be included, that must be clearly justified.

Finally, many funding agencies seek partnerships (e.g., with industry) in order to amplify the impact, or expedite commercialization efforts. Again, it is critically important to pay attention to the eligibility criteria (e.g., sometimes, donors or philanthropy can serve as partners), which might be an alternative to an industry partner, although each situation would be different and unique. These partnerships occasionally can be complicated by the need for data transfer agreements, protection of personal health information (PHI), or sharing of intellectual property (IP). By all means, one should not avoid these opportunities, but additional vigilance would be required; ideally, the host institution has offices with such expertise to facilitate such partnerships, which oftentimes can be extremely fruitful.

Once a grant is obtained successfully, this is the moment for celebration, and breaking out that bottle of champagne! Unfortunately, this moment of elation usually only lasts a few days, followed by the realization that now the hard work has just started, new data must be churned out, in preparation for the next grant. This is the true challenge of this academic path – running an independent laboratory is essentially like running a small business. One becomes an entrepreneur (like it or not); one needs to be opportunistic in pivoting to areas where there are sources of funding (e.g., breast or prostate cancer). One needs to be able to develop a budget skillfully to leverage the precious research dollars already captured. As an example, if there are opportunities for graduate students to obtain scholarships, such awards must be capitalized for the students – creating obvious win–wins! Developing effective collaborations is absolutely necessary in this competitive world of science. Just as no business can be successful *in silo*, neither can research. From a research budget perspective, if there is a neighboring collaborator with whom a research personnel (e.g., graduate student, animal technician) can be shared, then these are the partnerships, which will be of mutual benefit. Pursuing an academic career and running a successful laboratory program are decisions, which I have made early in my own career, that I have found to have been immensely gratifying. I would not have traded this for any other choices, and watching my graduate students and other trainees who have now carved out their own careers successfully brings me boundless joy and satisfaction.

Reviewing a Manuscript

Peer review is foundational to high-quality scientific advancement of the field of radiation oncology. Published literature becomes a permanent scientific record that will be referenced by future studies. Publications also help set the agenda for further areas of exploration. Peer review relies on a principle of reciprocal altruism [4]. There is often no recognition or monetary compensation and it costs the reviewer time and effort; nonetheless, it is a necessary responsibility for all researchers to help guide what scientific content gets published [5]. The quality of peer review depends on both the regularity of engagement of altruists and the contributions of each altruist in providing careful, constructive, objective criticism [4].

We acknowledge, however, that most of us have never been trained on how to perform peer review [6]. Engaging in peer review activities, reading the comments of other reviewers, and seeking guidance from researchers actively engaged on editorial boards of journals may be helpful to develop these skills [7]. Additionally, this section focuses on some key items to attend to as a reviewer to help facilitate and encourage your involvement in this important activity. There are many types of manuscripts that are submitted to journals for publications. We will focus on the peer review of original research articles (i.e., those articles publishing empirical findings).

Preparing to Review a Paper

Prior to accepting a review, all potential reviewers should ensure that they are free from conflict of interests with the authors of the paper and equipped with sufficient expertise to perform a quality review [6]. Without these two basic elements, the reviewer should decline and await future opportunities where they may be better suited to engage as a peer reviewer.

Without obvious conflicts of interest, reviewers may still be affected by some common biases. For example, for a given paper, if the authors of a manuscript are well known or from well-recognized institutions, there is often an increased rate of acceptance of those papers by reviewers [8]. One way to decrease this bias is blinding. Typically, authors are blinded to the reviewers (single-blind), but in double-blind review, reviewers are also blinded to the authors. This has been implemented by some journals to reduce three types of biases that result from knowing the manuscript's authors and affiliations: the Matilda effect (bias toward valuing contributions from males over females) [9], the Matthew effect (crediting collaborative papers mainly to the well-established researchers on a paper) [10], and the famous institution effect [8, 11]. In absence of a double-blind review process, we hope that awareness of these effects may better help you avoid these tendencies and achieve objectivity in your reviews. With the right mind set, you can now begin the review!

The Beginning and End

Every paper is constructed with a beginning and an end. It should start with an introduction that includes two to three paragraphs providing context and support for the hypothesis and goals of the study, and end with a discussion section that reviews and summarizes the study findings in the context of the greater literature [7]. Together, these sections should communicate the originality and importance of the results. Originality could come in the form of a conceptual, analytical, technological, or translational advancement in the field. Discussing the timeliness of the article results in addressing an urgent need, and/or direct implications on clinical practice are critical to include. As a reviewer, evaluating the logical flow of ideas and writing will help the investigator communicate their findings clearly and maximize their impact. Suggestions could include expanding or limiting the text in these sections to address the above items or improve the succinctness of their manuscript.

Methods

Next, reviewing the methods of a study is foundational. The design and methodology need to be able to test the proposed hypothesis for the results to be reliable and meaningful. The Enhancing the QUAlity and Transparency Of health Research (EQUATOR) network has established reporting guidelines for different types of health research studies that could be used as a checklist to understand if a study has been designed and conducted in a manner that is acceptable to the health research community [12]. For example, Consolidated Standards Of Reporting Trials (CONSORT) guidelines can be used for evaluating randomized trials, Strengthening the Reporting of Observational Studies in Epidemiology (STROBE) for observational studies, Standards for Reporting Diagnostic accuracy studies (STARD) for diagnostic or prognostic studies, and Preferred Reporting Items for Systematic Reviews and Meta-Analyses (PRISMA) for systematic reviews and meta-analyses. An additional way to assess appropriateness of design would be to evaluate how the manuscript you are currently reviewing compares to other published articles on similar topics in the field. Additionally, registration of prospective trials is recommended by the International Committee of Medical Journal Editors (ICMJE), which helps facilitate transparency, validity, and dissemination of results [13]. The World Health Organization (WHO) has further provided guidance on acceptable registries and trial data that are important to report [14]. Additionally, ethical and safety considerations should be addressed including a statement on ethical approval, if applicable. Further details are discussed in the institutional review board (IRB) section below.

   In addition to the above, descriptions of methods should be written to allow for reproducibility [15]. Sample sizes and statistical analyses should be clearly stated and justified. For laboratory science experiments, assays, controls (positive and negative), and outcomes are important to include. As well, deposition of materials, data, and protocols into accessible databases (e.g., genetic sequence in GenBank) are recommended to further facilitate transparency and reproducibility.

Analysis and Interpretation of Data

A proper study design will facilitate interpretation of data. Some common pitfalls in analysis have been previously described including inadequate controls, indirect comparisons, multiple comparisons, reporting correlation versus causation, p-hacking, and poor interpretation of nonsignificant data.

Firstly, the purpose of a control in a study is to account for effects of an intervention that are unrelated to the research question [16]. Inappropriate controls or inadequate controls can prevent researchers from making certain claims regarding the results of an intervention. Conclusions derived from analysis of a single group is an example where there is a missing second experimental control group [16]. Should this be the case in a manuscript, limitations in the study should be stated as well as a rationale as to why a control group was not included.

Making inferences without performing a statistical analysis has been another commonly identified pitfall [17]. For example, Makin et al. [16] describe a scenario whereby there is a significant effect measured before and after an intervention in one group, but a nonsignificant effect in another group. Does this mean that there is a greater effect in the former group? To make a firm claim, a statistical analysis must be made between groups rather than in each group individually. Additionally, in the scenario of many comparisons taking place, an astute reviewer should note the number of independent variables measured and the number of analyses performed, and recommend correction for multiple testing if this were not already addressed by the authors [16]. Otherwise the study could suffer from an increased risk of a Type I error (false positivity) [18].

Confusing correlation with causation is another classic misstep by investigators [19]. Reviewers should suggest rewording of claims if no interventional experiment was performed to help facilitate clarity of results. Randomized controlled trials have long been perceived as an approach that is amenable to causal conclusions compared to other types of clinical studies [20, 21].

Furthermore, p-hacking is a bias in the literature that occurs when there is selective reporting of significant results [22]. P-hacking has been described as an issue particularly when studies are not registered or preplanning on an analysis is not completed [23]. In these scenarios, it is recommended that the selection of variables to analyze be justified in the text. In the vein of p-value interpretation, another issue is that nonsignificant p-values are often disregarded or assumed to have no effect [16]. However, insufficient evidence to conclude an effect is not necessarily the same as providing support for a null hypothesis. In these scenarios, suggesting additional testing (e.g., Bayesian statistics [24] or equivalence tests [25]) may help the author decipher the difference between those two possibilities.

Lastly, knowing the limits of your own knowledge is very important. Commonly, researchers are asked to review a paper based on their expertise of specific subject matter. Nevertheless, the statistical analysis can be a crucial part of the paper and your role as a reviewer could be recommending that a manuscript to undergo additional review by a statistics expert [5]. Greenwood et al. [26] have put together a helpful checklist of general questions to ask to assess the methods, presentation, and interpretation of data; this framework can help decide whether an additional statistical review by an expert in the field may be helpful.

Understanding Publication Rules

Some additional strategies to assist in the peer review process in a timely fashion is to respond to peer review invitations quickly [27], complete your review as soon as possible, and take the time to familiarize yourself with the publication requirements. In particular, identifying any missing elements or formatting errors can help streamline the publication process and reduce time to publication [7]. For example, understanding the number of tables or figures permissible by the journal will allow you to comment on the appropriateness of the selected display items in supporting the main message of the article. Additionally, it would help you as the reviewer to provide precise and constructive suggestions on how the authors could incorporate additional main or supplementary figures to support their research claims. Depending on the audience of the journal, you could also suggest how the investigators could improve or tailor their writing to most effectively communicate with the target audience of the journal (e.g., clinicians, scientists, educators, or administrators).

Finally, reviewer comments should summarize the importance of the work being reviewed, the strengths and weaknesses of the study, and major/minor suggestions for improvement. Reviews should be written in a collegial manner [28]. As some have stated, "*you should review for others as you would have others review for you*" [4]. Together, we can work collaboratively to advance the field of radiation oncology through peer-reviewed publications.

Writing and Publishing a Manuscript

Academic radiation oncologists have the duty and privilege to contribute to the advancement of knowledge for our field. A major component of this endeavor is through writing and publishing of manuscripts. Manuscripts can take many different forms. New study results, meta-analyses, comprehensive reviews, and commentaries each have their place in the scientific process. It is of the utmost importance that scientific findings and opinions are communicated in a clear and balanced manner when disseminated to the research community. Equally important is execution of a plan for manuscript writing and strategy to get manuscripts published in an appropriate venue. This section will address important topics in scientific writing, including tips for effective communication, collaborative manuscript writing, and submission strategy.

How to Communicate Science through Writing

Writing skills do not always come naturally to clinicians and scientists. High-quality formal instruction in scientific writing is hard to come by during postgraduate training. Instead, it is often left to the individual to teach oneself the tricks of the trade of effective scientific writing. Authors must balance many competing demands when writing manuscripts. They must adhere to rigid formats without seeming dry. Technical details need to be conveyed, but the message should be accessible to a broader audience. While this can seem daunting, a few guiding principles can ensure the maximum possible impact of scientific manuscripts.

Authors should write with the reader in mind. By taking into account how manuscripts are read, authors are better able to communicate their findings as opposed to simply presenting results [29]. A focus on clarity, narrative structure, and creativity improves the impact of scientific writing. The first-person active voice is more direct and easier for the reader to follow. Appropriate use of punctuation and conjunctions can help the reader navigate the meaning of otherwise complex concepts. If executed effectively, the reader will come away with a clearer understanding of the author's research, which will ultimately lead to more citations and wider recognition in the field [30].

The reader expects to encounter information in a certain order. Forcing the reader to seek information in unexpected locations introduces unnecessary barriers to straightforward interpretation. This pertains to multiple aspects of manuscript writing including data presentation, manuscript organization, paragraph structure, and sentence structure [29]. Clear presentation of experimental data within manuscripts is critical for proper interpretation. Likewise, when a manuscript is structured with sections for introduction, methods, results, and discussion, misplacing components in the wrong section increases the workload for readers.

Appropriate paragraph structure can be challenging for beginning writers. Effective writing creates clear divisions between paragraphs. Paragraphs should be able to stand alone to communicate a point or group of points around a common theme [31]. The opening sentence of each paragraph gives an overview of the theme to be explored in the remainder of the paragraph. If multiple points are made in the same paragraph, it should be apparent how they relate to one another.

Proper sentence structure helps the reader find the desired information where he/she expects it. For instance, readers expect to find the subject and predicate in close proximity in the sentence. If, instead, the predicate is placed at the end of the sentence far away from the subject, the reader is forced to do extra work to link the two. Other important considerations in sentence structure include where the topic of the sentence is introduced (*topic position*) and where the emphasis is placed (*stress position*) [29]. The *topic position* provides the reader with context that is necessary for interpreting the point of the sentence. The reader expects the topic of a sentence to appear at the beginning, so any deviation from this can lead to misinterpretation by the reader. Conversely, the reader expects the emphasis to appear at the end of the sentence. The stress position should provide the reader with closure with respect to the point made by the sentence. In general, the topic position includes information that the reader is already familiar with, whereas the stress position introduces new information that the reader is meant to take away as important.

To summarize, scientific writing is among the most important tasks of an academic radiation oncologist. A useful framework for guiding authors is to focus on assisting readers interpret their writing. To this end, we find it helpful to read one's own writing after stepping away from a draft for a period of time. This allows an author to approach the writing fresh and from the reader's perspective. Authors can employ rhetorical devices that assist readers to link concepts across sentences and paragraphs. Parallel sentence structures can guide the reader by emphasizing common points. Special attention should be placed on transitions between sentences and paragraphs to guide the reader through the manuscript. With these concepts in mind, authors should feel confident that they can communicate their research findings to a broad audience of clinicians and scientists, thus augmenting the impact of their academic product.

The Abstract

The abstract is the most important means for efficiently communicating the content and impact of a scientific study. It is often the basis on which the work is judged by journal editors and other audiences [32–34]. Many scientific journals have specific guidelines for abstracts that must be abided. Some require structured abstracts with distinct headers (e.g., background, methods, results, and conclusions), but even unstructured abstracts should follow a similar formula. The most effective abstracts summarize abstract the study rationale, methods, and results, and then place the findings in a broader context to highlight the overall impact.

Bear in mind that the readership of the abstract often comes from a broad range of disciplines. Thus, emphasis should be placed on keeping the abstract accessible. To deliver the primary message of the manuscript in a clear and concise manner, authors should use present tense and pay close attention to sentence structure [35]. In place of long compound sentences, shorter sentences are generally easier to follow. Technical jargon and excessive use of adjectives and adverbs should be avoided if possible.

The reader abstract should come away from the abstract with a clear understanding of the impact of the study. This can be achieved by having a consistent message reiterated in the background and conclusion of the abstract. Alignment with keywords used throughout the manuscript can also be helpful. Finally, authors should avoid words that introduce vagueness or that minimize impact. Direct and confident language will help the reader take away the most important points of the manuscript.

Data Presentation

Science is driven by data. It is critical that data is presented in a manner that can be appropriately interpreted by the reader. In scientific manuscripts, data can be presented within the text of the results section as well as within standalone display items (i.e., tables and charts). Authors should be cognizant of readers who consume information in different manners. Some readers focus primarily on the text of the manuscript, whereas others focus primarily on the display items. Therefore, a robust manuscript will be able to communicate the major findings in both forms. This layer of redundancy also helps to reinforce important messages of the manuscript.

Display items (with their associated captions) must be able to stand alone in conveying the research findings. Jargon and abbreviations (if necessary) should be explained in the caption or footer. For tables, information that is familiar to the reader should appear on the left, and new information introduced to the reader should appear on the right. This organization of data aligns with the expectation of readers and allows for ease of interpretation. For graphs, titles of axes should be labelled, and the number of observations and results of statistical tests should be specified. Axes should be scaled appropriately without distortion.

As you prepare your data, you may wonder which elements need to be made available to peer reviewers. This depends on the nature of the data (clinical vs. nonclinical, proprietary, consent) and any restrictions on its use. It is important to understand policies of specific journals with regard to data publication. The academic mission depends on the veracity of published data and honesty of its analysis and interpretation. By adhering to the above principles, authors can avoid misleading presentation of data. Data transparency is garnering increasing attention across all health research fields [36], leading many journals to require datasets and analysis methods to be made available to the research community at the time of publication. This movement underscores the importance of clear and accurate communication of science across disciplines and highlights the need for specialized training on this topic for academic radiation oncologists.

Strategy in Manuscript Writing, Submission, and Peer Review

Before embarking on writing a manuscript, plan ahead for each step of the process, including: (1) data collection and analysis, (2) collaborative writing, and (3) manuscript submission. Strategizing for each of these steps will help ensure a smooth process and ultimate success for journal publication.

For any manuscript that includes primary data, consider how data is to be managed during manuscript preparation as well as after publication. A data management plan ensures that collaborators have access to and agree upon the main data elements and their use [37]. Ideally, the plan should be put in place prior to or early on during the writing process if not beforehand. If there are specific requirements for data handling and publication by ethics boards or funding agencies, this should be explicitly addressed in the plan.

The vast majority of manuscripts in our field include multiple authors. Collaborative manuscript writing has never been easier due to digital platforms specifically geared toward this purpose. Despite the technical ease, collaborative manuscript writing can still present some delicate issues. To avoid confusion, it is best to agree on authorship criteria and order before manuscript writing commences [38]. All authors must contribute meaningfully to manuscript writing and/or supervision, and lead authors may have extra responsibilities in drafting the manuscript, adhering to timelines, and assigning tasks to coauthors. While there is no singular approach to collaborative manuscript writing, the most important principle is transparency and open communication between coauthors, as without this, misunderstandings can lead to disagreements and conflict.

The manuscript is written, and you are ready for submission to journals. While this may seem like the end of the process, publishing original research in peer-reviewed journals has become increasingly complex. There are more journals than ever, so selecting the appropriate journal for the manuscript can be challenging. In addition to the scope and audience of the journal, one must consider article format, journal impact factor, listing on public servers, open access options, and author processing charges. Some journals have formal mechanisms for pre-submission inquiry to gauge the editor's interest, which can be useful even before the manuscript has been finalized for submission. Preprint server submission is increasingly popular, and some journals even have their own preprint servers for articles undergoing peer review. The decision to post a preprint may depend on many factors including the desire to create a public record of ongoing research or the need to cite the work for grant applications [39]. Once the appropriate venue is selected, include a concise cover letter to highlight the importance of your work. After feedback from reviewers is received, you will hopefully have the opportunity to respond and resubmit your work. If so, it is highly likely your manuscript will be accepted if you follow some simple rules. Be sure to be respectful in your response-to-reviewers by considering each and every comment and request [40]. Organize the responses in such a way that the editor and reviewers can easily navigate the document. The responses should be self-contained and include any new results that may also be included in the revised manuscript. As with the writing of the manuscript, be sure to engage collaborators and coauthors on the response-to-reviewers when appropriate.

Scientific publishing is a prerequisite for a career as an academic radiation oncologist. The process may seem overwhelming at first, but with practice, you can learn to refine your writing style and become an effective communicator. Thankfully, the cycle of academic activities – from grants to peer review to manuscript writing – is mutually reinforcing such that your skills in one domain will benefit all others.

IRB Process

History of Research Ethics

The origins of medical ethics began as early as the fifth to third centuries BC with the Hippocratic Oath to *"first do no harm*," from which the principle of non-maleficence was derived [41]. Later in 1620, the *Novum Organon* was published by Francis Bacon, introducing the idea that research should be beneficial to society [42]. However, it was the mistreatment of human subjects through experimentation on wartime prisoners during the twentieth century that led to the formalization of a code of ethics. In the 1947 Nuremberg trials (i.e., "the Doctors' Trial"), Nazi physicians and medical administrative personnel were found guilty of murder and torture [43]. This led to the Nuremberg Code mandating research to adhere to certain principles including voluntary consent of subjects, experimental validity with societal benefits, scientifically qualified researchers, avoidance of harm, and proper termination principles [44]. In 1964, the Declaration of Helsinki was created by the World Medical Association, which provided specific guidance on consent in therapeutic research [45]. Additionally, in 1979, the National Commission for the Protection of Human Subjects of Biomedical and Behavioral Research published the Belmont Report. This report outlined three foundational ethical principles including respect for persons, beneficence, and justice, which govern the field of biomedical research [46].

Of note, during the 1940s to 1970s, past human experimentation with radiation occurred in vulnerable persons from lower socioeconomic status, mental retardation, a terminal illness, or from minority groups or prisons. Experiments included feeding or injecting radioactive materials (minerals [47], plutonium [48]) and irradiating body parts (testicles [49], brain [50]) to examine their effects on the human body. These past historical events as well as those mentioned in the previous paragraph necessitate diligence in maintaining high standards of research ethics in radiation oncology.

Principles of Human Research

The purpose of human subject research is to obtain knowledge relevant to science or medicine through systematic investigation. To perform this, careful scientific review is required. In the modern era, Institutional Review Boards (IRBs in the US) and Research Ethics Boards (REBs in Canada) are the research ethics committees that help examine the benefits and harms of the proposed research. These reviews are based on the guidelines in the Belmont Report [46]. Depending on the jurisdiction, US Federal Regulations or Canadian Tri-Council Policy may be additionally considered [51].

Consent in Human Research

One of the foundational aspects of the Belmont Report focuses on respect for the autonomy of participants [46]. This is addressed through research consent, which is the communication and decision-making that occurs between a participant and the researcher proposing the study. This requires the ability for the patient (or substitute decision maker) to understand the information presented, appreciate the benefits and drawbacks of participating, and communicate that decision.

Valid consent includes being informed and deciding voluntarily [52]. Informed consent requires the researchers to communicate in lay language what is required in the study, the rationale behind the requirements, and when the study procedures will occur in addition to responding fully to all the questions posed by the eligible participants [53]. Participants need to be able to weigh the study risks, benefits, and alternatives as they relate to their own values, how the research could affect their quality of life, and be cognitively intact to be able to understand and remember the information during the decision-making time period [54]. Voluntary consent occurs in the absence of coercion or misrepresentation of the study information; the patient must also be capable to perform the steps of the decision-making process described above [55, 56].

The informed and voluntary nature of consent allows for reduction of harm and support of patient's rights in personal decision-making. It is important to note that consent is an ongoing process and should be obtained each time there is a change in a condition, treatment, or if research findings arise that could affect the decision to participate in the research [51]. The consent form documents the consent process, but is not the only aspect of the process [57]. Consent forms are reviewed by IRB/REBs; they commonly outline the investigators involved, purpose of research, potential harms and benefits, alternatives to participation, procedures for confidentiality, reimbursement, sponsorship, and conflicts of interest [51].

In general, a patient is presumed to be capable unless there are reasonable grounds to believe otherwise [58]. However, capacity is not static and can change over time, and depend on the complexity of decision-making. It is the responsibility of the researcher proposing the study to evaluate that capacity. One tool that can help with capacity assessment is the Aid to Capacity Evaluation (ACE) Tool [59]. This tool contains questions that can help decipher if the participant understands the proposed intervention, alternative options, consequences of accepting the intervention, and whether comorbid conditions may affect their judgement [59]. The need for research in vulnerable populations (e.g., children, elderly, mentally ill) or incapable persons have additionally allowed for the introduction of substitution decision maker to act on behalf of a participant in the decision-making process [60].

The Regulatory Environment

International Conference on Harmonization Tripartite Guideline: Good Clinical Practice (GCP) is an ethical and scientific quality standard for designing, conducting, recording, and reporting clinical trials of new healthcare interventions for human subjects [61]. Clinical trials are also registered after IRB/REB approval, prior to starting the research activity. Furthermore, there is an International Compilation of Human Research Standards that outline laws, regulations, and guidelines on protection of human subjects across 133 countries [62]. This document discusses principles for drugs and devices, clinical trial registries, research injury, social behavioral research, privacy/data protection, human biological materials, genetic, embryos, stem cells, and cloning.

National and international guidelines on membership of the review board recommend a minimum of five members with expertise to review the research including a scientist, a person with knowledge of the relevant law, and a non-scientist [51]. The research protocol is reviewed for scientific merit and equipoise of the research question [63]. More invasive research will require increased examination at review based on the concept of proportional review [51, 64]. The board will also review procedures of ongoing research including adverse event reporting, annual reports, and monitoring of research (data safety monitoring boards, audits of research documents, consents and results, monitoring of informed consent process) [65].

Conflicts of Interest

There are three types of conflicts of interest in research: conflict of interest, obligation, and bias [66]. Conflicts of interest include personal or financial interests of a researcher that can prevent them from satisfying their obligations to the participant [67]. Conflicts of obligation include two or more moral or legal responsibilities that inherently prevent fulfilment of the other responsibility(ies) without compromise [67]. Conflict of bias are psychological factors that stop a researcher from fulfilling their obligation toward a participant [68].

To manage conflicts of interest, conflicts must first be identified. Conflicts can be actual, potential, or perceived [51]. Once identified, they are to be disclosed to institutions, sponsors, peer reviewers, co-investigators, and/or research participants; this may lead to withdrawal from a role that is creating the conflict [51]. The goal of conflict-of-interest management is to support informed decision-making and participant welfare, ensure transparency and accountability, and minimize legal risks [51]. These principles are outlined by Tri-Council Policy Statement: Ethical Conduct for Research Involving Humans (TCPS 2) in Canada and other documents [51].

Special Issues Relevant to Radiation Oncology

In the field of radiation oncology, two common questions that are scientifically asked include: "Which is the better dose and fractionation of radiotherapy to administer?" and "What modality of radiotherapy is better?" As part of the scientific process, radiation doses that might lead to inferior disease control could be delivered to a proportion of patients during early-phase dose escalation studies. To reduce harm (or suboptimal benefit), early phase studies should limit the number of such participants and also directly inform the design of later studies. This situation has been described by Koyfman et al. [69], in relation to an example of a Phase 1 trial for stereotactic body radiotherapy for early-stage non-small cell lung cancer directly informing the dose used in a subsequent Phase 2 trial [70, 71]. Additionally, radiation oncology is a highly technological and dynamic discipline with quick adoption of new techniques of enhanced conformality or improved dosimetry. Koyfman et al. [69] remarked that trials comparing older to newer technologies are rare. Due to perceived lack of equipoise, questions on the superiority of new treatments or their cost–benefit compared to standard treatments may not be definitively answered in this field prior to proceeding with novel treatments.

Progress in radiation oncology requires careful consideration of the ethical principles of study design and consent similar to other fields of medical research. In particular, historical ethical violations in human experimentation with radiation in the twentieth century underscore the importance of continued diligence in providing ethical management of research in this discipline.

Conclusion

This chapter summarizes some foundational activities that all academic researchers in radiation oncology will engage in during their careers, including how to write grants, budgets, and manuscripts; review manuscripts; and how to navigate the ethics and review board process. We hope that our overview of these essential topics will facilitate a greater understanding of not only how to perform each of these activities well, but also provides the context on why these activities are important. We encourage you to use this text to help improve your academic research skillsets. Regular engagement in these activities with guidance and feedback on your performance by trusted advisors will help develop a basis for a successful academic career.

For Discussion with a Mentor or Colleague

- What are the critical elements to a successful research grant application?
- How do I build a budget for my upcoming grant application?

- How do I submit an REB application for my upcoming project?
- How do I structure my first major research paper for publication?
- What are the key steps in reviewing a manuscript?

References

1. Molldrem JJ. Preparing basic and translational grant proposals: thoughts from the trenches. Hematol Am Soc Hematol Educ Program. 2010;2010:181–4.
2. Wisdom JP, Riley H, Myers N. Recommendations for writing successful grant proposals: an information synthesis. Acad Med. 2015;90:1720–5.
3. Proctor EK, Powell BJ, Baumann AA, Hamilton AM, Santens RL. Writing implementation research grant proposals: ten key ingredients. Implement Sci. 2012;7:96.
4. McPeek MA, DeAngelis DL, Shaw RG, Moore AJ, Rausher MD, Strong DR, Ellison AM, Barrett L, Rieseberg L, Breed MD, Sullivan J, Osenberg CW, Holyoak M, Elgar MA. The golden rule of reviewing. Am Nat. 2009;173:E155–8.
5. Alam S, Patel J. Peer review: tips from field experts for junior reviewers. BMC Med. 2015;13:269.
6. Jericho BG, Simpson D, Sullivan GM. Developing your expertise as a peer reviewer. J Grad Med Educ. 2017;9:251–2.
7. Brown LM, David EA, Karamlou T, Nason KS. Reviewing scientific manuscripts: a comprehensive guide for peer reviewers. J Thorac Cardiovasc Surg. 2017;153:1609–14.
8. Tomkins A, Zhang M, Heavlin WD. Reviewer bias in single-versus double-blind peer review. Proc Natl Acad Sci U S A. 2017;114 https://doi.org/10.1073/pnas.1707323114.
9. Knobloch-Westerwick S, Glynn CJ, Huge M. The Matilda effect in science communication. Sci Commun. 2013;35:603–25.
10. Merton RK. The Matthew effect in science. Science (80-). 1968;159:56–62.
11. Blank RM. The effects of double-blind versus single-blind reviewing: experimental evidence from the American Economic Review. Am Econ Rev. 1991;81:1041–67.
12. The EQUATOR Network. Enhancing the QUAlity and Transparency Of Health Research. Available at https://www.equator-network.org/.
13. ICMJE. Recommendations. About the recommendations. Available at http://www.icmje.org/recommendations/browse/about-the-recommendations/.
14. WHO. WHO data set. WHO 2020. Available at http://www.who.int/ictrp/network/trds/en/.
15. Bishop D. Rein in the four horsemen of irreproducibility. Nature. 2019;568:435.
16. Makin TR, De Xivry JJO. Ten common statistical mistakes to watch out for when writing or reviewing a manuscript. Elife. 2019;8 https://doi.org/10.7554/eLife.48175.
17. Nieuwenhuis S, Forstmann BU, Wagenmakers EJ. Erroneous analyses of interactions in neuroscience: a problem of significance. Nat Neurosci. 2011;14:1105–7.
18. Cramer AOJ, van Ravenzwaaij D, Matzke D, Steingroever H, Wetzels R, Grasman RPPP, Waldorp LJ, Wagenmakers EJ. Hidden multiplicity in exploratory multiway ANOVA: prevalence and remedies. Psychon Bull Rev. 2016;23:640–7.
19. Stigler SM. Correlation and causation: a comment. Perspect Biol Med. 2005;48:88–S94.
20. Cartwright N. Are RCTs the gold standard? BioSocieties. 2007;2:11–20.
21. Listl S, Jürges H, Watt RG. Causal inference from observational data. Community Dent Oral Epidemiol. 2016;44:409–15.
22. Wicherts JM, Veldkamp CLS, Augusteijn HEM, Bakker M, van Aert RCM, van Assen MALM. Degrees of freedom in planning, running, analyzing, and reporting psychological studies: A checklist to avoid P-hacking. Front Psychol. 2016;7 https://doi.org/10.3389/fpsyg.2016.01832.

23. Forstmeier W, Wagenmakers EJ, Parker TH. Detecting and avoiding likely false-positive findings – a practical guide. Biol Rev. 2017;92:1941–68.
24. Dienes Z. Using Bayes to get the most out of non-significant results. Front Psychol. 2014;5:781.
25. Lakens D. Equivalence tests: a practical primer for t tests, correlations, and meta-analyses. Soc Psychol Personal Sci. 2017;8:355–62.
26. Greenwood DC, Freeman JV. How to spot a statistical problem: advice for a non-statistical reviewer. BMC Med. 2015;13:270.
27. Kahn CE. Be an all-star manuscript reviewer! Radiol Artif Intell. 2020:1–49.
28. Stiller-Reeve M. How to write a thorough peer review. Nature. 2018; https://doi.org/10.1038/d41586-018-06991-0.
29. Gopen GD, Swan JA. The science of scientific writing. Am Sci. 1990;78:550–8.
30. Freeling B, Doubleday ZA, Connell SD. How can we boost the impact of publications? Try better writing. Proc Natl Acad Sci U S A. 2019;116:341–3.
31. Plaxco KW. The art of writing science. Protein Sci. 2010;19:2261–6.
32. Lilleyman JS. How to write a scientific paper - a rough guide to getting published. Arch Dis Child. 1995;72:268–70.
33. Van Way CW. Writing a scientific paper. Nutr Clin Pract. 2007;22:636–40.
34. Alexandrov AV. How to write a research paper. Cerebrovasc Dis. 2004;18:135–8.
35. Weinberger CJ, Evans JA, Allesina S. Ten simple (empirical) rules for writing science. PLoS Comput Biol. 2015;11:1004205.
36. Haibe-Kains B, Adam GA, Hosny A, Khodakarami F, Shraddha T, Kusko R, Sansone SA, Tong W, Wolfinger RD, Mason CE, Jones W, Dopazo J, Furlanello C, Waldron L, Wang B, McIntosh C, Goldenberg A, Kundaje A, Greene CS, Broderick T, Hoffman MM, Leek JT, Korthauer K, Huber W, Brazma A, Pineau J, Tibshirani R, Hastie T, Ioannidis JPA, Quackenbush J, Aerts HJWL. Transparency and reproducibility in artificial intelligence. Nature. 2020;586:E14–6.
37. Michener WK. Ten simple rules for creating a good data management plan. PLoS Comput Biol. 2015;11 https://doi.org/10.1371/journal.pcbi.1004525.
38. Frassl MA, Hamilton DP, Denfeld BA, de Eyto E, Hampton SE, Keller PS, Sharma S, Lewis ASL, Weyhenmeyer GA, O'Reilly CM, Lofton ME, Catalán N. Ten simple rules for collaboratively writing a multi-authored paper. PLoS Comput Biol. 2018;14 https://doi.org/10.1371/journal.pcbi.1006508.
39. Bourne PE, Polka JK, Vale RD, Kiley R. Ten simple rules to consider regarding preprint submission. PLoS Comput Biol. 2017;13:–e1005473.
40. Noble WS. Ten simple rules for writing a response to reviewers. PLoS Comput Biol. 2017;13:–e1005730.
41. Edelstein L. The Hippocratic oath, text, translation and interpretation. Baltimore: Johns Hopkins Press; 1943.
42. Bacon F. Novum Organum. London: William Pickering; 1620.
43. Trials of war criminal before the Nuremberg military tribunals under control council law 10 (Superintendent of Documents, US Government Printing Office, Washington, 1950).
44. Annas G. The Nazi Doctors and the Nuremberg Code: human rights in human experimentation: Annas, George J., Grodin, Michael A.: 9780195101065: History: Amazon Canada. New York: Oxford University Press; 1995.
45. World Medical Association declaration of Helsinki: ethical principles for medical research involving human subjects. JAMA J Am Med Assoc. 2013;310:2191–4.
46. U. States National Commission for the Protection of Human Subjects of Biomedical, B. Research, The Belmont Report Ethical Principles and Guidelines for the Protection of Human Subjects of Research The National Commission for the Protection of Human Subjects of Biomedical and Behavioral Research. 1978.
47. Hornblum A, Newman J, Dober G. Against their will: the secret history of medical experimentation on children in cold war America: St Martin's Press; 2013.
48. Kaufman SR. The world war II plutonium experiments: contested stories and their lessons for medical research and informed consent. Cult Med Psychiatry. 1997;21:161–97.

49. Mccally M, Cassel C, Kimball D. Government-sponsored radiation research. Med Glob Surviv. 1994;1
50. Szetela C. Toward increased public representation on bioethics committees: lessons from judging the cold war human radiation experiments. Account Res. 1999;6:183–203.
51. C. I. of H. R. N. S. and E. R. C. of C. and S. S. and H. R. C. of Canada, Tri-Council Policy Statement: Ethical Conduct for Research Involving Humans. Government of Canada, Ottawa, 2018. www.nserc-crsng.gc.ca.
52. Holm S. In: Beauchamp TL, Childress JF, editors. Principles of biomedical ethics. 5th ed: Oxford University Press; 2001, pound19.95, pp 454. ISBN 0-19-514332-9. J Med Ethics. 2002;28:332-a-332.
53. Iltis A. Lay concepts in informed consent to biomedical research: the capacity to understand and appreciate risk. Bioethics. 2006;20:180–90.
54. Lloyd A. Informed consent: what did the doctor say? Lancet. 1999;353:1713.
55. Wertheimer A. *Coercion*: Princeton University Press; 1988. https://press.princeton.edu/books/hardcover/9780691637143/coercion.
56. Faden R, Beauchamp T. A history and theory of informed consent. New York: Oxford University Press; 1986.
57. WHO, WHO. Templates for informed consent forms. 2015. Available at: https://www.who.int/ethics/review-committee/informed_consent/en/.
58. Roberts LW. Reviews and overviews informed consent and the capacity for voluntarism. 2002.
59. Etchells E, Darzins P, Silberfeld M, Singer PA, McKenny J, Naglie G, Katz M, Gordon G, Molloy HDW, Strang D. Assessment of patient capacity to consent to treatment. J Gen Intern Med. 1999;14:27–34.
60. Bravo G, Gagnon M, Wildeman S, Marshall DT, Pâquet M, Dubois M-F. Comparison of provincial and territorial legislation governing substitute consent for research. Can J Aging/La Rev Can du Vieil. 2005;24:237–49.
61. ICH harmonised tripartite guideline: Guideline for good clinical practice. J Postgrad Med. 2001;47:264–267.
62. International compilation of human research standards 2020 edition. Office for Human Research Protections U.S. Department of Health and Human Services, 2020.
63. Miller FG, Brody H. Clinical equipoise and the incoherence of research ethics. J Med Philos. 2007;32:151–65.
64. Tansey CM, Herridge MS, Heslegrave RJ, Lavery JV. A framework for research ethics review during public emergencies. CMAJ. 2010;182:1533–7.
65. Chaddah MR. The Ontario Cancer research ethics board: a central REB that works. Curr Oncol. 2008;15:49–52.
66. Institute of Medicine (US) roundtable on environmental, conflicts of interest, bias, and ethics. Natl Acad Sci. 2009. Available at: https://www.ncbi.nlm.nih.gov/books/NBK50715/.
67. Komesaroff PA, Kerridge I, Lipworth W. Conflicts of interest: new thinking, new processes. Intern Med J. 2019;49:574–7.
68. Cain DM, Detsky AS. Everyone's a little bit biased (even physicians). JAMA J Am Med Assoc. 2008;299:2893–5.
69. Koyfman SA, Yom SS. Clinical research ethics: considerations for the radiation oncologist. Int J Radiat Oncol Biol Phys. 2017;99:259–64.
70. McGarry RC, Papiez L, Williams M, Whitford T, Timmerman RD. Stereotactic body radiation therapy of early-stage non-small-cell lung carcinoma: phase I study. Int J Radiat Oncol Biol Phys. 2005;63:1010–5.
71. Timmerman R, Paulus R, Galvin J, Michalski J, Straube W, Bradley J, Fakiris A, Bezjak A, Videtic G, Johnstone D, Fowler J, Gore E, Choy H. Stereotactic body radiation therapy for inoperable early stage lung cancer. JAMA J Am Med Assoc. 2010;303:1070–6.

Radiation Oncology Career Development in an Academic Satellite Network

Stephen G. Chun, Valerie I. Reed, Charles R. Thomas Jr., and Timur Mitin

Background

In the United States, roughly half of all cancer patients are treated in the community setting. As academic radiation oncology programs look to grow programmatically, off-campus community satellite centers will play an increasing role in both the clinical and academic mission at cancer centers. Integrated academic radiation oncology satellite campuses have become commonplace at major cancer institutions such as Massachusetts General Hospital, M.D. Anderson, Memorial Sloan-Kettering, Johns Hopkins, the Mayo Clinic, Stanford University, Oregon Health & Sciences University, the University of Pennsylvania, and many others.

Recognizing that the academic mission and patient values go hand in hand is crucial to build a successful academic satellite career. The appropriate alignment of professional goals with clinical care in a satellite campus is fundamental to bring focus to what can be a diffuse array of opportunities. Satellite campuses bring patients value in terms of quality of care along with timely access and convenience at a most challenging time in their life. Particularly for fractionated radiation therapy, treatments near home enhance quality of life by easing the burden of commuting. Efforts to brand and clinical integrate satellite practices embody substantial career opportunities to protect patient safety and improve outcomes. With the rising

S. G. Chun (✉) · V. I. Reed
Division of Radiation Oncology, The University of Texas, M.D. Anderson Cancer Center, Houston, TX, USA
e-mail: sgchun@mdanderson.org

C. R. Thomas Jr. · T. Mitin
Department of Radiation Medicine, Knight Cancer Institute, Oregon Health & Science University, Portland, OR, USA

© Springer Nature Switzerland AG 2021
R. A. Chandra et al. (eds.), *Career Development in Academic Radiation Oncology*, https://doi.org/10.1007/978-3-030-71855-8_15

cost of healthcare, the lower cost structure of satellites also has potential to reduce the financial toxicity to patients. Moreover, with the COVID-19 pandemic, there has been renewed interest in care delivery through satellite campuses to limit spread of COVID-19 and facilitate social distancing in overcrowded central urban campuses [1].

As major cancer centers continue to expand their radiation oncology satellite networks, it is an opportune time for career development in this setting. As such, physicians primarily working in these settings be regarded on the same par as main campus faculty in the department. Furthermore, it is imperative that these physicians have opportunities for face time at the main campus aside from the annual holiday parties and/or the summer picnic. Improvements in information technology (IT) infrastructure have come a long way to facilitate inclusion of offsite physicians in main campus endeavors. While a traditional academic career may be more challenging in a satellite campus, there are many opportunities in the areas of quality assurance, clinical integration, and community research. With the rise of burgeoning academic radiation oncology satellite networks throughout the United States, it is conceivable that opportunities for leadership and professional development in satellite campuses could equal or surpass main campus sites in the future. This chapter will focus on career and leadership opportunities in an off-campus satellite setting for radiation oncologists in an academic network.

Career Opportunities in Quality Assurance and Safety

When implementing an off-campus satellite program, the highest institutional priority is to maintain quality assurance (QA) and mitigate risk by creating a high reliability center and establishing a culture of safety. In this process, a collaborative effort between off campus and main campus faculty is key to building a new practice while maintaining quality control. Radiation oncologists with interest and expertise in quality and safety provide enormous value as there are unique challenges in establishing an offsite radiation oncology practice. This section will highlight the unique professional advancement and leadership opportunities in satellite campuses in the area of quality and safety.

Although the overarching principles of quality and safety are similar between main and satellite centers, there are unique challenges in satellite campuses. Identifying means to integrate human resources requires leadership, particularly when satellite personnel such as radiation therapists, physicists, nursing, and referring physicians have a different reporting structure (or even different employer). Depending on setup and resources, the electronic medical records (EMRs) may differ from the main hospital resulting in significant information technology (IT) challenges. Furthermore, community radiation oncology centers often lack emergency rooms or inpatient services requiring integration with other hospital networks for urgent and inpatient care. Potential avenues to address these issues of safety and integration include participation in institutional quality and safety committee or the quality and safety committee at referring community hospitals. Physicians can also show leadership by modifying safety policies specific for the community radiation oncology clinic. IT issues can be a formidable problem particularly if different EMRs are in use, but this also results in significant opportunities for the physician to become involved in the clinical informatics field as discussed later in this chapter.

To maintain quality of care and branding of a satellite radiation oncology service line, there are multiple QA processes that require leadership to create a robust peer review process. Peer review can be conducted in person on-site and/or remotely. IT investments in remote-conferencing capabilities are ever the more important to promote social distancing with COVID-19 [2]. Another opportunity is in the development of clinical guidelines/procedures regarding peer review process. The process of formalizing the peer review process and monitoring the outcomes is an area of increasing interest in the medical literature with opportunities for peer-reviewed publications on the subject for satellite physicians [3].

Establishing a culture of safety is requisite for a high reliability organization and requires implementation of a transparent safety incident review process with root cause analysis with the goal of having continuous improvement. A safety incident management system plays a key role in monitoring near misses as well as actual safety events. Both radiation-specific safety incidents as well as general clinic incidents should be formally reported and reviewed on a regular basis. Some hospitals may report both general clinic and radiation-specific incidents into one institutional safety reporting system while others may use a different safety reporting system for radiation-specific incidents. The Radiation Oncology Incident Learning System (RO-ILS) initiated by the American Society of Radiation Oncology (ASTRO) is a radiation-specific safety incident reporting system available free of charge to radiation oncology practices in the United States (https://www.astro.org/Patient-Care-and-Research/Patient-Safety/RO-ILS). A satellite radiation oncologist can take the lead in reviewing safety events at their clinic and developing programs, providing opportunities to interface with institutional leaders of risk management, clinical operations, and quality control.

With the increasing regulatory burden placed on healthcare institutions, knowledge of local and national quality metrics are particularly valuable to a radiation oncology satellite. Opportunities for formal certifications in this area are also available from organizations such as the American Board of Medical Quality (ABMQ). As radiation oncology involves the interconnection of complex multidisciplinary oncologic care with advanced radiation technology, radiation oncology practices are subject to audit by multiple agencies such as the Joint Commission (JC), the Centers for Medicare and Medicaid Services (CMS), and the Nuclear Regulatory Commission (NRC). The JC and CMS are charged with determining minimum standards deemed status for Medicare and Medicaid reimbursement. Deemed status from the JC is based upon rigorous record review and an on-site survey showing substantial evidence of compliance standards. CMS has also developed minimum standards known as the conditions of participation and CMS contracts with state agencies to inspect facilities to ensure they meet these standards. The United States Nuclear Regulatory Commission (NRC) is responsible for formulating policies governing nuclear reactors and radioactive materials, including materials used in the diagnosis and treatment of disease. Depending on state-specific laws, certain safety incidents may need to be reported to the state health department and the radiation oncologist managing quality and safety should be acquainted with this requirement. There are also radiation oncology-specific accreditations including Accreditation Program for Excellent (APEx) offered through ASTRO and Radiation Oncology Practice Accreditation (ROPA) through the American College of Radiology (ACR) (https://www.acraccreditation.org/modalities/radiation-oncology-practice). Due to the increasing regulatory complexities inherent to the delivery of modern radiation therapy, familiarity with regulatory requirements provides great value to radiation oncology departments. A summary of resources to better understand the field of medical quality are provided in Table 1.

IT plays a fundamental role in quality and safety, providing opportunities in clinical informatics. The emerging field of clinical informatics evaluates the way IT can be applied to improving efficiency and outcomes by structuring data to create an "information-based" approach to healthcare that is similar in conception to the principles of "evidence-based" medicine. In radiation oncology where multiple planning systems and EMRs often exist and the need to develop software intermediaries that integrate multiple software applications known as application program interfaces (API) has been increasingly recognized. APIs decrease the need for multiple manual inputs of the same information into different computer systems, thereby decreasing risk of error as well as clinician burnout due to less repetitive manual entry. Radiation oncologists with basic informatics knowledge can give valuable clinical input to the IT team on development of such programs. Additionally, radiation oncologists that participate in institutional informatics committees will be able to provide guidance on which IT issues should be given priority for implementation. Multiple clinical informatics resources are listed at the end of this chapter. For those who want to learn principles of database science and/or computer programming, multiple free online courses (MOOCs) courses are available through multiple platforms as described in the resources section.

In summary, there are numerous career and professionalism opportunities in quality and safety for radiation oncologists in a satellite campus. These opportunities exist both at the institutional and national levels. Additionally, it may also be possible for radiation oncologists to have major roles in institutional collaborations with outside vendors such as health information technology companies or radiation oncology vendors. Educational courses and certifications and even graduate degrees are increasingly available to facilitate a career in quality and safety.

Table 1 Resources in medical quality and safety and clinical informatics

Textbooks	Quality and safety websites	Clinical informatics websites	Multiple massive free online courses
American College of Medical Quality. *Medical Quality Management: Theory and Practice*. Jones & Bartlett Publishers; 2010.	American Board of Medical Quality. http://www.abmq.org	American Medical Informatics Association. https://www.amia.org	Coursera. https://www.coursera.org
Dlugacz YD. *Introduction to Health Care Quality: Theory, Methods, and Tools*. Jossey-Bass; 2019.	Institute for Healthcare Improvement. http://www.ihi.org	Healthcare Information and Management Systems Society. https://www.himss.org/	edX. https://www.edx.org
Nash DB, Joshi MS, Ransom ER, Ransom SB. *The Healthcare Quality Book: Vision, Strategy, and Tools, Fourth Edition*. Health Administration Press; 2019.	American Society for Healthcare Risk Management. https://www.ashrm.org	Department of Medical Informatics and Clinical Epidemiology, Oregon Health and Sciences University. https://www.ohsu.edu/school-of-medicine/medical-informatics-and-clinical-epidemiology	Udacity. https://www.udacity.com
Wager KA, Lee FW, Glaser JP. *Health Care Information Systems: A Practical Approach for Health Care Management 4th Edition*. Jossey-Bass; 2017.	Agency for Healthcare Research and Quality. https://www.ahrq.gov	The University of Texas Health Science Center at Houston School of Biomedical Informatics. https://sbmi.uth.edu	
Hoyt R, Muenchen R. *Introduction to Biomedical Data Science*. Lulu.com; 2019	National Quality Forum. http://www.qualityforum.org/Home.aspx	American Board of Preventive Medicine, Clinical Informatics Board Certification. https://www.theabpm.org/become-certified/subspecialties/clinical-informatics	

Clinical Research at a Satellite Campus

Clinical trial enrollment remains a major challenge throughout the United States despite evidence that majority of cancer patients are interested in clinical trial participation [4]. Currently, it is estimated that less than 5% of adult cancer patients are enrolled on therapeutic clinical trials [5]. The potential to improve adult cancer clinical trial participation is suggested by the pediatric cancer trial participation rate of 50% [6]. Not only are clinical trials a vital tool to advance cancer care, but better survival rates in clinical trial participants suggest that trials improve quality of care [7]. It is estimated that it takes an average of 17 years to translate a clinical finding into clinical practice [8], and trials provide a means to efficiently advance clinical care in a radiation oncology practice.

There are a number of logistical advantages provided by radiation oncology satellite campuses that directly facilitate trial participation. While availability of a clinical trial for a disease site is the most commonly cited reason for nonparticipation, transportation cost, and availability of childcare are also major factors that can impede trial participation [9]. For elderly and low-income patients, lack of transportation not only obstructs clinical research participation, but to oncologic care in general. Satellite campuses have a major logistical advantage in this regard, allowing trial participation closer to place of residence or work. Additionally, patients living near a satellite may be more willing to do the long-term follow-up required on many trials than international or out of town patients seen at main campus centers.

In terms of practice development, clinical trials provide a means of differentiating an academic satellite practice from other competing centers. As over 70% of cancer patients are interested in clinical trial participation, trials provide a potential competitive advantage in the healthcare marketplace. While advanced LINAC technology has become widely available in both academic and community practices, clinical trials mostly remain unique to the academic setting. At the M.D. Anderson Cancer Center, there has been success in implementing clinical trials in Houston Area Location (HAL) satellites. The earliest success of a radiation oncology clinical trial at M.D. Anderson was a randomized trial of standard versus hypofractionated radiation for early-stage breast cancer [10], where roughly half of patients were enrolled from satellite locations. M.D. Anderson has since published a successful strategy used to enhance trial enrollment in satellite campuses [11]. To date at M.D. Anderson, there has been a track record of robust HAL satellite participation in trials for disease sites including breast cancer [12], bone metastases [13], lung cancer [14], head and neck cancer, and prostate cancer.

Clinical trial participation also opens doors to opportunities at the national level. The NRG Oncology group, for example, is specifically interested in building community participation through a Community Oncology Research Program (NCORP) from the National Cancer Institute (NCI). Several career development opportunities through NCORP are listed on the NRG Oncology website (https://www.nrgoncology.org/Scientific-Program/NRG-NCORP-Research-Base/NCORP-Resources).

High-accruing physicians on cooperative group trials will naturally have opportunities to be coinvestigators on developing cooperative group concepts and conduct secondary analyses of prospective trials [15].

In addition to clinical trial participation, it is not impossible for satellite-based faculty to engage in collaborative clinical research by taking advantage of interactive video technology and video conferencing. With COVID-19, IT infrastructure investments can no longer be just an optional part of a radiation oncology strategic plan, but are now of vital public health interest for social distancing and curbing the pandemic. The sudden interest in remote IT solutions provides great opportunity to democratize and level the playing field for satellite faculty in terms of inclusion and research. Any physician regardless of location can conduct analyses, serve as a principal investigator of a trial, or mentor trainees with fairly small investments in interactive video technology.

National and Institutional Service

Faculty at satellite campuses frequently have broad practical knowledge of multiple disease sites, providing unique insights to the institution compared to main campus physicians who might focus on one or two disease sites. Establishing a presence in institutional and national leadership is a long-term task will require considerable patience and perseverance by satellite faculty over a career. Advocacy from departmental and institutional leaders is crucial to overcoming the entry barriers for national and institutional leadership.

Early career radiation oncologists may have vast opportunities to serve on various institutional committees. For junior faculty, institutional committee involvement provides vast opportunities to create personal and professional connections with local providers and to advance the department's footprint in the hospital. Serving on local Institutional Review Boards can be particularly useful to junior faculty to better understand the clinical research infrastructure of the institution, advocate for incorporation of radiation into clinical trials, and to observe the art of clinical trial development. Another area where satellite radiation oncology faculty can be particularly useful to institutions is in the growth of global outreach programs. Due to the broad experience in satellite campuses that requires pragmatism and understanding of practice building, satellite faculty can provide unique insight for large institutions looking to further build their oncology network internationally.

Service on national committees can be a rewarding and fruitful experience, but there can be substantial entry barriers to involvement. Without mentorship, this initial phase of career development can be challenging, especially for community-based radiation oncologists without disease site specialization. It is vital to seek the mentorship of department leaders to overcome barriers to involvement in national committee assignments. Additionally, clinicians can also seek these independently volunteer to participate in committees of the American Society of Radiation

Oncology (ASTRO), American College of Radiation Oncology (ACRO), and the American Radium Society (ARS). While there has been diminishing presence of radiation oncology with the Radiologic Society of North America (RSNA) there remain educational lecture and committee opportunities for radiation oncologists. Radiation oncology journals also represent opportunities to provide service as a reviewer with some providing recognition for service. For example, the Editorial Board of the *International Journal of Radiation Oncology, Biology and Physics* provides awards for excellence in reviewing annually.

Educational Service

The paucity of radiation oncology trainees rotating through satellite campuses can pose a challenge to a career in educational leadership, but there are other opportunities for career development in education. It should be emphasized to department leadership that most trainees will go on to practice in the community setting, underlying the educational value of rotating in satellites. Additionally, education goes two ways, with trainees bringing knowledge of main campus practices and paradigms that can indirectly facilitate clinical integration of a satellite practice.

Academic institutions often struggle with placement of student learners, such as medical school, nursing school students, and even college and high school students who are eager to participate in summer programs. Satellite clinics can add to the educational capacity for these student learners with fewer other competing learners compared to main campuses. Satellite campuses also allow a comprehensive exposure to disease sites in radiation oncology. Furthermore, close engagement with the multidisciplinary team can provide students a high-quality educational experience and comprehensive exposure to the multidisciplinary management of oncology patients.

In addition to opportunities with student learners and residency training programs, satellite faculty can also take the lead in developing a continuing medical education (CME) program in the satellites. With limited ability to attend main center conferences, satellite physicians have unique challenges to obtain CME credit requisite for American Board of Radiology (ABR) maintenance of certification (MOC). Particularly with COVID-19, the creation of virtual CME-self assessment module (SAM) sessions can bring tremendous value to all physicians in the department for MOC. CME programs need not be focused on radiation oncology and can also be used as a means to network with referring physicians. Multidisciplinary CME programs provide value in terms of networking, education, and clinical integration with best evidence-based practice.

At the national level, there are a number of educational service activities well suited to radiation oncologist at satellite campuses. Organizations such as ASTRO, ACRO, ARS, and the American Society of Clinical Oncology (ASCO) specifically aim to include community-based physicians in the leadership of educational programs. Volunteering educational opportunities through these organizations allows practitioners to create professional and personal connections with national and international experts. Many organizations regularly solicit proposals for educational sessions for their annual meetings. Community-based radiation oncologists with generalist practice experience are poised to ask most practical and timely questions and put together educational sessions that are well received by selection committees and ultimately audiences.

A unique and highly rewarding opportunity is professional engagement at the international level. The field of radiation oncology is not uniformly developed across the world, and in many countries physicians lack formal didactic education and/or lengthy dedicated clinical training. For radiation oncologists who are fluent in foreign languages, there is an even greater opportunity and impetus to organize lectures, seminars, contouring, and planning workshops in foreign countries, eventually participate in formulation of clinical guidelines of these countries. Because of generalist background and experience, these educational opportunities do not end after few lectures on the same disease site topic, and allow for a longitudinal cooperation. Oregon Health and Science University has been involved in educational sessions organized by the Russian Society of Clinical Oncology (RUSSCO) for Russian oncologists since 2015. Over these years, majority of educational sessions were accompanied by audience surveys, which were analyzed and published and established a peer-reviewed track record of educational involvement combined with measurement of effectiveness [16–18]. Similarly, at MD Anderson faculty in the radiation oncology satellite campuses are routinely utilized for education at international sites and tasked with developing disease site guidelines for the international network.

Hurdles to Career Development Satellites

Historically, radiation oncology practices in satellite campuses have not been conducive to academic career development. Perhaps, the biggest historic hurdle to career development has been the view of satellites primarily in terms of clinical mission rather than as part of an integrated academic mission. Cultural challenges may exist in radiation oncology departments where satellite providers are not viewed inclusively. Differences in physician contracts and benchmarks can also create a disincentive for academic involvement in the satellites. Participation in education leadership can also be challenging if trainees do not rotate in the satellites. Many satellites lack the clinical resources and budget to implement clinical research. Some of these challenges can take years and require substantial perseverance to address, particularly with regards to culture.

It is critical that radiation academic satellite network: oncology department leadership set a tone of inclusivity and a shared vision with the satellites. A dedicated session that highlighted multiple successful dyads (satellite junior faculty along with main campus department chair) took place at the 2018 annual meeting of the Society of Chairs of Academic Radiation Oncology Programs (SCAROP). It is the duty of the chair to make it clear to all stakeholders that satellite-based investigators are not second-class citizens in the department. The tone is set not only by interpersonal interaction, but also by physician salary structure and evaluation criteria that allow satellite physicians to align with the academic mission. While satellite physicians have historically faced challenges in getting meaningful and regular face time at the main center, interactive video technology and teleconferencing can now be leveraged to maintain a "virtual" presence in main center conferences and academic satellite network: research meetings. In terms of trainee education, the importance of satellite exposure should be emphasized as most radiation oncology residents graduates go on to practice in the community setting. Although lobbying for clinical research resources is a formidable task, prospective clinical trial enrollments are a major component of Cancer Center Support Grants for which satellites can often contribute to at a lower cost structure than main campus counterparts.

Summary

We have provided an overview and framework for career development in an academic radiation oncology satellite setting. With complex regulatory standards that are constantly evolving, there are major opportunities for career advancement in radiation oncology medical quality. Satellites are also emerging as a setting for clinical research with a lower cost structure than the traditional centralized cancer center setting. In some cases, it is actually the satellite site that can become a major focus of excellence with respect to program development within the umbrella of the main campus program. With rapid expansion of telemedicine, the reach and scope of satellite campuses is expected to grow, making it an opportune time for career advancement in the satellite setting. While unforeseen, the push for IT solutions for remote working during COVID-19 may prove be a major unforeseen benefit to satellite radiation oncologists, helping to level the playing field for an academic radiation oncology career.

For Discussion with a Mentor or Colleague

- What are the expectations for quality assurance and how can a culture of safety be established off campus?
- How can IT resources be leveraged to maintain a presence in the department?
- How can career development in a satellite be focused without disease site specialization?
- What are effective strategies do manage cultural elitism from the main campus toward satellite practices?
- What is an appropriate balance of practice development and career advancement in a satellite campus that is in alignment with institutional vision?

- How can a shared vision for success be fostered between a satellite and main campus?
- What potential institutional and national leadership opportunities are well suited to radiation oncologists located off campus?
- How do you encourage staff engagement when implementing new programs?
- How can I stay connected to major decision makers that do not work at my locations?
- What strategies can be used to build a satellite clinical trial program that is in the shared interest of all stakeholders?
- How can a start-up package to support clinical research coordinator/biostatistics/research nurse be obtained at the institutional and national levels?

Acknowledgments We would like to acknowledge Mr. Tadd Pullin, Mr. Kyle Taylor, Ms. Audrey Trevino, Ms. Marcel Lake, and Ms. Juliana Purvis for their assistance in the development of this chapter.

Conflicts of Interest Dr. Chun is a consultant for AstraZeneca, P.L.C., and Norton Healthcare, Inc. Dr. Reed is a consultant for Varian Medical Systems, Inc. Dr. Mitin is a consultant for AstraZeneca, P.L.C., and Novocure, Inc.; receives clinical research funding from Novocure, Inc.; and receives royalties from UpToDate, Inc.

References

1. Noticewala SS, Koong AC, Bloom ES, et al. Radiation oncology strategies to flatten the curve during the coronavirus disease 2019 (COVID-19) pandemic: experience from a large tertiary cancer center. Adv Radiat Oncol. 2020;5(4):567–72.
2. Ning MS, McAleer MF, Jeter MD, et al. Mitigating the impact of COVID-19 on oncology: clinical and operational lessons from a prospective radiation oncology cohort tested for COVID-19. Radiother Oncol. 2020;148:252–7.
3. Ballo MT, Chronowski GM, Schlembach PJ, Bloom ES, Arzu IY, Kuban DA. Prospective peer review quality assurance for outpatient radiation therapy. Pract Radiat Oncol. 2014;4(5):279–84.
4. Comis RL, Miller JD, Aldige CR, Krebs L, Stoval E. Public attitudes toward participation in cancer clinical trials. J Clin Oncol. 2003;21(5):830–5.
5. Unger JM, Cook E, Tai E, Bleyer A. The role of clinical trial participation in cancer research: barriers, evidence, and strategies. Am Soc Clin Oncol Educ Book. 2016;35:185–98.
6. Bond MC, Pritchard S. Understanding clinical trials in childhood cancer. Paediatr Child Health. 2006;11(3):148–50.
7. Unger JM, LeBlanc M, Blanke CD. The effect of positive SWOG treatment trials on survival of patients with cancer in the US population. JAMA Oncol. 2017;3(10):1345–51.
8. Morris ZS, Wooding S, Grant J. The answer is 17 years, what is the question: understanding time lags in translational research. J R Soc Med. 2011;104(12):510–20.
9. Rivers D, August EM, Sehovic I, Lee Green B, Quinn GP. A systematic review of the factors influencing African Americans' participation in cancer clinical trials. Contemp Clin Trials. 2013;35(2):13–32.
10. Shaitelman SF, Schlembach PJ, Arzu I, et al. Acute and short-term toxic effects of conventionally fractionated vs hypofractionated whole-breast irradiation: a randomized clinical trial. JAMA Oncol. 2015;1(7):931–41.

11. Ludmir EB, Adlakha EK, Chun SG, et al. Enhancing clinical trial enrollment at MD Anderson Cancer Center satellite community campuses. Acta Oncol. 2019;58(8):1135–7.

12. Shaitelman SF, Lei X, Thompson A, et al. Three-year outcomes with hypofractionated versus conventionally fractionated whole-breast irradiation: results of a randomized, noninferiority clinical trial. J Clin Oncol. 2018:JCO1800317.

13. Nguyen QN, Chun SG, Chow E, et al. Single-fraction stereotactic vs conventional multifraction radiotherapy for pain relief in patients with predominantly nonspine bone metastases: a randomized phase 2 trial. JAMA Oncol. 2019;5(6):872–8.

14. Chun SG, Liao Z, Jeter MD, et al. Metabolic responses to metformin in inoperable early-stage non-small cell lung cancer treated with stereotactic radiotherapy: results of a randomized phase II clinical trial. Am J Clin Oncol. 2020;43(4):231–5.

15. Chun SG, Hu C, Choy H, et al. Impact of intensity-modulated radiation therapy technique for locally advanced non-small-cell lung cancer: a secondary analysis of the NRG oncology RTOG 0617 randomized clinical trial. J Clin Oncol. 2017;35(1):56–62.

16. Mitin T, Degnin C, Chen Y, et al. Radiotherapy for hepatocellular carcinoma in Russia: a survey-based analysis of current practice and the impact of an educational workshop on clinical expertise. J Cancer Educ. 2020;35(1):105–11.

17. McClelland S 3rd, Chernykh M, Dengina N, et al. Bridging the gap in global advanced radiation oncology training: impact of a web-based open-access interactive three-dimensional contouring atlas on radiation oncologist practice in Russia. J Cancer Educ. 2019;34(5):871–3.

18. Mitin T, Dengina N, Chernykh M, et al. Management of muscle invasive bladder cancer with bladder preservation in Russia: a survey-based analysis of current practice and the impact of an educational workshop on clinical expertise. J Cancer Educ. 2020.

When Life Happens: Parental Leave, Part-Time Schedules, and Flexible Workplace Strategies

Emma B. Holliday

Introduction

Over the past 50 years, the United States (US) workforce has undergone some progress with regard to gender parity. According to the US Census Bureau, women made up 38% of the workforce in 1970 and 47% of the workforce in 2010 [1]. The physician workforce has seen more striking trends. In 1970, women made up only 11% of medical students, while in 2017, the number of women entering medical school exceeded that of men for the first time [2]. The influx of women into the field of medicine has been unequally distributed among specialties. Radiation oncology has been traditionally male dominated, but representation of women among full-time academic radiation oncology faculty has been increasing slowly. In 1985, approximately 16% of faculty were women compared with 28% in 2015. The representation of women among radiation oncology resident physicians is also increasing; approximately 25% of radiation oncology residents in 1985 were women compared with 35% in 2007 [3].

As trends from Northern European countries have shown, increasing numbers of women into a field can bring increased discussion of issues and challenges related to balancing responsibilities at work and at home. Historically, a successful career in academic radiation oncology as well as academic medicine more broadly required dedication to clinical duties during business hours as well as countless hours spent during nights and weekends pursuing grants, manuscripts, and collaborative networking activities. In the mid- to late-twentieth century, work–life balance was achieved within families by division of labor into two categories: inside the home and outside the home. However, the rise of the dual-career family necessitated

E. B. Holliday (✉)
Radiation Oncology, The University of Texas MD Anderson Cancer Center,
Houston, TX, USA
e-mail: ebholliday@mdanderson.org

© Springer Nature Switzerland AG 2021   201
R. A. Chandra et al. (eds.), *Career Development in Academic Radiation Oncology*, https://doi.org/10.1007/978-3-030-71855-8_16

reevaluation of this system, which typically put working women at a disadvantage. While only about 50% of male faculty in STEM fields have spouses who work full time, 90% of female faculty do [5]. Furthermore, studies of successful physician scientists and academicians show that women take on a disproportionate amount of domestic labor and caregiving responsibilities even when both partners work outside the home [4].

Although the issues of "work–life balance" had been relegated to the realm of women's issues, men are increasingly participating more actively in parenting, caregiving, and other responsibilities outside the workplace. Therefore, discussion of issues and policies related to the more successful balance of work and nonwork priorities is pertinent to both men and women and may also have the desired downstream effect of improving workforce diversity. This chapter will seek to explore variations in current parental leave policies within and outside of the US and discuss strategies of how best to discuss this sensitive topic with current and/or potential employers. Next, we will outline and discuss ways individuals and institutions can best balance responsibilities at work and home while maintaining desired forward academic progress.

Parental Leave

In a Pew Research poll, the US ranks last out of 41 countries when it comes to paid parental leave [6]. Data from the Organization for Economic Cooperation and Development (OECD) list several European countries that mandate a year or more of parental leave at the federal level. Japan has a similarly generous policy. In 34 of 41 countries listed, paid leave is allocated for mothers and fathers, though in most cases mothers receive the majority [6]. The health benefits of paid maternity leave for both mothers and infants have been well documented and include decreased rehospitalization rates for mothers and infants [7], decreased rates of postpartum depression [8], improved duration of breastfeeding [9, 10], and overall maternal health [11]. There are economic benefits to offering paid parental leave as well including enabling women to stay in their jobs and reducing employee turnover [12].

Five US states (California, New Jersey, New York, Rhode Island, and Washington state) and the District of Columbia have state-mandated paid leave policies in place, but the only national standard is the Family and Medical Leave Act (FMLA) which allows eligible employees to 12 weeks of leave in a 12-month pay period to either take care of a child (within 1 year of birth, adoption or foster placement), take care of a spouse, child, or parent with serious health conditions or for a serious health condition which makes the employee unable to perform essential functions of their job [13]. Important limitations of FMLA are that employees must have worked 12 months for their employer to be eligible. Additionally, FMLA only mandates that an eligible employee's job be protected while they are out on *unpaid* leave. Therefore, newly hired faculty or trainees may not be able to access FMLA. Additionally, trainees or young faculty with student loan debt, bills, and other financial obligations may not have the luxury of taking 3 months without pay. Trainees may face delayed graduation from residency or fellowship if they take the 12 weeks allowed under FMLA, and young faculty may fear retribution, implicit or explicit bias from leadership or peers.

For trainees, there is no standard policy per the Accreditation Council for Graduate Medical Education (ACGME) [14]. Policies vary widely with eight of the top 50 medical schools with graduate medical education programs offer an average of 6.6 weeks paid parental leave for residents and 25 programs offer none at all [15]. Some programs offer flexibility such as reordering or combining research blocks or other rotations that do not require a new parent's physical presence. Others offer nothing other than 2–4 weeks of combined sick and vacation time and require new parents to return to work 2 weeks after birth [16]. Some also require "payback" for call and other duties missed during postpartum recovery which simply shift increased stress later during the child's first few months of life [17].

Radiation oncology, specifically, has developed a reputation for being one of the more family-friendly specialties both during training and beyond. The American Board of Radiology requires 36 months of clinical radiation oncology experience over the usual 4-year residency period [18]. This allows for more flexibility than specialties such as internal medicine, which only allows 4 weeks leave per year without having to repeat that year of training [19]. However, recent job market stressors has placed additional emphasis on research, networking and studying for multiple board exams which can require significant extracurricular time commitment [20]. A 2014 study of radiation oncology residents showed 52% of respondents were parents and 44% had a child during residency. Men were more likely to have children than women (65% vs 47%), and were much more likely to have a partner who did not work (25% vs 2%). Of female trainees who were pregnant during training, one-third reported feeling their pregnancy resulted in increased workload for their coresidents, one-quarter reported feeling they received less clinical experience, and nearly half reported feeling they obtained less research experience compared to their colleagues without children. Fewer than half of all respondents reported that they were aware of the parental leave policy at their institution. None of the male parents took more than 1 month of leave, but nearly one-quarter of female parents took between 2 and 6 months of leave [21]. Figure 1 provides a snapshot of the experiences of radiation oncology residents with pregnancy and parenthood during training.

For academic faculty, a 2018 study outlined policies for US medical schools listed on top-10 lists for both National Institutes of Health (NIH) funding as well as the US News and World Report academic ranking. For these institutions, the mean length of full salary support for faculty was 8.6 weeks, but most formal policies had stipulations that allowed for discretion on the part of individual departmental leadership. Additionally, many also included constraints that parental leave could only be taken by the primary caregiver providing >50% care to the child, which prevents mothers and fathers from both taking this benefit [22]. Since, for many families, the logistics of postpartum recovery and breastfeeding cause >50% of newborn care to be performed by the mother, policies such as these may lead to continued

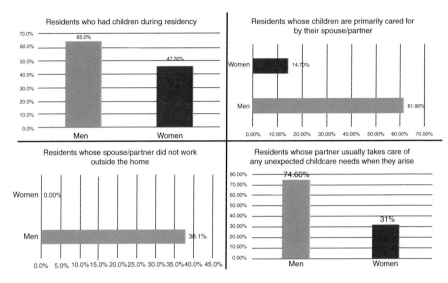

Fig. 1 Experiences of radiation oncology residents who had children during residency by gender. Holliday et al. [21]

disproportionate use of parental leave by women and propagation of parental leave and family-friendly policies as a "woman's issue."

Best practices may vary by situation and individual comfort level, but prospective faculty and trainee candidates should be encouraged to ask directly about the parental leave policies during the recruitment/interview process [23]. It is important to know not only what the official policy is regarding how much leave is available and with what pay, but also to know how commonly this policy has been utilized in the recent past. If 12 weeks of leave are available at the institution but if 8 of 10 recent new parents returned to work after 1 month, that may provide valuable insight into the culture of the institution and/or department (Table 1).

Part-Time Careers

In 1993, only 13% of clinical faculty and 6% of basic science faculty at US medical schools worked part time [24]. In contrast, in 1995, 29% of the Dutch physician workforce worked part-time (12% of male physicians and 63% of female physicians) [25]. In Germany, it is common for a residency position or a faculty position to be "shared" by two physicians wishing to work part-time. It is considered a common and desirable way to achieve work–life balance during childrearing years. In fact, the demand for part-time contracts is outpacing the number of available positions for male and female physicians [26].

In the US, interest in part-time clinical work has increased dramatically [27] and has been touted as an option to promote work–life balance and reduce burnout [28].

Table 1 Questions to ask when evaluating parental/familial leave policies

Issue	Specific questions to ask
Time and pay	1. What is the maximum amount of leave available for my specific situation (birth-giving parent, non-birth-giving parent, adoptive/foster parent, family member who requires temporary full or part-time care for illness or injury, etc.)? 2. Is leave paid? If so, must sick and vacation time be exhausted before dedicated parental leave monies can be utilized? 3. What portions of my salary will I receive on leave? Base (or a percentage of base), incentive, bonus, etc.? 4. Will I retain my full benefits while out of leave including any retirement matching or other programs?
Productivity and academic advancement	5. Will my clinical productivity benchmarks be prorated for the time I am out? 6. How will my weekend/overnight/call responsibilities be effected for the year? 7. If applicable, are there resources or programs available to support my lab or other clinical research activities while I am out on leave?
Return to work	8. If applicable, what accommodations are available for breastfeeding/pumping mothers? Is there dedicated space convenient to clinical and administrative areas? Can clinic templates be adjusted to allow for adequate breaks for pumping? 9. Are there flexible workplace policies that will allow me to attend necessary doctor's appointments or other responsibilities after returning to work? 10. Is onsite childcare available? What do other young parents in the institution/department use for childcare?
Workplace culture	11. How does the institution/department support faculty to take parental/familial leave? 12. How many faculty utilized parental/familial leave in the last 5 years? How many were women versus men? 13. How much leave did they take? 14. How was clinical and administrative coverage arranged for the faculty who were on leave? 15. Has the academic/professional trajectory of faculty who have taken leave been effected negatively?

Certain shift-work specialties such as emergency medicine and hospitalist medicine are considered more "family-friendly" and amenable to part-time work. Radiology, pathology, and other specialties without direct patient care responsibilities also lend itself well to a part-time model [29]. There is some debate whether or not a part-time model works well for specialties requiring longitudinal patient care. Perceived negatives toward part-time oncology in the US include worse communication and contact with colleagues and threatened continuity of care and compromised patient–doctor relationship. For hospital- or private practice–employed physicians, there is a concern about the ability of part-time oncologists to effectively build a network of referring physicians. For academic institutions, there is concern of creating "second-class citizens" with respect to career trajectory, promotional clocks, and research opportunities. All institutions that employ physicians worry about the increased costs associated with a larger workforce and what to do about the costs of benefits [28].

There are few published data on the number or percentage of radiation oncologists working part-time in the US. However, a survey study in Australia and New Zealand published in 2002 reported 5.3% of all radiation oncology physicians worked less than 0.5 FTE; 14.6% of women and 2.3% of men. Overall, 61% of women and 11% of men in training in Australia and New Zealand stated that they desired part-time work in a parallel survey [30]. For part-time work in radiation oncology to work effectively, the authors of this study made several specific recommendations. First, job descriptions should be explicit with regard to what an equitable pro-rated distribution of clinical and nonclinical responsibilities between full- and part-time radiation oncologists. Second, clear job expectations and timetables should be set so part-time radiation oncologists complete all time-sensitive work prior to "off days." Third, a clear mechanism needs to be in place for patient and other queries to be addressed when a part-time radiation oncologist is off. Next, part-time radiation oncologists should be reachable to urgent queries even when they are off. Finally, the group emphasized that good communication between the part-time radiation oncologist, clinic staff, and patients is critical to making this model work [30].

Flexible Workplace Policies

In addition to part-time employment models, there have been other flexible work hour policies evaluated to help physicians more effectively balance demands of work and home. According to a 2018 survey by the *Harvard Business Review*, 96% of white-collar workers in the US need flexibility in the workplace, but only 47% have it. The flexible work policies described in this study included not only part-time schedules, but also flexible working hours, the ability to step away from work for unexpected events or needs and make up the time/work later, the ability to work remotely for all or part of their workweek, and the opportunity to travel minimally for work [31]. Flexible workplace policies have commonly been referred to as "family-friendly" policies, although increasingly flexibility is being prized even by those without children or familial responsibilities.

On average, the majority of childcare, eldercare, and other domestic responsibilities has fallen disproportionately on the shoulders of women. Therefore, most studies show women are more likely to seek out and utilize flexible workplace policies. While touted as a way to promote gender diversity and support mothers in the workplace, flexible workplace policies can actually lead to increased stigma and decreased career advancement to women who seek to utilize them [32]. If utilization rates of such policies by men remain low, a "femininity stigma" is allowed to propagate for men who do request family leave or other flexible workplace accommodations [33, 34]. A workplace culture that rewards overtime, 24-hour availability, and "face time" at work will necessarily discourage utilization of flexible workplace policies.

Within academic medicine, utilization rates of flexible workplace policies have been low even when they exist on paper. The University of California Davis published their flexible work policies available to faculty of the School of Medicine in 2017. These included 12 weeks paid leave for childbearing; 12 weeks unpaid leave for FMLA; part-time appointment at the chair's discretion with retained benefits if ≥50% appointment, as well as tenure clock extension or deferral of advancement for those with 50%+ responsibility for a child under 5 years of age, on medical leave, or who have other significant reasons that impact productivity [35]. Shauman et al. surveyed medical school faculty at the University of California Davis and found that nearly 40% of 472 responding faculty reported considering utilizing flexible workplace policies. Reasons for not utilizing such policies included lack of information and awareness, unsupportive departmental culture and norms, interdependence of faculty within departments, and lack of supports from managers/chairs. Respondents described hostility or resentment on the part of those not using flexible workplace policies for having to "pick up the slack."

Within radiation oncology there is a worry that, in a field full of high-achievers and hard-workers, if you are not willing to stay late, come in early, be available and put work first, there will be a dozen others behind you who will be. The current employment climate for new graduates may intensify these fears. However, there are several potential opportunities to incorporate flexible working policies into a clinical radiation oncologist's workflow so that they benefit all faculty, not just mothers and fathers.

The COVID-19 outbreak in particular has accelerated the development and adoption of processes at many workplaces that may improve workplace flexibility in the years to come [36]. Radiation oncology departments are no exception. Steps taken to improve physical distancing within clinics during the pandemic may be continued to improve flexibility for physicians moving forward. Departments have learned that templates can be consolidated so that fewer physicians are in clinic at the same time. Telemedicine options for on-treatment visits or select follow-ups and consults can be performed from home with a reliable internet connection, secure virtual private network, and user-friendly platform [37]. Those same IT tools allow for notes, contours, and plan, evaluate, and care coordination for patients to be effectively conducted remotely. Online meeting platforms reduce the need for in-person meetings for operations, education, or tumor boards. "Doc of the day" systems allow for clinical cross-coverage of simulations, stereotactic radiation treatments, and walk-in visits, which enable physicians to work from home or protect time in a lab or other research setting. Physical-distancing aside, better separation of clinical and administrative or research duties have the potential enhance academic productivity.

While some worry that extensive cross-coverage may leave the door open for miscommunication, errors, or a disrupted doctor–patient relationship [38], effective communication and structured hand-off tools can help make such policies a success.

All things considered, allowing for a more predictable work week is desirable regardless of what one's nonclinical responsibilities include. More widespread adoption of flexible work policies at the department level may also reduce the stigma women or faculty with young families may feel when inquiring about or seeking to utilize such policies.

Additional Policies to Promote Academic Success for Caregivers

Multiple studies have shown a disproportionate number of women in the upper echelons of medical academia, suggesting that female faculty are not hitting promotion and tenure milestones at the same frequency or on the same timeline as their male counterparts [3, 39–44]. Although the myriad of potential contributing factors to gender disparities within academic radiation oncology are beyond the scope of this chapter, they have been discussed elsewhere [45]. As discussed in the sections above, caregiving responsibilities and other domestic labor still fall disproportionately on the shoulders of women for the majority of physician household [4]. The collision between biological and tenure clocks is unavoidable for many female faculty.

The early years of a successful academic physician's career are typically spent in the "building phase." They are building mentorship and collaborative networks; they are building their reputation and establishing themselves as experts in their field; they are building the foundation for their research career, seeking grant funding, or other support. Leaves of absence or competing familial priorities during this phase can lead to missed opportunities that impact a faculty's entire career trajectory. For example, many career development programs and sources of seed grant funding are time-limited to a certain number of years postgraduation. Most American Society for Radiation Oncology (ASTRO) career development grants are limited to those within 5 years of their first faculty appointment [46]. Some American Society of Clinical Oncology career development awards are only available in the first 3 years of faculty appointment [47]. With some exceptions, most prestigious National Institutes of Health (NIH) K-awards are designed for early- to mid-assistant professor-level faculty [48].

With reduced time to lay this foundation, many academicians worry that it is impossible to succeed in academia if they cannot maintain high levels of publication and grant writing [35]. This can become a self-fulfilling prophesy; risks of attrition are particularly high for clinician-scientists during the phase of life where physicians may have to balance a busy clinical load, familial responsibilities, and establishing their research career. Programs and policies targeted to help with this balance may help to keep promising junior faculty in the academic pipeline. The Doris Duke Charitable Foundation has one such program called the Fund to Retain Clinical Scientists (FRCS), which provides financial support to physician-scientists facing caregiving challenges. The program offers grants from $30,000 to $50,000 per year to cover research support of buyout clinical duties [49]. With increased research-assistant personnel in the lab or extra time out of clinic, grant recipients were able to spend more time writing grants, bringing projects to completion, and writing manuscripts without as much encroachment into personal and family time.

In addition to funding and research career support, another gaining popularity among academic medical institutions is a "stop the clock" policy for promotion and tenure. This type of policy allows faculty to extend the time they have before going up for promotion without being subject to "up or out" rules. At some institutions, this policy applies not only to those who have primary responsibility of care for a child under 5 years of age, but also for those who have had significant illness or provide significant care for ailing family members. A survey of faculty affairs leadership from 126 US medical schools indicated that 79% had a tenure-stopping policy available [50]. However, similar to the familial leave policies discussed above, having such a policy on the books does no good if faculty are not aware of it or are afraid to use it. Results from the same faculty affairs survey showed that at 75% of institutions, between zero and five faculty members utilized tenure-stopping policies [50]. A survey study from the University of California Davis showed similarly low utilization rates with only 6.7% among female School of Medicine faculty and 0% of male faculty [51]. Barriers to utilization may include a fear of perceived weakness or inferiority for taking a longer road to promotion and tenure. Departmental culture change including promotion and normalization of such policies by leadership is necessary to improve utilization.

Other programs designed to help improve academic promotion and career development of female junior faculty do focus on institutional/departmental culture using a more holistic approach. One such program was tested in a randomized controlled trial at the University of Pennsylvania. This study randomized 27 departments either to the control arm or to participation in a three-tiered program with specific interventions aimed at the development of women assistant professors, faculty-led task forces to effect changes at the departmental level, and engagement of institutional leaders. This program included professional development courses for women including a semester-long manuscript writing program, a seminar-style total leadership program, as well as other peer-support and mentorship sessions. Concurrently, an outside facilitator worked with department leadership and other stakeholders to brainstorm and implement policies that would improve their local environment for women's career success [52]. This program both helped women "work smarter not harder" but also helped emphasize the critical role of departmental culture in the amount of work–family conflict seen even with equivalent work demands [53].

Although programs and policies such as these are geared toward women in academic medicine, all faculty engaged in the care of young children, aging parents, or an ailing family member stand to benefit from improvements to the traditional system of promotion, tenure, and academic career development. As work–life balance becomes less of a gendered issue, we can see continued improvements in both the diversity of our physician workforce as well as job satisfaction for all.

Summary Points

- Parental and family leave policies in the US vary widely by state and institution. Physician applicants should be encouraged to ask prospective institutions/departments both about their written policies as well as how they are utilized.
- Interest in part-time work opportunities for physicians is increasing. With careful attention to continuity of patient-care, this may be possible within radiation oncology.
- Flexible workplace policies are desirable for physicians with caregiving responsibilities. Such policies include the ability to work from home for part of the workweek, the ability to step away from work if needed for urgent caregiving situations, and a robust cross-coverage or "doc of the day" system.
- Additional policies to support the academic career development of academic faculty with caregiving responsibilities include "stop the clock" policies with regard to promotion, tenure, and extended eligibility for research/grant funding. Skills building seminars may also help, but participation and buy-in from leadership are vital.
- Although "family-friendly" initiatives are often touted as "pro-woman," familial leave, part-time opportunities, and flexible workplace policies can benefit working mothers and fathers as well as physicians without children who have interests and/or responsibilities outside of medicine.

For Discussion with a Mentor or Colleague

- Brainstorm with a mentor or colleague what your priorities are for the next year, 5 years, and 10 years. Include things you would like to prioritize and accomplish both at work and in your familial/personal life. Honestly evaluate your current/potential job position to determine how compatible it is with those priorities.
- Review the questions in Table 1 with a mentor or colleague and see if she or he has any other recommendations for questions to ask when evaluating a position with regard to parental/familial leave policies
- Brainstorm with a mentor or colleague what your ideal work schedule would be with regard to hours in clinic as well as hours spent on other work activities. Discuss strategies to negotiate with your current/potential employer on how to achieve your preferred schedule.
- Brainstorm with a mentor or colleague whether or not you would like to incorporate working from home or other flexible workplace policies into your current/potential position. Discuss strategies to negotiate with your current/potential employer on how to achieve your preferred balance.

References

1. US Census. United States Census Bureau: women in the workforce 1940–2010.
2. Heiser S. American Academy of Medical Colleges. AAMC.
3. Ahmed AA, Hwang W-T, Holliday EB, et al. Female representation in the academic oncology physician workforce: radiation oncology losing ground to hematology oncology. Int J Radiat Oncol Biol Phys. 2017;98:31–3.
4. Jolly S, Griffith KA, DeCastro R, et al. Gender differences in time spent on parenting and domestic responsibilities by high-achieving young physician-researchers. Ann Intern Med. 2014;160:344–53.
5. National Academy of Sciences (US), National Academy of Engineering (US), and Institute of Medicine (US) Committee on Maximizing the Potential of Women in Academic Science and Engineering. Beyond bias and barriers: fulfilling the potential of women in academic science and engineering. Washington, DC: National Academies Press (US); 2007.
6. Livingston G, Thomas D. Among 41 countries, only U.S. lacks paid parental leave. *FacTank*. 2019.
7. Jou J, Kozhimannil KB, Abraham JM, et al. Paid maternity leave in the United States: associations with maternal and infant health. Matern Child Health J. 2018;22:216–25.
8. Kornfeind KR, Sipsma HL. Exploring the link between maternity leave and postpartum depression. Womens Health Issues. 2018;28:321–6.
9. Navarro-Rosenblatt D, Garmendia M-L. Maternity leave and its impact on breastfeeding: a review of the literature. Breastfeed Med. 2018;13:589–97.
10. Monteiro FR, Buccini GDS, Venâncio SI, et al. Influence of maternity leave on exclusive breastfeeding. J Pediatr. 2017;93:475–81.
11. Aitken Z, Garrett CC, Hewitt B, et al. The maternal health outcomes of paid maternity leave: a systematic review. Soc Sci Med. 2015;130:32–41.
12. Barron D. The economics of paid parental leave: a California experiment shows it can actually save businesses money. 2017.
13. Department of Labor. Family and Medical Leave Act FAQ. *Department of Labor: FMLA FAQ*.
14. Ortiz Worthington R, Feld LD, Volerman A. Supporting new physicians and new parents: a call to create a standard parental leave policy for residents. Acad Med. 2019;94:1654–7.
15. Gottenborg E, Rock L, Sheridan A. Parental leave for residents at programs affiliated with the top 50 medical schools. J Grad Med Educ. 2019;11:472–4.
16. Shifflette V, Hambright S, Amos JD, et al. The pregnant female surgical resident. Adv Med Educ Pract. 2018;9:365–9.
17. Hariton E, Matthews B, Burns A, et al. Pregnancy and parental leave among obstetrics and gynecology residents: results of a nationwide survey of program directors. Am J Obstet Gynecol. 2018;219:199.e1–8.
18. ABR. The American Board of Radiology: initial certification for radiation oncology certification requirements. 2019.
19. American Board of Internal Medicine. Special training policies for certification.
20. Kahn J, Goodman CR, Albert A, et al. Top concerns of radiation oncology trainees in 2019: job market, board examinations, and residency expansion. Int J Radiat Oncol Biol Phys. 2020;106:19–25.
21. Holliday EB, Ahmed AA, Jagsi R, et al. Pregnancy and parenthood in radiation oncology, views and experiences survey (PROVES): results of a blinded prospective trainee parenting and career development assessment. Int J Radiat Oncol Biol Phys. 2015;92:516–24.
22. Riano NS, Linos E, Accurso EC, et al. Paid family and childbearing leave policies at top US medical schools. JAMA. 2018;319:611–4.

23. Weaver AN, Willett LL. Is it safe to ask the questions that matter most to me? Observations from a female residency applicant. Acad Med. 2019;94:1635–7.
24. Froom JD, Bickel J. Medical school policies for part-time faculty committed to full professional effort. Acad Med. 1996;71:91–6.
25. Heiliger PJ, Hingstman L. Career preferences and the work-family balance in medicine: gender differences among medical specialists. Soc Sci Med. 2000;50:1235–46.
26. Ziegler S, Krause-Solberg L, Scherer M, et al. [Working hour preferences of female and male residents: developments over 4 years of postgraduate medical training in Germany]. Bundesgesundheitsblatt Gesundheitsforschung Gesundheitsschutz. 2017;60:1115–23.
27. Darves B. Part-time physician practice on the rise. N Engl J Med Career Center. 2011. https://www.nejmcareercenter.org/article/part-time-physician-practice-on-the-rise/.
28. McMurray JE, Heiligers PJM, Shugerman RP, et al. Part-time medical practice: where is it headed? Am J Med. 2005;118:87–92.
29. Miller CC. How medicine became the stealth family-friendly profession. The New York Times. 2019.
30. Vinod SK, Jalaludin BB, Rodger A, et al. Part-time consultants in radiation oncology. Australas Radiol. 2002;46:396–401.
31. Dean A, Auerbach A. 96% of U.S. professionals say they need flexibility, but only 47% have it. Harvard Business Review. 2018.
32. Rogier S, Padgett M. The impact of utilizing a flexible work schedule on the perceived career advancement potential of women. Hum Resour Dev Q. 2004;15:89–106.
33. Rudman L, Mescher K. Penalizing men who request family leave: is flexibility stigma a femininity stigma? J Soc Issues. 2013;69:322–40.
34. Coltrane S, Miller E, DeHaan T, et al. Fathers and the flexibility stigma. J Soc Issues. 2013;69:279–302.
35. Shauman K, Howell LP, Paterniti DA, et al. Barriers to career flexibility in academic medicine: a qualitative analysis of reasons for the underutilization of family-friendly policies, and implications for institutional change and department chair leadership. Acad Med. 2018;93:246–55.
36. Kramer A, Kramer KZ. The potential impact of the Covid-19 pandemic on occupational status, work from home, and occupational mobility. J Vocat Behav. 2020;103442
37. Lewis GD, Hatch SS, Wiederhold LR, et al. Long-term institutional experience with telemedicine services for radiation oncology: a potential model for long-term utilization. Adv Radiat Oncol. 2020;5(4):780–2.
38. Marks LB, Jackson M, Xie L, et al. The challenge of maximizing safety in radiation oncology. Pract Radiat Oncol. 2011;1:2–14.
39. Jena AB, Olenski AR, Blumenthal DM. Sex differences in physician salary in US public medical schools. JAMA Intern Med. 2016;176:1294–304.
40. Wright AL, Schwindt LA, Bassford TL, et al. Gender differences in academic advancement: patterns, causes, and potential solutions in one US College of medicine. Acad Med. 2003;78:500–8.
41. Ash AS, Carr PL, Goldstein R, et al. Compensation and advancement of women in academic medicine: is there equity? Ann Intern Med. 2004;141:205–12.
42. Ahmed AA, Egleston B, Holliday E, et al. Gender trends in radiation oncology in the United States: a 30-year analysis. Int J Radiat Oncol Biol Phys. 2014;88:33–8.
43. Beeler WH, Griffith KA, Jones RD, et al. Gender, professional experiences, and personal characteristics of academic radiation oncology chairs: data to inform the pipeline for the 21st century. Int J Radiat Oncol Biol Phys. 2019;104:979–86.
44. Holliday EB, Jagsi R, Wilson LD, et al. Gender differences in publication productivity, academic position, career duration, and funding among U.S. academic radiation oncology faculty. Acad Med. 2014;89:767–73.
45. Holliday EB, Siker M, Chapman CH, et al. Achieving gender equity in the radiation oncology physician workforce. Adv Radiat Oncol. 2018;3:478–83.
46. Anon. American Society for Radiation Oncology. *American Society for Radiation Oncology.*

47. Anon. American Society for Clinical Oncology.
48. Anon. National Institute of Health.
49. Jones RD, Miller J, Vitous CA, et al. The most valuable resource is time: insights from a novel national program to improve retention of physician-scientists with caregiving responsibilities. Acad Med. 2019;94:1746–56.
50. Bunton SA, Corrice AM. Evolving workplace flexibility for U.S. medical school tenure-track faculty. Acad Med. 2011;86:481–5.
51. Villablanca AC, Beckett L, Nettiksimmons J, et al. Career flexibility and family-friendly policies: an NIH-funded study to enhance women's careers in biomedical sciences. J Womens Health (Larchmt). 2011;20:1485–96.
52. Grisso JA, Sammel MD, Rubenstein AH, et al. A randomized controlled trial to improve the success of women assistant professors. J Womens Health (Larchmt). 2017;26:571–9.
53. Westring AF, Speck RM, Dupuis Sammel M, et al. Culture matters: the pivotal role of culture for women's careers in academic medicine. Acad Med. 2014;89:658–63.

Part IV
Mid and Senior Career

Professionalism: Instincts Below the Surface and Environmental Influences

Introduction

Definitions of professionalism commonly invoke themes of competence, skill, and focus on the performance expected for a given set of responsibilities in a work environment. For most occupations—and especially for physicians and others in the health care arena—layered atop these basic expectations for professionalism is the assumption that behaviors will conform to a set of ethical and behavioral guidelines applicable to relationships with the client/patient, other professionals in the same space, and society at large.

One of the most frequently cited papers in the canon of literature pertaining to professionalism in medicine is the work of Hickson and colleagues from Vanderbilt University, "A complementary approach to promoting professionalism: identifying, measuring, and addressing unprofessional behaviors" [1]. The article begins with an all-too-familiar anecdote wherein a physician loses their cool in a stressful situation to the detriment of patient care, disrespecting the support staff, and generally behaving in a fashion unbecoming a hangry two-year-old. Hickson offers a practical roadmap for the proper administrative response to such circumstances, beginning with an informal dialogue with a physician who suffers a momentary lapse in good manners to more stringent disciplinary interventions for repeat offenders or those whose transgressions are more egregious.

All physicians are human, and it is possible for any of us in a moment of frustration to act in a way that is immediately regretted. Fortunately, as Hickson notes, most individuals respond well to a so-called "cup of coffee" intervention in which an isolated sentinel incident is reviewed during an even-tempered dialogue, the momentary stressful context is considered, and forward-looking solutions are

B. D. Kavanagh (✉)
Department of Radiation Oncology, University of Colorado, Aurora, CO, USA
e-mail: BRIAN.KAVANAGH@CUANSCHUTZ.EDU

© Springer Nature Switzerland AG 2021
R. A. Chandra et al. (eds.), *Career Development in Academic Radiation Oncology*, https://doi.org/10.1007/978-3-030-71855-8_17

identified to reduce the risk of recidivism. Most such events are isolated and unlikely to reoccur. However, a pattern of repeated egregious behavior calls for analysis and interventions scaled up in proportion to the magnitude of the problem. Furthermore, heightened awareness in recent years of cultural–environmental influences that operate in sometimes subtle but often insidious ways illuminates so-called "hidden curricula" in medical education that can negatively impact a physician's level of professionalism. Finally, the current age of social media calls for special reflection by physicians in terms of how they can best project themselves toward colleagues and patients in that forum.

Challenging Drivers of Habitually Unprofessional Behavior

In 2007 Roback and colleagues reported an analysis of a cohort of 88 physicians who had been referred to a multidisciplinary program that provides evaluations for severe complex problems such as mental health challenges, substance dependence, compulsive sexual behavior, and other counterproductive behaviors [2]. The subjects were categorized according to the nature of the offensive behavior that prompted referral to the program into three groups: behaviorally disruptive subjects with repeated instances of uncontrolled anger or conduct demeaning others, sexual boundary violators who had had inappropriate communication or action with patients or staff members, and all others (substance abuse, emotional instability, professional irresponsibility, etc.). The investigators reviewed the results of one or more validated personality evaluation instruments to look for correlations with the different categories of offensive behavior. While the cohort of sexual boundary violators were more likely to have profiles indicative of character deficits such as impulsiveness or anger or extreme defensiveness, overall there were no consistent indicators that could reliably serve as screening tools to predict serious problems with professional behavior.

Hickson and colleagues identify common drivers and environmental conditions that can lead to unprofessional behaviors [1]. Physicians can be compromised by substance abuse, narcissism, selfishness, poorly controlled anger, and spillover tensions from acute or chronic family/home life problems. Exacerbating or enabling conditions can include insufficient clinical or administrative support, poorly performing colleagues, and an existing system in which bad behavior (e.g., yelling at the practice director) has been rewarded with desired outcomes (e.g., more favorable on-call schedule). Unraveling the intertwined contributing factors can be challenging, and in the ideal situation an institution would have expertise and resources in place to facilitate appropriate corrective changes in the environment and individual rehabilitative interventions. Few physicians are trained to work with peers in need of such help, and so in general it is best whenever possible to communicate concerns about a colleague to the Human Resources or Professionalism office so that the troubled individual can receive the necessary guidance and support.

Hidden Curricula Impacting Professionalism

The concept of a "hidden curriculum" impacting education in medicine was advanced in 1982 by Haas and Shaffir in the context of discussing *professionalization*, also called professional socialization, the process whereby medical students transition from simply having a relevant fund of knowledge to projecting their competence to others [3]. The focus of Haas and Shaffir's work was a comparison of how students in a traditional versus nontraditional curriculum navigate the unwritten rules about various rites of passage that—rightly or wrongly—are common in both domains and seem essential for creating the "cloak of competence" that is fundamental to achieving self-confidence in the practice of medicine. In retrospect it is ironic that the authors mentioned that their students expected a "gentleman's agreement" among peers to collude regarding assessments of each other's work.

The irony for that specific choice of words, of course, relates to the more recent focus on hidden curricula in medical education that prop up various forms of institutional sexism and racism, and an example would be the selection of a gender-favoring term to describe a typical medical student and "his" inclination to be a team player. While this particular cliché might be a rather mild offense at worst, word and phrase choices in day-to-day conversation can constitute nuanced microaggressions. Examples cited in an essay about microaggressions in the field of Radiology include a statement to a female radiologist such as, "You are too pretty to be a radiologist and sit in the dark, you should be in pediatrics" or a comment to a minority physician that "It is really impressive how well you are doing considering your background" [4]. In each case there is a passive–aggressive undertone of intellectual superiority or personal entitlement that has the effect of diminishing the accomplishments, autonomy, and/or legitimacy of the targeted individual. Perhaps not surprisingly, in a multi-institutional study of medical school faculty, male physicians were less likely to recognize gender-directed microaggressions toward women than their female counterparts [5].

The American College of Physicians (ACP) characterizes "hidden curricula" as the lessons that are not explicitly taught but, rather, are learned by virtue of being embedded in the culture of medicine [6]. Not all of these are negative: the ACP position statement on optimizing clinical learning environments offers the example of a primary care physician visiting her hospitalized patient after hours pro bono out of concern for the patient's well-being, thus acting as a positive role model for professionalism that trainees should emulate. The problematic aspects of hidden curricula are instances in which in which sexist, racist, or otherwise objectionable behaviors by individuals in positions of authority and influence are normalized to a point where they are seen as acceptable or even preferable to those under their tutelage, who will then likely repeat the same transgressions.

Leaders from within the field of radiation oncology and the larger house of medicine have called for an end to entrenched inequities across the spectrum of health care that perpetuate sexist and racist abuses. Sexual harassment and flagrant discriminatory treatment of women in medicine prompted the emergence of the TIME'S UP movement as a possible paradigm for remedy [7]. Chapman and colleagues provided an overview of the structural racism present within society at large that bleeds over into all of healthcare, including radiation oncology, with adverse consequences for patients and providers [8]. These authors endorse a proactive strategy of rejecting anti-Black microaggressions and policies that propagate inequities and ensuring appropriate representation in leadership roles from groups who are underrepresented in medicine.

Professionalism in the Era of Social Media

High-speed digital communications are a part of modern life. For the practicing physician, advantages include quick access to online medical information sources and multiple options for remote networking with colleagues. The world of social media opens up many more opportunities, ranging from real-time updates from scientific meetings [9] to direct interactions with patients and other healthcare stakeholders.

Within the field of radiation oncology, Dr. Matthew Katz has been at the forefront of social media, embracing the various available computer apps to promote new forms of journal clubs and connect communities of physicians across specialty and geographic boundaries. In a 2014 essay, Katz pointed out some important considerations for physicians as they choose to engage in or abstain from social media and other online communications forums [10]. First of all, it is widely known that many patients seek medical information through online sources, and doctors might wish to participate in social media for no other reason than to help combat the misinformation and quackery that is ubiquitous on the web. Secondly, the fact that patients can always access postings on public social media sites is important to remember, and so physicians should be mindful of what they post online.

Because so many of its members are now electing to enter the realm of social media, the American Society for Radiation Oncology (ASTRO) has recommended a list of Social Media Best Practices that include six specific suggestions [11], paraphrased here:

1. Establish an online identity, but consider separate professional and personal accounts if there is a desire to have private contacts with family and friends that will not be scrutinized by patients or coworkers.
2. Protect physician–patient confidentiality, and avoid giving personalized medical advice via social media.
3. Engage in real time, for example by posting updates from live meetings (if the presenter has given permission) and by participating in journal clubs and other live discussions.

4. Use social media as an educational tool and possibly also a means of boosting awareness of ongoing clinical research to enhance accrual to important trials.
5. Be transparent about conflicts of interest, and be aware of your institution's policy on social media.
6. Respect the platform in terms of official unofficial rules that may apply. It is advisable to observe interactions on Twitter, LinkedIn, or other platforms before jumping in. Although the interactions are not face-to-face, it is usually advantageous to maintain the same collegial and courteous manners used in ordinary offline meetings. Patients and patient advocacy groups following the discussions will form impressions based on the tone as much or perhaps more than the content of the commentary.

Additional details are available from the ASTRO website. Another good resource is the guidance offered by Bibault and colleagues [12].

Conclusions

Long-established core values in medicine, sometimes expressed as the three As (availability, affability, and ability), remain essential building blocks for physician professionalism. Patients expect and deserve skill and high-quality care, doctors must be personable with patients and colleagues, and the job calls for commitment that often extends beyond what is typical for other vocations. Achieving a high level of professionalism requires not only a strong fund of medical knowledge but also self-awareness and emotional intelligence. As role models for others in society, physicians especially need to cultivate sensitivity about gender and racial biases that can lead to disparities in healthcare outcomes and unfair consequences for coworkers. Finally, in an internet-based world, physicians are not only evaluated by their bedside manner and talent but also by their online social media presence, and as a result they should be mindful of the appearance and words of their avatars in that space.

For Discussion with a Mentor or Colleague

- Have you observed situations in which my reaction under stress could have been improved? If so, how?
- Have you observed instances in which I did not appear to recognize the mood or meaning of another person in the context of a disagreement or other stressful situation or a non-stressful situation?

- Have you noticed examples of written communication from me (email, social media, or other) in which my tone or word choice was either likely misunderstood or was somehow less effective in the communication that it should have been?
- Have you observed instances in which I did not appear to understand how my actions or words or tone of voice were received by another person during an in-person encounter?

References

1. Hickson GB, Pichert JW, Webb LE, Gabbe SG. A complementary approach to promoting professionalism: identifying, measuring, and addressing unprofessional behaviors. Acad Med. 2007;82(11):1040–8.
2. Roback HB, Strassberg D, Iannelli RJ, Finlayson AR, Blanco M, Neufeld R. Problematic physicians: a comparison of personality profiles by offence type. Can J Psychiatry. 2007;52(5):315–22.
3. Haas J, Shaffir W. Ritual evaluation of competence: the hidden curriculum of professionalization in an innovative medical school program. Work Occup. 1982;9(2):131–54.
4. DeBenedectis CM, Jay AK, Milburn J, Yee J, Kagetsu NJ. Microaggression in radiology. J Am Coll Radiol. 2019;16(9 Pt A):1218–9.
5. Periyakoil VS, Chaudron L, Hill EV, Pellegrini V, Neri E, Kraemer HC. Common types of gender-based microaggressions in medicine. Acad Med. 2020;95(3):450–7.
6. Lehmann LS, Sulmasy LS, Desai S. Hidden curricula, ethics, and professionalism: optimizing clinical learning environments in becoming and being a physician: a position paper of the American College of Physicians. Ann Intern Med. 2018;168(7):506–8.
7. Choo EK, Byington CL, Johnson NL, Jagsi R. From# MeToo to# TimesUp in health care: can a culture of accountability end inequity and harassment? Lancet. 2019;393(10171):499–502.
8. Chapman CH, Gabeau D, Pinnix CC, Deville C Jr, Gibbs IC, Winkfield KM. Why racial justice matters in radiation oncology. Adv Radiat Oncol. 2020. https://doi.org/10.1016/j.adro.2020.06.013.
9. Knoll MA, Kavanagh B, Katz M. The 2017 American Society of Radiation Oncology (ASTRO) annual meeting: taking a deeper dive into social media. Adv Radiat Oncol. 2018;3(3):230.
10. Katz MS. Social media and medical professionalism: the need for guidance. Eur Urol. 2014 Oct;66(4):633–4.
11. https://www.astro.org/Meetings-and-Education/SM-Best-Practices. Accessed 11 July 2020.
12. Bibault J-E, Katz MS, Motwani S. Social media for radiation oncologists: a practical primer. Adv Radiat Oncol. 2017;2(3):277–80.

Promotions

Charles R. Thomas Jr.

Overview

The primary mission of academic medical center is to improve the overall health of the human condition. This is based upon the need to develop programs of excellence within the submissions of education/teaching, research/scholarly activity, patient-directed health care, and other service (including intramural and extramural). The major tools for executing these responsibilities rest with the faculty. Hence, faculty success depends, in essence, on a system that provides recognition and rewards for work done in promoting the multiple missions of the school.

The major keys to successful promotion are self-discipline, self-awareness, social intelligence, and documented accomplishments that contribute to one or more of the missions of your radiation oncology department, affiliated cancer center, as well as the broader institution.

Promotion and appointments in academic medicine are based upon a number of factors, some of which are under control of the person being considered and others that are beyond one's control. Some of the reasons why individuals are or are not successfully promoted include components of both the official criteria that are stated in the written guidelines of the institution and a set of unofficial guidelines, the latter of which is, at least, as important if not more so than the former.

For individuals who require a more nuanced discussion regarding P&T, please contact the author of this chapter to set up a counseling session.

C. R. Thomas Jr. (✉)
Department of Radiation Medicine, Knight Cancer Institute, Oregon Health & Science University, Portland, OR, USA
e-mail: thomasch@ohsu.edu

© Springer Nature Switzerland AG 2021
R. A. Chandra et al. (eds.), *Career Development in Academic Radiation Oncology*, https://doi.org/10.1007/978-3-030-71855-8_18

A key for success in the promotion ladder is to understand the importance of cultivating and sustaining respectful relationships across the academy. While this may seem rather intuitive, many individuals have experience unnecessary difficulty in navigating the promotion process due, in large part, to not appreciating the importance of relationship building.

The promotion and tenure (P&T) process involves a number of items that are assembled to comprise the dossier that will undergo serial consideration by players from both intramural (including within the division, the larger academic department, and extra-departmental) and extramural (including extra-institutional) units. Some of the individuals are may be known to the candidate, such as the membership of the departmental P&T committee as well as membership of the medical school and/or graduate school P&T committees. Within academic radiation oncology, the comparatively smaller size of specialty is such that the department chair may serve de facto in the dual capacity as chair of the departmental P&T committee.

It is critical that all faculty review the promotion and tenure guidelines, preferably during the recruitment process, again during as part of the on-boarding process as employment commences, and as part of the regular (annual or semiannual) faculty review process. The guidelines will describe the different academic tracks and associated expectations for achieving promotion in sequential academic ranks. In addition, they describe the recommended time in rank before most promotions are considered. Most P&T guidelines allow for a limited provision of switching between academic tracks.

We will only briefly discuss tenure. The first thing to understand is that this designation is not a lifetime job guarantee. This is similar to ABR board certification prior to the 1990s, which many older diplomats feel is a lifetime guarantee of certification. The ABR has never guaranteed lifetime certification as the rules can always be changed. Moreover, while most medical schools have a tenure track, no more than one-quarter of full-time faculty are tenured. Basically, tenure is a contract between the faculty member and the institution. As such, a faculty member has earned an "indefinite" term of employment following a predefined probationary period. Such faculty members can be terminated only for cause and following an established procedure. The AAUP (American Association of University Professors) has been updating tenure practices for nearly 8 decades [1, 2]. For academic radiation oncologists, most associate and full professors are not tenured. Walling has summarized the salient points on tenure for the academic physician.

The timetable of events is especially crucial understand. The COVID pandemic may result in some institutions modifying their timelines. Some institutions have a mandatory time by which a faculty member must be either go up for promotion or, in some instances, successfully achieve the promotion to the next academic rank.

Tracks

There are multiple tracks that one can be hired into. It is critical that the areas of emphasis for a given track be consistent with the abilities and desire of the faculty as well as the needs of the radiation oncology program. Most medical schools have between 2 and 4 tracks that can be considered for full-time and part-time academic radiation oncologists. Most tracks with the exception of the pure research track require some degree of regular engagement in the clinical mission. As the average salary of an academic radiation oncologist is higher than most other specialties, a robust clinical engine is required. The terms clinician-educator, physician-educator, physician-investigator, academic clinician, academic investigator, community academician, etc. may have different definitions within the P&T committee bylaws between institutions; we urge all faculty to periodically review the formal track descriptions to make sure that there is alignment of expectations and interests with the department and larger institution.

The most important point for the academic radiation oncologist is to appreciate that no matter what track one is one, meaningful contributions to multiple department and institutional missions can occur. Basically, it's not so much what formal track you are on but what are and your department chair poised to do so that you're successful – plain and simple.

Dossier Essentials

The essential components of the promotion packet include the curriculum vitae (CV) (per the institutional recommended format), NIH biosketch, time-effort, statement, Personal Statement, educator's portfolio, and letters of support.

At some institutions, the annual faculty performance reviews are required.

(Editor's Note: while a dedicated chapter about the academic CV is covered in another chapter of this book, the promotion CV may benefit from annotation and highlighting in 1–2 sentences, the main impact of select publications. Also, see section "Personal Statement".)

Time-Effort Statement

This is usually a short form which describes the proportion of time spent in the different categories of work activity in the prior since the last promotion or appoint, whichever is most recent. This often assumes a full 1.0 FTE. Specifically, a percentage designation of time spent in the scholarly, teaching, and service (intramural and extramural) missions. A short description of the candidate's position description and how it has changed (or not) will help to place the time-effort statement information into proper perspective for the P&T committee.

Personal Statement

This is an opportunity for the candidate to describe to the evaluating committee and potential letter writers why she/he deserves the appointment and/or promoting being sought. Quite frankly, this *is not* a time to be reserved, shy, or coy, regarding one's contributions. The Personal Statement tells the world why the candidate meets and, more often than not, exceeds the formal criteria for promotion at the institution. This an opportunity to highlight contributions that are not properly appreciated within the traditional CV format. Now is the time for the candidate to clearly elucidate the contributions to the scholarly, education, and service missions.

It is allowable to include website hyperlinks to lab or instructional pages that further showcase the candidate's horsepower. For example, the UCSD Department of Radiation Medicine and Applied Sciences has long maintained a high-quality template of faculty lab page hyperlinks, https://medschool.ucsd.edu/som/radiation-medicine/research/labs/Pages/default.aspx. There are others of course.

Moreover, some of the most impactful Personal Statements that I have seen have included a career timeline, sometimes with a color matrix, which allows the evaluator to appreciate the evolution of the candidate's career.

At my institution, I encourage my faculty to include a brief statement on their individual contributions to diversity and equity. I consider this a normative part of faculty development and should be included into the annual faculty reviews.

Educator's Portfolio

As the scholarship of education becomes more critical in academic medicine and especially radiation oncology, it is important to consistently document these contributions [3, 4]. I encourage keeping a separate document for all learners, starting medical school and certainly by starting residency, as it's never too soon begin this process. By doing so, the rewarding and often very time-consuming contributions to educational activities can be kept to date.

Educator contribution areas are multifold and include the following major areas: (1) direct instruction, (2) curriculum development, (3) advising and mentoring, (4) educational leadership and administration, and (5) learner assessment.

For radiation oncology, *direct instruction* (or teaching) activities are most common in the daily clinic where patient care is delivered. The institution that is provided throughout the delivery of clinical care, including teaching others by role modeling how to perform a directed history and physical exam, simulation, treatment planning, and chart documentation, is a highly valued teaching contribution. Other activities include giving lectures, workshops, small group sessions, and facilitation of online courses. I recommend that all academic faculty immediately request for the objective feedback from learners within a couple days of giving singular teaching presentation such as a lecture.

Curriculum development is a longitudinal set of systematically designed, sequenced, and evaluated teaching activities that learners are subjected to. The recommended documentation includes the course title, role (i.e., course director, financier, founder, etc.), learner gap/purpose, target learners (i.e., PGY2 radiation oncology residents, M4 radiation oncology clerkship enrollees, etc.), length (hrs., frequency), and methods and design (i.e., ROVER, a Virtual Radiation Oncology for Medical Students online course, https://www.radoncvirtual.com/rover).

Advising and mentoring, when effective, can be the backbone of a successful career in academic radiation oncology. Mentoring is a more involved and reciprocal process. Advising can be more limited. It is entirely possible that an advisor can serve as a mentor and vice versa. In addition to listing an advisees and mentors, which may include a broad spectrum of learners, it is important to include evidence of quality or effectiveness as well as quantity. (Editor's Note: a separate chapter on mentoring is in this book.)

Educational leadership and administration would include the candidate's role as radiation oncology medical student clerkship director, residency and/or fellowship program director, graduate program director, and training grant principal investigator (i.e., K12 or R25 NIH grant). Again, while quantity is admirable, evidence of quality or effectiveness is equally important.

Leaner assessment may include practices involved in measuring just how did learner knowledge change (or not) following the specific educational intervention of the candidate. Pre-test and post-test questions are very common.

A more detailed example of best practices in documenting an educator's portfolio is in the Appendix of this chapter.

Letters of Support

The letters are expected to be from both intramural and extramural investigators. The exact number of required letters is listed in the institutional P&T website. Ultimately, the department P&T committee and/or department chair will determine which investigators will be approached to provide a letter in support of the faculty candidate for promotion. While I and other department chairs are often approached by junior (Instructor or Assistant Professor) faculty to write letters on their behalf, it is not *their* job to do that. In fact, some academic institutions consider such actions antithetical to the process.

The institutional P&T committee chair, associate deal for faculty affairs, and/or the radiation oncology department chair will formally send out a short letter to prospective referees asking for their assistance in the P&T for a specific candidate. The letters should be accompanied by a signed and dated referee form seeking to determine (1) whether the relationship, in any, has or currently exists between the letter writer (referee) and the candidate as well as (2) the basis of the letter referee's knowledge of the candidate's work. For example, the relationship should confirm whether the referee is a present or past colleague (at the same institution as a student, postdoctoral fellow, or faculty member), a past mentor, a collaborator (worked with and/or co-authored papers), or none of the above. The issue of how the referee is aware of the candidate's contributions seeks to determine the sources of that knowledge. Sources might include the candidate's publications (H-index, M-index, I-index), CV/biosketch, grants via NIH reporter [https://projectreporter.nih.gov/reporter.cfm], scientific or educational presentations, personal knowledge, or participation in review panels (i.e., study sections, advisory board, etc.).

In addition, intramural letters from the faculty member's immediate supervisor (i.e., division or section chief), chair of departmental P&T committee (for appropriately sized programs), and department chair are required.

For candidates at institutions located with a NCI-affiliated cancer center, the director, associate director, and research program leader are welcome intramural sources of letter.

It is important that some letter of the letters be considered non-conflicted. Finally, a candidate's residency training director is not considered a non-conflicted letter and will likely carry little weight within the evaluation process.

Referees who are asked to write letters on behalf of a candidate for promotion should carefully review the details of the invitation letter, the accompany dossier, the deadline requested for the letter to be submitted, and, more importantly, a self-evaluation as to whether the referee is even qualified to comment on the merits of the candidate's contribution. If all of the aforementioned are met, then it is critical that the referee make an informed decision as to whether she/he has the requisite time to devote to (1) digesting the P&T guidelines from the requesting institution, (2) reviewing the candidate's dossier, (3) writing a professional letter, and (4) maintaining confidentiality. If any of these four areas is problematic for the referee, then it is best for all parties to respectfully decline the invitation to participate.

Team Science

Over the past two decades, it has been recognized that in order for progress to be made in scientific inquiry, the model of a single PI driving all aspects of an idea from start until publication is an outdated model [5]. In fact, the individual PI model was never a transparent model since critical collaborations were often barely acknowledged if at all. Most medical school P&T committees now recognize team-based investigation as being normative within collaborative research. The NIH is clearly committed to team science.

There are certainly a number of fruitful collaborations within the realm of academic radiation oncology, including but certainly not limited to the Radiation Oncology Education Collaborative Study Group (ROECSG), the Joint Head and Neck Radiotherapy-MRI Development Cooperative, and the consortium on Validating Predictive Models and Biomarkers of Radiotherapy Toxicity to Reduce Side-Effects and Improve Quality of Life in Cancer Survivors (REQUITE) [2]. The academic climate in our specialty is actually stronger in large part to the appreciation of the team science concept.

It is critical that individuals being evaluated for promotion clearly outline their specific contribution to the project. This can be articulated in the Personal Statement as well as the department chair letter, so that there is no ambiguity as to the importance of one's contribution to a collaborative project.

I believe that an appreciation of team science is long overdue. This approach allows there to be multiple winners in the pursuit of scientific inquiry and doesn't require single person or group to be further marginalized within the academy.

Objective Criteria for Promotion

This section will summarize what is generally expected to achieve promotion in academic radiation medicine. While all academic institutions have official criteria, some departments of radiation oncology, including the University of Washington, have crafted granular criteria that provide further guidance for our specialty [6]. The major missions for which a decision to approve or deny an application for promotion from Assistant Professor to Associate Professor and then from Associate Professor to Full Professor at most western medical schools. For the purposes of distinguishing different levels of achievement, I will use the following specific terms: satisfactory, substantial, and outstanding. These terms all have synonyms, and different institutional P&T committee guidelines may describe such. Nevertheless, the sequential increase in achievement from satisfactory to substantial to outstanding is a very reasonable standardization.

These levels of achievement are applied to each of the major missions that are being evaluated for by the P&T committee: scholarship/research, education/teaching, and service (intramural and extramural). The matrix below provides a clear set of goal-driven contributions that are considered in the decision process.

For evaluation of scholarship/research contributions, the matrix below provides a description of criteria and milestones that sequentially differentiate the levels of achievement from satisfactory to substantial to outstanding (adapted from OHSU P&T public access site).

Scholarship Research Excellence	Satisfactory	Substantial	Outstanding
	• Individually or as a team, peer reviewed high quality publications • Original work: theoretical, applied • Inventions, methodology advances • Individual or collaborative local or institutional funding • Mentored career development award • Serve as a journal reviewer • Local or state peer presentations • Dissemination of curriculum through peer reviewed abstracts and curriculum repositories • Participate in creation of clinical guidelines or clinical evidence reviews	• Continuing individual or collaborative publications in peer-reviewed journals o f high quality with substantial role • Develop new methods or tools that add to research capacity in one or more fields • Develop and disseminate innovative learner assessment tools • Achieve independent f unding • Obtain funding for collaborative efforts • Be invited to present work at regional level • Lead Departmental research program • Journal review or editorial board member • National grant reviewer (NIH, NSF, VA, etc.) • Peer reviewed publication of educational materials in journals or repositories • Leadership role in the creation/dissemination of clinical guidelines or evidence reviews, implemented regionally	• Scholarship recognized at the national and international level • Maintain sustained extra mural funding in independent or collaborative grants • Member of professional society committees • Leadership, innovation in collaborative research • Develop industry partnerships, patents, disclosures, licenses • Leadership and innovation in the development of educational materials disseminated and used at other institutions • Leadership roles in national scientific committees, organizations • National or international Invited presentations • National recognition/awards from professional or public groups • National implementation of clinical guidelines or evidence reviews

For evaluation of education/teaching contributions, the matrix below provides a description of criteria and milestones that sequentially differentiate the levels of achievement from satisfactory to substantial to outstanding.

| Teaching Educational Excellence | • Teaching at a level typical for peers (lectures, labs, small groups, clinic/ward, supervising research)
• Satisfactory or better evaluations
• Mentees completeprogram,participate in presentations & publications, and accomplish goals
• Serve on depart mental educational committees
• Participate in learner assessment at a level typical for peers | • Sustained (years) teaching a ta level greater than peers
• Course or departmental teaching awards
• Consistently excellent evaluations from peers
• Invitations to teach in other departments
• Significant role in innovative curriculum/course design
• Improved outcomes due to curricular change
• National accreditation of newt raining program
• Mentees with significant accomplishments, awards
• Participate in developing effective mentoring activities, lead improving department mentoring
• Sustained service: institutional education committees
• Course program director, Department educational leadership
• Develop, implement innovative assessmen ttools | • Institutional, regional or nationalt eaching awards
• Consistently excellent learner, course director, peer evaluations
• Peer- reviewed dissemination of educational materials in journals or national curriculum repositories
• Regional/national presentation ofi nstructional materials or curriculum
• Instructional materials disseminated and used at other institutions
• Invitations to provide curriculum consultation to other institutions
• Quantity of mentoring exceeding most peers with evidence of mentoring effectiveness as measured by mentees' accomplishments
• Mentoring consultant to ther departments or leads initiatives to improve mentoring in the institution
• Multiple sustained educational leadership roles in the institution
• Leadership roles in national educational organizations |

For evaluation of service contributions, the matrix below provides a description of criteria and milestones that sequentially differentiate the levels of achievement from satisfactory to substantial to outstanding.

Service — Clinical Excellence

• Membership on departmental committees at level of peers • Membership on institutional committees • Participation in educational, scientific, healthcare related community organizations • Journal reviewer • Multi-center collaborative clinical research studies • Clinical service at a level commensurate with clinical FTE • Satisfactory or better evaluations for clinical performance • Participate in the development of innovative, clinical initiatives or shared scientific resources • Local or state presentations	• Leadership of departmental committees • Institutional committee service sustained over years • Leadership of educational, scientific or healthcare community organization • Lead department clinical, educational, research program • Leads development of a new institutional shared scientific resource • Leadership in regional committees/organizations, or active membership nationally with an impact level greater than peers • National credentialing activity (board exam questions) • Clinical Expertise recognized awarded locally or regionally • Regional presentations (within Oregon or the Northwest) • Lead development of innovative clinical initiatives • Receive institutional funding for innovative or complex clinical initiatives or shared scientific resources • Participate in practice initiatives that demonstrate an impact on quality • Collaborate in initiation of effective, innovative interdisciplinary practice-related activities	• Institutional high-intensity committee service at a level significantly greater than peers and/or serve as committee chair • National reputation for leadership activities in educational, scientific or healthcare related community organizations • Multiple sustained administrative leadership roles in the institution • Leadership roles in national committees/organizations • Membership on interdisciplinary health care-related work groups or committees at the national level • Receive national recognition/awards for clinical expertise from professional and public groups • National or international level presentations of novel synthesis of knowledge or new techniques and/or procedures • Invitations for clinical program consultation to other institutions • Produce innovative clinical programs that are disseminated and serve as models for other institutions • Obtain external funding for practice innovations, new clinical initiatives or innovative or complex shared scientific resources

Depending on the current job description and time-effort, including time devoted to the different missions, some of these missions may not be required for select faculty. In most cases, some measurable commitment and achievement in all of the three major missions are required. Satisfactory performance is required in all. Unsatisfactory performance in any of the missions will preclude further consideration until evidence of improvement is demonstrable.

Promotion from Assistant Professor to Associate Professor requires substantial achievement in at least one of the missions for medical schools. A minority of institutions require the equivalent of substantial achievement in multiple mission areas to be promoted to the Associate Professor level. In fact, a faculty who is receiving high-quality and sustained mentoring as part of their career development often is not put up for promotion without having demonstrated clear evidence of achieving more than the bare minimum requirements for promotion regardless of the medical school affiliation.

Promotion from Associate Professor to Full Professor requires Outstanding achievement in one or more of the core missions. There is usually a 4–7-year requirement that a faculty be in-rank at the Associate Professor level prior to becoming a Full Professor. *Of course, it only takes one Nobel Prize for a candidate to immediately get promoted to Full Professor with indefinite tenure.*

Summary

The promotion, appointment, and tenure process is a continuum that actually begins well before that actual year the formal packet is assembled. An understanding of the public criteria (discussed above) as well as the invisible criteria, that latter which necessitates health mentorship and relationship cultivation, is critical to success. We recommend that you update your CV, biosketch, and educator portfolio, at least, quarterly. The future is bright for pipeline of high-quality investigators who seek careers in academic radiation oncology.

Take-Home Messages

- The promotion and appointment process is mean to acknowledge faculty contributions to the multiple missions of the radiation oncology program and the broader institution.
- No particular academic track should carry more prestige than any other.
- Time-effort reality must become aligned with the primary expectations of the given academic track for a given faculty member.
- The official (public) and unofficial (not public) criteria for promotion should be appreciated by faculty and their respective career development committee.

For Discussion with a Mentor or Colleague

- Can you please share with me examples of well-crafted Personal Statements for successfully promoted faculty in our specialty?
- Can you please help me develop a career development committee? If so, are you able and willing to lead the committee?
- What are some creative strategies to engage as a way to mitigate some of the COVID-19-related challenges to the traditional geographic work environment within academic radiation oncology?
- Based on what you've observed as to my strengths and weaknesses, can you please advise me how to discern which committee service obligation are potentially high-impact and which ones are likely to be an unrewarding time sink for me?
- Can you please help evaluate and re-evaluate my short-term, intermediate-term, and long-term career development plan so that it's aligned with metrics for promotion at my current and/or future radiation oncology department?

Appendix

OHSU Educator's Portfolio [permission has been granted by the OHSU Legal Counsel]

University of Washington Department of Radiation Oncology promotion and tenure document [permission has been granted courtesy of Ramesh Rengan]

OHSU Educator's Portfolio

Note: This model was influenced by the AAMC's Group on Educational Affairs Consensus Conference on Educational Scholarship (2/06, Charlotte, NC). Findings published in: Simpson D, Fincher RM, Hafler JP, Irby DM, Richards BF, Rosenfeld GC, Viggiano TR. Advancing Educators and Education: Defining the Components and Evidence of Educational Scholarship. Medical Education 2007:41(10):1002-1009.

Educator Activity Categories. These five educator activity categories emerge from the literature as common formats in presenting educational contributions for academic promotion. They define the contents appropriate for inclusion in academic promotion documents.

a. **Direct Teaching:** Any activity that fosters learning, including direct teaching and creation of associated instructional materials. Examples of direct teaching include lectures, workshops, small-group facilitation, role modeling in any setting (such as ward attending), precepting, demonstration of procedural skills, and facilitation of online courses.
b. **Curriculum Development:** A longitudinal set of systematically designed, sequenced and evaluated educational activities occurring at any training level or venue.
c. **Mentoring and Advising:** Mentoring: a sustained, committed relationship from which both parties obtain reciprocal benefits. Advising: a more limited relationship than mentoring that usually occurs over a limited period, with the advisor serving as a guide.
d. **Educational Leadership and Administration:** Leadership of educational programs which involves achieving results through vigorous pursuit of excellence such as ongoing evaluation, dissemination of results, and maximization of resources. Examples include positions such as director of courses, clerkships, residencies, fellowships, graduate programs and leadership of education committees such as curriculum and course committees, admissions committees, and accreditation committees.
e. **Learner Assessment:** All activities associated with measuring learners' knowledge, skills, and attitudes which includes one or more of the following: development, implementation, analysis, or synthesis and presentation of the assessment tool or strategy.

Two overriding principles for documenting educator's activities cross all five categories:

- **Excellence:** *Quantity* – descriptive information regarding the types and frequencies of education activities and roles; and *Quality* – evidence of effectiveness and excellence in the activity, using comparative measures when available
- **Engagement with the education community:** Engagement is demonstrated by a scholarly approach to the education activity (i.e. learning from relevant education literature and best practices) and scholarship (i.e. creating a product that is reviewed by peers for quality and made public for others to learn from and build upon).

The purpose of this document is to assist faculty in documenting educational activity for promotion and tenure through an Educator's Portfolio (EP) approach. Your EP should present a summary of your contributions in education and should not be longer than necessary to paint a picture of the quantity and quality of work, generally not exceeding 10 pages. Note: Supporting materials such as teaching evaluations will be uploaded as part of your promotion packet and do not need to be included in your EP document.

Presenting Evidence of Quantity, Quality, and Engagement for Educator Activities

Suggested documentation templates and examples are included in the **Appendix** in the following five Educator Portfolio categories: **Direct Teaching, Curriculum Development, Mentoring and Advising, Educational Administration and Leadership,** and **Assessment of Learner Performance.** The examples in the Appendix are intended to provide a broad range of possible contributions and accomplishments in each category.

Use **only** applicable categories and emphasize activities of the last 5 years. For each applicable category, provide evidence of: Quantity, Quality and, if appropriate, Evidence of Engagement with the Community of Educators.

NOTE: Faculty are NOT expected to contribute in all categories but for those with education as a prominent aspect of their job, more than one category is expected in their promotion portfolio.

Direct Teaching

Educator's Portfolio Format

1. Evidence of Quantity:
   a. Document the frequency and duration of teaching along with a description of your role. Indicate the type and number of learners involved in the activity. For consideration of OHSU faculty promotion, the recipients of the teaching activities would be trainees in any of OHSU's training programs. For faculty members who have recently transferred from another school of medicine, the recipients can be trainees at the prior institution.
   b. Summarize teaching activities that are ongoing or recurrent rather than listing them separately each year
   c. Separate learner categories if you teach at multiple levels (e.g., students, residents/fellows, faculty/peers)
   d. Some continuing professional education activities may be more appropriately listed as a Scholarship activity depending on the venue and the sponsorship of the event.
   NOTE: Some education provided to patients or community groups may be more appropriately listed as a Service activity rather than a Teaching activity.
2. Evidence of Quality:
   a. Summarize learner evaluations using standard rating scales or narrative comments; comparative ratings for each year should be given and compared to peer group/normative data whenever possible
   b. Indicate when additional details are available in Teaching Quality Documents
   c. Include *internal* peer review of specific teaching activities by members of your division, department or course director/committee, if available
   d. Invitations to teach outside department or school
   e. Repeat invitations to teach to the same group or in the same course
   f. Teaching awards, including criteria for judgment and selection
3. Evidence of Engagement with the Community of Educators
   a. Descriptions of how teaching approach or uses of instructional materials are informed by educational literature or "best practices"
   b. Presentation in a peer-reviewed or invited forum at a regional/national meeting

    c. *External* peer review of teaching and/or instructional material (cite where and how peer reviewed)
    d. Data demonstrating adoption by other faculty
    e. Inclusion in a national repository of teaching materials, e.g. AAMC MedEdPORTAL

Curriculum Development

Definition: Curriculum is defined as a longitudinal set – that is, more than one or two teaching sessions – of designed educational activities that includes evaluation. To include an activity in the curriculum category, educators must define the purpose (goals) and describe the specific methods chosen to maximize the learning experience and evaluate effectiveness of the curriculum. Curriculum includes both the content of the training activity and the methods for helping learners develop the important knowledge and skills. It is not simply a set of written materials used in a course. The description of the curriculum must include a description of how the educational goals will be met and how learner success will be evaluated.

Educator's Portfolio Format

1. Evidence of Quantity:
    a. Describe your role and contribution to the curriculum. If the curriculum was co-authored include your role, content contributed and expertise provided.
    b. Include description of curriculum purpose, intended audience, duration, design and evaluation.
    c. Summarize methods used including innovative approaches or techniques for teaching or evaluating learners
2. Evidence of Quality:
    a. Summarize learner reactions or ratings of curriculum
    b. Outcomes, including impact on learning (e.g. pre- and post- curriculum knowledge/skill acquisition)
    c. Include peer review by members of your division, department or curriculum committee, if available
    d. Invitations to develop or collaborate on similar curriculum outside department or school
3. Evidence of Engagement with the Community of Educators
    a. Descriptions of how curriculum approach or uses of instructional/evaluation materials are informed by educational literature or "best practices"
    b. Presentation of curriculum work in a peer-reviewed or invited forum at a regional/national meeting
    c. Peer review of curriculum (cite where and how peer reviewed)
    d. Data demonstrating adoption of curriculum by other departments or schools
    e. Invitations to provide curriculum consultation for other departments or schools
    f. Inclusion in a national repository of curriculum, e.g. AAMC MedEdPORTAL

Advising and Mentoring

Definitions:
- *Advising*: a more limited relationship than mentoring that usually occurs over a limited period, with the advisor serving as a guide.
- *Mentoring:* a sustained, committed relationship from which both parties obtain reciprocal benefits.

Educator's Portfolio Format

1. Evidence of Quantity:
   a. List each advisee or protégé, his/her level of training or rank, purpose or specific goals of the relationship
   b. Describe the process of advising/mentoring (duration, frequency and nature of contact
   c. Include current status of advisee or protégé
2. Evidence of Quality:
   a. Evaluations of advising and mentoring effectiveness from advisees/protégés
   b. Numbers of advisee or protégés choosing you to assist them in accomplishing their goals.
   c. Listing of advisees'/protégés' significant accomplishments including publications, presentations, grants, awards, goal attainment, resolution of problem
3. Evidence of Engagement with the Community of Educators
   a. Participation in professional development activities to enhance skills in advising and mentoring
   b. Developing or leading initiatives that improve departmental or institutional advising and mentoring practices
   c. Conducting mentor skill enhancement training sessions that advance the field of mentoring or assist other individuals in being more effective in their mentoring
   d. Serving as a mentoring consultant to departments
   e. Secure program development funding for advising and mentoring

Educational Administration and Leadership

Definition: Activities associated with leadership of educational programs which involves achieving results through vigorous pursuit of excellence such as ongoing evaluation, dissemination of results, and maximization of resources.

Educator's Portfolio Format

1. Evidence of Quantity:
   a. Describe your educational administrative roles, responsibilities and the duration. Include positions as director of courses, clerkships, residencies, fellowships, graduate programs.

   b. Describe the nature of the educational leadership projects you have undertaken including your role and their duration (e.g. residency program task force to develop competency-based evaluation tools).

    c. Include service or leadership on education committees such as curriculum and course committees, admissions committees, ad-hoc committees that advise on education programs, institutional education committees, accreditation committees.
2. Evidence of Quality:
    a. Data demonstrating achievement of goals
    b. Evaluations of your performance as a leader with peer comparisons, if available
    c. Program or project outcomes such as learner evaluations of training program, accreditation results
3. Evidence of Engagement with the Community of Educators
    a. Documentation of ongoing quality improvement
    b. Evidence of innovative approaches used in program or project management
    c. Resources garnered for program enhancements or expansion
    d. Presentation of program or project in a peer-reviewed or invited forum at a regional/national meeting
    e. Data demonstrating adoption of program or project innovation by other departments or schools
    f. Invitations to provide consultation to other departments or schools

Learner Assessment

Definition: Activities associated with developing or improving a learner assessment process or instrument.

Educator's Portfolio Format

1. Evidence of Quantity:
    a. Provide a brief description of the assessment activity.
    b. Describe your role in the development, implementation, analysis or synthesis and presentation of the assessment activity.
    c. Document the size and nature of the learner population being assessed, the scope of the assessment and the intended uses of the information.
2. Evidence of Quality and Engagement with the Community of Educators:
    a. Measures of reliability and validity appropriate to the type of assessment
    b. Evidence that the new approach improves upon previous approaches
    c. Presentations on the assessment process or outcomes to local audiences, such as curriculum committees
    d. Peer-reviewed presentations and workshops at professional meetings about the assessment strategy
    e. Acceptance of the assessment tool in a peer-reviewed repository

APPENDIX

Educator's Portfolio Documentation Examples for Direct Teaching:

STUDENTS

Teaching Activity/Role	Year	Quantity	# Learners	Quality	Evidence of Engagement with the Community of Educators
Student Lectures/Small Group Seminars/Practicum					
Required Clerkship Seminar Leader	2004-05	16hrs per rotation; 8 rotations per year	8-12 per rotation	For 2004-2005: "Was an effective seminar leader"; Mean rating = 5.41 on a 7-point scale (mean for all clerkship faculty = 4.89)*	Presented methods used in this seminar to teach student use of EBM at national society meeting
Epidemiology I	2004-present	3 lectures/yr	30 students per course	Course director invited me to include my lectures in another course at Portland State	
Physiology Lab Course	2005-present	4hrs/week during12 week course	12 per course	"Outstanding teaching reviews" as reported by course director	
Research Practicum Experience	2006	100 hrs of research internship each	2 MPH students	One student submitted manuscript, "Medical Debt and Access to Health Care"	
Student Clinical Teaching					
Principles of Clinical Medicine Preceptorship	2006, 2007	120hrs/yr	One MS1 student	4.4 average student rating on a 5-point scale (mean for all preceptors = 4.7)*	
Inpatient Attending	2002-present	6 weeks/yr	12/yr	4.7 average student rating on a 5-point scale	Developed new evaluation tool adopted by other inpatient faculty to assess student oral presentation skills
Clerkship Lectures	2007, 2008	2 lectures per rotation; 8 rotations per year	8 per rotation	No formal evaluations	

RESIDENTS & FELLOWS

Teaching Activity/Role	Year	Quantity	# Learners	Quality	Evidence of Engagement with the Community of Educators
Resident & Fellow Lectures/Small Group Seminars					
Noon Conferences	2004-present	6 lectures/yr on clinical topics	20 per lecture	No formal evaluation	
Journal Club Presenter	2006-present	4/year	10 per session	Residents identify this as an important part of their overall residency training	
Ethics Seminar	2007	2 half-day workshops per yr	20 per workshop	Time allotted expanded from 1 to 2 half days due to resident demand	Developed 4 instructional cases that have been adapted by 2 other departments for resident education
Resident & Fellow Clinical Teaching					
Clinic Precepting	2006, 2007	2 ½ days per week	3-4 residents per clinic	See Teaching Quality Documents 2007 Resident Teacher of the Year Award	
Inpatient Attending	2002-present	6 weeks/yr	12 residents per yr	See Teaching Quality Documents	

OTHER LEARNERS

Teaching Activity/Role	Year	Quantity	# Learners	Quality	Evidence of Engagement with the Community of Educators
Multiple Level Learners					
Interdisciplinary Surgery Conference	2006 - present	monthly	Students, residents, fellows, faculty	Increased attendance by multiple members of health care team from 5 departments	
Department Grand Rounds	2005, 2007	1/year	Students, residents, fellows, faculty	4.8 average rating on a 5-point scale	Invited to give 2007 topic at 2 other regional hospital Grand rounds
ACLS Course instructor	2007, 2008	2 lectures and 2 workshops per course	30 per course	Invited to become certified as a course director	
CME					
Statewide Ethics Conference (one day conference)	2008	Conference Director	250 participants from all sectors of health care	Conference was over subscribed; overall conf ratings very high	Funding obtained from sponsoring institutions to support this as an annual conference

Educator's Portfolio Documentation Examples for Curriculum Development:

Example #1
Title: Evidence-Based Medicine (EBM) series within PCM course

Role: Series Coordinator - responsible for organizing instruction and recruiting small group leaders. Collaborated with faculty from 2 other departments to develop learning objectives and instructional materials

Purpose/Need: Develop a new EBM series for all first year students that is clinically relevant

Intended Audience: First year medical students

Duration: 12 week course held each year

Methods/Design: Multi-method approach including interactive lecture series and clinical vignettes (6 two-hour sessions), small group projects spanning 12 weeks (format and materials developed for use by groups culminating in brief group presentations to entire class). Projects scored using a novel Impact Checklist.

Significant Results & Outcomes: Rated as one of the best components of the first year PCM course. Improved GOSCE performance on EBM module.

Dissemination: Impact Checklist for evaluating EBM student projects accepted for presentation (peer-reviewed) at 2009 Educational Society Meeting

Example #2
Title: Ultrasound Rotation for Emergency Medicine residents

Role: Rotation Coordinator - responsible for organizing instruction and schedule. Collaborated with faculty from radiology and emergency medicine departments to develop competencies and instructional materials. Accumulated a library of images for teaching cases

Purpose/Need: The curriculum is intended to teach emergency medicine residents about the use of diagnostic ultrasound in the emergency department setting

Intended Audience: 2nd year emergency medicine residents; elective chosen by 6 residents per year on average

Duration: 4 week rotation

Methods/Design: 1:1 instruction with radiologist; self- directed learning using teaching cases

Significant Results & Outcomes: Favorable ratings from residents. Working with Emergency Medicine Program Director to incorporate teaching cases as standard part of their conference series.

Dissemination: none

Example #3

Title: Self-learning CD-Rom on Cardiac Physiology

Role: Co-designer - responsible for content and developing interactive lecture. Collaborated with Information Technology department to produce CD.

Purpose/Need: The CD is intended to give medical students additional instructional materials to learn cardiac physiology

Intended Audience: 1st and 2nd year medical students

Duration: NA

Methods/Design: CD includes 4 lectures with slide notes, illustrative cases followed by questions for self discovery and appropriate current medical literature. A pre and post assessment of learning is being developed.

Significant Results & Outcomes: Plan to study student performance on cardiac physiology segment of overall Physiology course.

Dissemination: Obtained a grant from a professional society to distribute the CD to all medical schools

Example #4

Title: Gross Anatomy for Graduate Students

Role: Course director

Purpose/Need: This course is designed to prepare graduate students to be able to teach Gross Anatomy in a professional school

Intended Audience: 3rd year and above graduate students

Duration: 12 week course, every year

Methods/Design: The course is a mixture of lectures, dissection laboratory sessions, and small group discussions on teaching methods

Significant Results & Outcomes: Graduate students who have gone on to become successful teachers in Gross Anatomy courses

Dissemination: None

Educator's Portfolio Documentation Examples for *Advising and Mentoring*:

Name of Advisee or Protégé	Level of Advisee or Protégé	Purpose of Relationship	Duration and Process	Current Status of Protégé	Outcome(s) of Relationship
Charles X (Protégé)	Medical Student	• Development of professional goals • Career guidance in service of minority health care	9/2001–present • Met 4-5 times per year • Edit paper, CV • Advocate for LCME liaison position • Provided shadowing clinical experience	Internal Medicine Resident	• MD received 2006 • Published essay in *Acad Medicine* • Appointment as AAMC Student Liaison to LCME
Kimberly Y (Advisee)	Junior Faculty	Preparation of academic promotion documents	8/05-12/05 • 1-on-1 + e-mail • Revise/reframe CV and portfolio • Consult with department chair re: letter of rec	Associate Professor	Promoted 6/06 to Associate Professor
Ron Z (Advisee)	Graduate student	• Masters Thesis advisor • Career guidance in biomedical research	7/2006 -10/2007 • 1-on-1 meetings • Review thesis • Collaborate on manuscripts	Enrolled in PhD program	• MS received 2008 • Nominated for Outstanding Master's Thesis Award • Published manuscript in J Biochemistry • Presented at the Society for Biochemistry Research Annual Meeting, Atlanta April 2007

Educator's Portfolio Documentation Examples for *Educational Administration and Leadership:*

Year	Time Commitment	Administrative or Leadership Role	Description of Activities	Quality	Outcomes
2006-07	0.2 FTE	Associate Residency Director	Develop curriculum, design educational methods and evaluation; oversee resident clinical schedules; liaison to community training sites	• Highly competitive residency with 100% fill rates • Invited to chair special Dean's task force on evaluation	• Co-authored RRC site visit document-achieved full accreditation • Procedure tracking system adopted by 3 other departments • 2 national presentations of community training programs
2007-present	Monthly meetings	MD/PhD Program Committee member	Sets policy and curriculum for MD/PhD program	Not assessed	Prepared materials for LCME site visit
2006	Task Force met for 6 months	Resident Evaluation Task Force member	Re-designed all resident evaluation tools to be aligned with ACGME competencies	Completed task force goals prior to start of academic year	New tools implemented beginning July 2007
2005-present	80 hours/year	Co-Director, Advanced Topics in Cancer Biology	Organize schedule and instructors, attend classes, review student work and grade students	Student ratings of overall quality = 4.2 on 5 point scale	Continues to be course offering each year in graduate program

Educator's Portfolio Documentation Examples for *Learner Assessment:*

Example #1
Assessment Activity: OSCE to assess mental health screening skills

Role: Collaborated with a multidisciplinary team to create 4 cases including clinical scenario and standardized patient roles/scripts. Performed a literature review on the use of OSCEs to teach mental health skills as a basis for the cases. Developed the observed behavior checklist tool for each case and oriented faculty evaluators to the tool.

Learner Population to be Assessed: First year residents at the start of their behavior health rotation (12 residents per year)

Methods/Design: Mental health OSCE is required component of Behavioral Health rotation. The four cases represent a spectrum of commonly encountered mood disorders in primary care. Each resident performs the OSCE, is rated by a faculty and a peer, and receives formative feedback on performance.

Significant Results & Outcomes: Residents and evaluators showed a high degree of satisfaction with the OSCE as a method to assess skills and highlight areas for improvement and learning

Dissemination: OSCE design and implementation presented as department Grand Rounds. Initial results of OSCE used in grant application to obtain funding to expand mental health training in residency

**University of Washington School of Medicine
Department of Radiation Oncology**

Guidelines for
Appointment and Promotion

Adopted by Radiation Oncology Department June 2012
Approved by UW A&P Committee June 2012

Revision Adopted by Radiation Oncology Department December 2018
Revision Approved by UW A&P Committee December 2018

**University of Washington School of Medicine
Department of Radiation Oncology
Guidelines for Appointment and Promotion**

Table of Contents

University of Washington School of Medicine
Department of Radiation Oncology
Guidelines for Appointment and Promotion

I.   Guidelines Overview

This document is used by the Department of Radiation Oncology to provide guidance for faculty members in understanding what is required for appointments and promotions within the department. In the initial part of the document (sections II – III) performance criteria for promotion are described. In the second part of the document (section IV) guidelines for appointment and promotion at specific ranks and titles are described. Appointments will be based on an assessment of the candidate's professional training, record of achievements, and level of peer recognition within his/her field of expertise. Assessments for promotion will be based on well-documented achievements in the areas of teaching, administrative service, clinical practice, research and professionalism that the faculty member has performed. A third part of the document (section V) describes how the faculty member's performance will be measured based on their level of performance, and allocation of effort, in the areas of their job focus.

In accord with the University's expressed commitment to excellence and equity, any contributions in scholarship and research, teaching, and service that address diversity and equal opportunity shall be included and considered among the professional and scholarly qualifications for appointment and promotion outlined below.

II. General Guidelines for Appointment and Promotion

Conferring a professorial rank is a means of acknowledging notable contributions of faculty members to the University and to their disciplines. Promotion is not granted as a reward for long-term service, but rather to recognize those who have excelled in specific aspects of the academic mission.

University guidelines for the appointment and promotion of faculty members are found in the University Policy Directory, and in particular Volume II, Part II, Chapter 24 of the Faculty Code found on-line at: http://www.washington.edu/admin/rules/policies/RoadMap.html and

http://www.washington.edu/admin/rules/policies/FCG/FCCH24.html

Listed below are further guidelines for promotion of faculty in the Department of Radiation Oncology. The general criteria of quality and productivity in each area of academic activity: *Teaching, Research/Scholarship, Clinical Practice, and Departmental Service* are described in this document. The criteria are applicable for regular and research faculty.

The criteria for appointment or promotion in the Department of Radiation Oncology are predicated on adoption of a single, broadly-based academic appointment that will encourage and reward performance in all aspects of the department's mission and achieve or exceed a standard in teaching, administrative service contributions, professionalism, research / scholarship, creativity, and clinical practice; recognizing that scholarly contributions as defined in this document are a requisite for academic appointment and promotion. Both quality of overall performance, admittedly a subjective measure, and quantity of achievement will be considered important determinants of a recommendation for promotion.

These Guidelines apply to all faculty (radiation oncologists, medical physicists, radiobiologists, radiochemists, and other non-physicians) within the Department of Radiation Oncology, School of Medicine. It is advisable that all faculty members within the department familiarize themselves with the content of these guidelines so as to begin the documentation of their activities in anticipation of applying for promotion at some time in the future.

General Criteria Considered in Promotion of a Faculty Member (adapted from the UW Faculty code) are as follows:

Effective Teaching: Originality, innovation, and creativity in teaching are highly prized and specially rewarded. The quality of teaching, along with scholarship, will be weighed heavily in determining eligibility for promotion. Effective teaching is evaluated by the ability to organize and promote learning at the appropriate level and with appropriate subject matter, to incorporate up-to-date information, to stimulate intellectual student discussion and debate, and the ability to test and use new approaches to education at the undergraduate, graduate and continuing education levels. A review of evaluation materials from the Department's teaching evaluation program will be considered. The opinions of students, and colleagues and student and resident performance, measured by the resident's score card, are important in this evaluation. Establishing a positive learning environment is required. A review of the number and quality of teaching interactions with students, residents, fellows, practicing physicians, and other healthcare providers will influence the rating of the individual seeking promotion. Any teaching performance that addresses diversity and equal opportunities shall be considered among the qualifications for appointment and promotion.

Competence in Administrative Service: Competence in administrative service is evaluated by demonstration of effective participation on committees, in administrative functions, clinical duties, special training programs, continuing education, and community services to schools, industry, and state, local, national and international organizations and governments. Administrative service is deemed of equal importance compared to other criteria.

The Department's success requires effective administration of its teaching and clinical programs. Hence, it is expected that a high percentage of key administrative positions within our Department, School of Medicine, and the faculty's site of practice will be filled with active faculty clinicians. At the time of promotion, each faculty member will provide a description of his/her activities relating to this type of service which will include committee membership.

Professionalism: Professionalism is valued by the University and Department and is expected to be evident among its faculty in carrying out UW Medicine's mission of improving the health of the public through teaching, research and patient care. Professionalism includes demonstrating excellence, integrity, respect, compassion, accountability, and a commitment to altruism in our work interactions and responsibilities. It is expected that faculty will conduct themselves in a professional manner in all of their interactions with patients, members of the public and the University community, and each other. This requirement is to promote excellence, integrity and altruism in all of our activities; to assure that all persons are treated with respect, dignity and courtesy; and to promote constructive communication and collaborative teamwork.

Research/Scholarship: Scholarship is evaluated by effectiveness of teaching, research, and contribution to knowledge through publications, lectures, and conference presentations. Its quality is reflected in the national and international scientific reputation of the faculty member and in the performance of his/her students or trainees. Evaluation of scholarship will be based upon review of the number and quality of journal publications, chapters, textbooks, contributions on clinical and/or educational research projects, and invited presentations at regional, national, and international meetings. Scholarly contributions may focus on clinical medicine, health services, applied clinical research, medical education, or other relevant fields. Objective evidence of scholarship will be required for advancement. Any research and scholarship that addresses diversity and equal opportunity shall be considered for among the qualifications for appointment and promotion.

Creativity: The University recognizes that clinicians and other academics may perform a number of time and energy consuming duties essential to the role of the University in relation to health professionals and the community. These activities contribute to the candidate's function as a role model to other members of the profession and the public as a recognized expert for trainees. Creativity is evaluated by quality and quantity of published work, range and variety of intellectual interests, grant and fellowship awards and success in training graduate and professional students. Creativity is manifested through professional innovation (inventions, patents and licenses, new techniques, conceptual innovations, etc.); exemplary professional practice (instrumental in the introduction and dissemination of an invention, new technique, conceptual innovation, educational program, etc.); or contributions to the development of professional practices (guidelines development, health policy development, government policy, diversity, equity and inclusion policy consensus conference statements, regulatory committees and setting of standards. Membership and holding office in professional organizations in itself is not considered evidence of creativity.

III. Performance Criteria for Promotion

Overview

Faculty members will be evaluated for promotion based on the percentage effort, as defined in their job description, in the categories of *teaching, clinical and administrative service, and Research/Scholarship*. All Faculty members are expected to spend a *minimum of 5% of their time on administrative service*. Except for Research Faculty and Clinical Faculty, all Faculty members are expected to spend *a minimum of 10% time on teaching*. The expectations for a Faculty member's effort (defined as a % time) in each of the four categories will be determined by his/her job description, outlined at the time of hire. It is expected that the job description outlining specific roles, responsibilities and duties will be reviewed during each performance evaluation. Changes in the job description, and % effort in the categories, will be negotiated between the Faculty member and the Department Chair.

Descriptions of what constitutes the specific measurements of performance are provided below. Specific examples of performance within each category are provided in Section II.1 – II.5

- **Superior Performance**: A Faculty member demonstrates superior performance by *exceeding expectations* in multiple areas of the specific category over a sustained period.

- **Satisfactory Performance:** A Faculty member demonstrates satisfactory performance if he/she consistently meets expectations in all areas of the specific category.

- **Unsatisfactory Performance:** A Faculty member demonstrates unsatisfactory performance if he/she fails to meet the expectations of that specific category.

- **Unacceptable performance:** A faculty member demonstrates unacceptable performance if he/she consistently under-performs in any of areas of the specific category.

Each Faculty member is expected to maintain at least a satisfactory rating in every category as defined by their faculty track/pathway.

III.1 Teaching

Promotion requires that the candidate has contributed in a meaningful way to the achievement of the Department's and the University's educational mission. This includes public and external education. The nature, quantity and quality of these contributions will be evaluated with reference to departmental norms, and expectations consistent with job descriptions and career pathways, and academic, and where applicable, clinical responsibilities.

The evaluation of teaching performance will be conducted in accordance with the standards outlined and be influenced by the percentage weighting of teaching in the Faculty member's job description. With the exception of Research Faculty and Clinical Faculty appointments, each Faculty member is expected to have a teaching component in the job description (minimum 10%) and is expected to engage in regular professional development for the purpose of enhancing their teaching skills. While a Clinical Faculty member is not expected to have a teaching component, there may be exceptions which will be specified in the faculty member's job description. In those occasions, the teaching component for that clinical faculty member will be adjusted based on their site of practice and may be greater or less than 10% depending on the opportunities available for teaching. Teaching shall include educational efforts directed at undergraduate, graduate, and continuing education. The effectiveness in the performance of teaching will be measured by teaching evaluations including evaluations by undergraduate students, medical students, residents, fellows, and peers. Ensuring documentation of teaching evaluation data is the responsibility of the faculty member and should include evaluation of hands-on patient-based teaching in the clinic, faculty-led resident didactic conferences and lectures, departmental lectures and grand rounds presentations, peer-to-peer reviews, and resident/fellow rotation instruction. Two trainees will be asked to submit a letter attesting to the faculty member's ability to teach as part of the promotion packet, if there is a teaching component in the faculty member's job description. The attestations should be from trainees within the last three years. Teaching evaluations are expected annually and peer evaluation are expected annually for Assistant Professors and at least every three years for Associate and full Professors and the year before promotion from Associate Professor to Professor.

Teaching will take many forms including, didactic lectures, small group or case-based learning, bedside clinical teaching, seminars, and/or research training. Candidates seeking promotion on the basis of excellence in education and teaching must demonstrate superior (significant and high quality) contributions to teaching and/or other education related activities.

Examples:

Superior Teaching Performance:
    a. Evaluations in the top 10% of teachers
    b. Nominations for and/or receipt of one or more departmental, institutional, local or national teaching awards
    c. Contributions to course and/or curriculum development
    d. Development and/or participation in professional development activities focusing on medical, physics, or biomedical education, including:
        i. Recognition of teaching talent by selection to a major educational postgraduate education and/or continuous professional learning
        ii. Directorship of a graduate training, residency, or fellowship program
        iii. Coordination or participation in an undergraduate, medical student, resident or fellow teaching block in the medical curriculum
        iv. Chairing of a major faculty, departmental or hospital education-related committee

Superior teachers will have published education-related research or experiences in prestigious medical or basic sciences journals, presented papers or posters at national and international educational/professional meetings and encouraged trainees in these endeavors. They will be regular and/or invited participants in the Faculty's continuous professional development efforts and/or actively participated in Faculty departmental or divisional continuing medical education events including departmental, multidisciplinary group or institutional presentations/lectures such as grand rounds.

Leadership in the educational forums shall be considered a measure of superior performance and include activities as identified above, but also the development, implementation and/or evaluation of innovative teaching methods. Superior teachers shall be identified by their role-modeling impact as evidenced by unsolicited testimonials from peers or trainees. They will have accepted formal or informal mentorship relationships with undergraduate students, medical students, residents, fellows or junior faculty.

Satisfactory Teaching Performance:
    a. Fulfillment of their assigned teaching duties within the context of their job description
    b. Satisfactory evaluations of their teaching activities by students, residents, fellows, and peers
    c. Participation in formal evaluations of students, residents, fellows, and peers
    d. Demonstrated commitment to personal professional development of their teaching skills by participation in teaching enhancement activities
    e. Consistent active participation in departmental teaching activities such as, didactic lectures, chart and QA rounds, when appropriate

Abstract presentations at educational meetings and participation in local professional development efforts are expected if the individual has a significant clinical educator/administrator role or if they are more senior educators.

An effective teacher will have the following attributes. One is not expected to have all of these attributes; however, candidates seeking promotion on the basis of excellence in teaching would be expected to show greater evidence of three or more of these attributes:
    a. Mastery of the subject area
    b. Skill in one or more of : lecturing to large groups, facilitation of small groups, one-to-one

teaching, and supervision and mentoring
- i. The ability to effectively employ appropriate educational methods
- ii. The ability to stimulate and challenge the intellectual capacity of learners
- iii. The ability to influence students' intellectual development and development of critical skills and critical thinking
- c. Be a professional and educational role model
- d. Professionalism in teaching that includes respect for students and colleagues, sensitivity to diversity; ability for self-assessment and participation in ongoing professional development and accessibility to learners.

Unsatisfactory Teaching Performance:
- a. Inconsistent teaching evaluations with several below average scores without consistent and sustained improvement over time.
- b. A lack of commitment to professional development in the area of teaching
- c. Lack of participation in mentorship activities with students, residents, fellows or other postgraduate trainees.
- d. Non-active participation in didactic lectures, chart and QA rounds, when appropriate

Faculty in this category may also have few scholarly contributions to local or national educational endeavors.

Unacceptable Teaching Performance:
- a. Consistent under-performance in teaching activities and duties
- b. Unwillingness to participate in teaching activities such as lectures, small group seminars and didactic sessions, clinical bedside teaching, mentorship activities
- c. Consistent poor evaluations of teaching activities, such as didactic presentations; poor evaluations of clinical or research trainee supervision
- d. Failure to participate in continuing medical education
- e. No evidence of scholarly contributions to educational endeavors.

Documented unprofessional or unethical behavior including discrimination or harassment of any group in the teaching role is considered unacceptable, as is unresponsiveness to recommendation for professional development of teaching or supervisory skills.

III.2 Administrative Service

Service within the University and to external agencies forms an important and often time-consuming aspect of many faculty members' academic careers. In providing this service, they contribute to the continued excellence of the academic environment and allow the University a voice and visibility in external agencies. Although service in itself cannot be the main criteria for promotion, the department may consider service in support of the mission of the University and Department.

The evaluation of a Faculty member's administrative service performance will be influenced by the negotiated percentage in the Faculty member's job description. Each Faculty member is expected to provide at least 5% administrative service to his/her professional discipline, the Department of Radiation Oncology, UW Medical School or the University of Washington. Administrative service to the discipline includes leadership responsibilities for professional societies (e.g., holding office, chairing committees, organizing meetings), responsibilities for review of research proposals (e.g., ad hoc external reviews, grants panels, site visits, advisory committees) and/or review of research publications (e.g., article reviews, editorial boards). Administrative service to the Department of Radiation Oncology includes membership and/or chairing of committees, running residency training programs, and/or leadership positions (e.g., Department Chair or Vice Chair). Administrative service to the School of Medicine or University includes serving as Associate/Assistant Deans, Division Leaders, Directors, or Program Directors. Administrative service to the public in a Faculty member's professional capacity include communication of expertise to government, lay audience education and voluntary professional services.

Examples:

Superior Administrative Service Performance: Contributions can be related to research or education and include contributions to the discipline such as
  a. serving as Chair of grants panel or site visit,
  b. serving as editor of a high-impact journal,
  c. organizing a major national or international conference, or
  d. serving as president of a professional organization;
  e. recognition by receipt of a service award from a professional society would be considered meritorious.

Superior effective leadership in coordination of teaching programs, chairing major committees, developing significant new educational or clinical initiatives and leadership of multidisciplinary tumor board groups is expected.

Satisfactory Administrative Service Performance:
  a. being a member of an ad hoc review of research proposals and articles
  b. serving on a grants panel, editorial board or conference organizing committee
  c. holding office or committee membership in a professional organization
  d. serving on teaching, administrative and/or quality-assurance committees
  e. participating in policy development
  f. organizing for the department

For a Faculty member whose job description is greater than 30% research, some administrative service to the discipline (e.g., journal or grant reviews, service on grant panels, a research ethics board and/or office in professional societies) is expected.

Unsatisfactory Administrative Service Performance:
  a. consistently failing to participate in discipline-related activities
  b. making minimal contributions to the organizational efforts of the Department; and/or
  c. having frequent absences from the departmental meetings

Unacceptable Administrative Service Performance:
  a. refuse to participate in at least one Department/Faculty/University committee
  b. refuse to peer review journal articles or grant applications
  c. refuse to contribute to quality assurance efforts
  d. being asked to withdraw from a review or other committee for ethical reasons (e.g., breach of confidentiality)
  e. providing inadequate supervision of a program resulting in loss of funding or accreditation, or

f.   providing inaccurate information to the public

III.3 Professionalism

It is the policy that all faculty members of the Department of Radiation Oncology should behave in a professional manner at all times. They will conduct themselves appropriately in interactions with patients, colleagues, trainees, staff, and students. Faculty should promote communication and teamwork in their interactions. Professionalism refers to demonstrating integrity, respect, dignity, courtesy, and a commitment to excellence. An individual's professional behavior will be an important factor in evaluation for appointment and promotion for all faculty appointment tracks. Interaction with other professionals includes, but is not limited to, front desk personnel, intake staff, medical assistants, nurses, therapists, dosimetrists, physician assistants, nurse practitioners, administrative staff, residents, and physicians.

Excellence represents a dedication to the continuous improvement of the quality of care, research inquiry, and teaching effectiveness. Pursuit of excellence should be accompanied by integrity, empathy, compassion, and respect for the diversity of values and opinions of others.

Accountability refers to taking responsibility for ones' behavior and activity.

Altruism reflects a commitment to advocate for the interest of others over ones' own interests.

Unprofessional behavior means behavior that violates laws or rules regarding discrimination and harassment; violates rules of professional ethics, including professionalism in clinical, educational, research or business practices; or is disrespectful, retaliatory or disruptive.

Discrimination and harassment means discrimination or harassment on the basis of race, color, creed, religion, national origin, citizenship, sex, age, marital status, sexual orientation, disability, or military status.

Professional ethics means ethical standards that have been established by external professional societies or associations, e.g., Joint Commission, American Association of Medical Colleges, National Institutes of Health, or by UW Medicine entities for various professions (e.g., physicians, physicists, nurses).

Professionalism in clinical practice settings includes, but is not limited to safeguarding the care needs and privacy concerns of patients and adherence to established standards on patient safety, timeliness of completing medical records, quality improvement initiatives, communication and follow-up with patients, reporting errors, and regulations governing billing practices.

Professionalism in the conduct of research includes, but is not limited to a commitment to intellectual integrity, welfare of human subjects and research animals, diligent and unbiased acquisition, evaluation, and reporting of scientific information, adherence to university research regulations, and collegial and fair treatment of trainees and research staff at all levels.

Professionalism in education includes, but is not limited to a commitment to the highest standards of scholarship, innovation in teaching methods, respect for the student-teacher relationship and learning environment, and leadership through modeling of life-long learning.

Ethical business practices means the wise use of resources and practices that are compliant with and appropriate under laws and regulations governing conflicts of interest, sponsored research, or the delivery of and reimbursement for healthcare services.

Disrespectful, retaliatory, or disruptive behavior includes, but is not limited to behaviors that in the view of reasonable people impact the integrity of the healthcare team, the care of patients, the education of trainees, or the conduct of research such as:

- Shouting or using profane or otherwise offensive language
- Degrading or demeaning comments
- Physical assault or other uninvited or inappropriate physical contact;
- Threats or similar intimidating behavior, as reasonably perceived by the recipient; unreasonable refusal to cooperate with others in carrying out assigned responsibilities; and
- Obstruction of established operational goals, beyond what would be considered respectful dissent.

III.4 Clinical Practice

The evaluation of clinical practice performance will be influenced by Faculty member's rank and the percentage in the Faculty member's job description. Evaluation of clinical competence will focus on two main areas: 1) fund of knowledge, technical expertise, problem-solving skills, management of complex patients, overall clinical skills, and mastery in implementation of evidence-based treatments; and 2) humanistic qualities, responsibility, compassion, integrity, professional behavior and attitudes, interpersonal skills, and effectiveness in working in multidisciplinary settings. The Faculty member must abide by the professional standards of his/her discipline. To demonstrate superior clinical practice, the candidate must show that his or her practice is recognized as exemplary by peers and has been emulated or otherwise had an impact on practice. Being a competent health care practitioner, while valuable to the public and profession, and for educational role-modeling, is not sufficient to meet the criterion of superior clinical practice performance.

Examples:

Superior Clinical Practice Performance:

a. Achieved substantive recognition at the regional, national and/or international level as a leader in his/her clinical area of expertise.
b. Exceptional recognition by peers or patient groups for exemplary patient care and/or clinical services
c. Exhibit a fund of knowledge, problem-solving skills, and the ability to successfully manage complex patients
d. Introduction or development of a new treatment approach or treatment paradigm, diagnostic or therapeutic strategy, procedure, or device
e. Evidence of initiative and leadership in clinical care such as leadership of multidisciplinary tumor board groups/teams, development of clinical programs, trials or research initiatives, participation in multi-institutional collaborations, coordination of efforts to improve quality of care through quality assurance (QA) measures, medical error reduction, or improved cost effectiveness
f. Serving as an advisor or resource or holding a leadership position in academic, national or government agencies/organizations (such as NIH/NCI, NCCN, RTOG, AMA, etc.)

g. Successful mentorship of junior faculty and trainees
h. The Faculty member is considered by their peers to be a role model of professional integrity and exhibit collegiality and cooperativeness

Satisfactory Clinical Practice Performance:

Providing the standard of care expected within their medical profession. This includes effective patient care and management of patient problems and clinical responsibilities on a day-to-day basis. It is the expectation that each Faculty member would be recognized as an expert in his/her area of expertise within the department and institution. Regular attendance and active participation in departmental meetings including faculty meetings, chart rounds, and grand rounds is expected. Faculty members are expected to work and interact in a collegial manner with staff within the department, through the institution and with others in the medical community. Participation and representation in multidisciplinary tumor board group conferences and clinics. The Faculty member does not have any formal complaints about them to the Department, Hospital or regulatory/licensing body and has demonstrated active participation in a regular maintenance of competence program and continuing professional development.

Unsatisfactory Clinical Practice Performance:

Demonstrated difficulties in performance of their clinical duties such as:
a. Significant gaps in one's fund of knowledge, technical expertise , overall clinical skills, or problem-solving skills
b. Delays or failures to complete medical records or other documents
c. Substantiated complaints filed about their interactions or communications with patients, families and/or colleagues
d. Failure to behave in a collegial manner and/or instances of significant conflicts with trainees, staff, or peers
e. Limited attention to maintenance of competence activities and continuing professional development

Unacceptable Clinical Practice Performance:

Egregious errors or behaviors; this would include:
a. Failure to exhibit a fund of knowledge, technical expertise, overall clinical skills, or problem-solving skills
b. Any form of substantiated unethical or unprofessional behavior
c. No evidence of activity dedicated to maintenance of competence and continuing professional development
d. Persistent failure to complete medical records or other documents
e. Persistent failure to interact with and communicate effectively with patients, families and/or colleagues, including clinical and administrative staff with numerous complaints and/or
f. Persistent failure to behave in a collegial manner or numerous significant conflicts with trainees, staff, or peers

Persistent, unjustified and significant deviation from generally-accepted practice guidelines or behavior, particularly after efforts of a remedial nature have been suggested or provided, would indicate that this categorization is appropriate.

III.5 Research/Scholarship Performance

Successful research leads to the advancement of knowledge through contributions of an original nature. Promotion to Associate or Full Professor based on research requires that the candidate has a record of sustained and current productivity in research and research-related activities. For the criterion of superior achievement in research to be met, the research should result in significant changes in the understanding of basic mechanisms of molecular or cellular function and disease, accuracy of predictive models, clinical care, health services delivery or health policy, or the social sciences and humanities as applied to health. The researcher's work should present creative insights, ideas or concepts, and must have yielded a significant quantity of information leading to new understanding. The new information may derive from the invention and/or application of new techniques, novel experimental approaches and/or the identification and formulation of new questions or concepts, those applicable to inclusion, diversity and equal opportunity. It is expected that research advances will be communicated through the publication of papers, reviews, books and other scholarly works.

Sources of funding may vary depending on the area of research. Not all research requires external funding. However, as a general rule, the individual seeking promotion on the basis of achievement in research should have a strong and continuing record of external funding commensurate with the type and area of research. Although usually recognition will be given to funding in the form of peer-reviewed grants, other sources may be appropriate. For example, funding from industry may be a major source available to basic and clinical scientists performing clinical trials, studying new drugs and developing new technologies. This funding is expected to comply with the conflict of interest guidelines in the School of Medicine.

The evaluation of Research/Scholarship performance will be conducted in accordance with the standards outlined below and will be influenced by Faculty member's rank and the percentage weighting of Research/Scholarship in the Faculty member's job description.

Examples:

Superior Research/Scholarship Performance: Publications of the research, obtaining research funding, presentations at professional meetings and supervising research efforts.

    a. having a substantial record of research productivity with either a landmark paper in a prestigious international journal or multiple papers in high-impact journals that make a significant impact on the field

    b. having a consistent successful record of funding in the form of multiple peer-reviewed national or international grants with substantial funding

    c. having a significant leadership role in obtaining major peer-reviewed or industrial funding

    d. obtaining recognition in the form of a major national or international award or invitation to present a keynote address at a major meeting with national or international participation, and

    e. taking on exceptional administrative service, such as serving as Chair or Deputy Chair of a grant review panel or editor of a high-impact journal.

Satisfactory Research/Scholarship Performance:

a. having continued publication productivity in respected journals in the field
b. having success at obtaining adequate funding to support the Faculty member's work
c. having an established or emerging national/international reputation with invited presentations in accordance with rank,
d. being invited to serve on national committees, grant review panels, or as a journal reviewer

Unsatisfactory Research/Scholarship Performance:
a. record of low publication output, in accordance with job description, over a number of years;
b. having a lack of or inadequate research funding; and
c. having few or no research trainees over a number of years

Unacceptable Research/Scholarship Performance:
a. having no publication over a number of years
b. having no (or minimal) research funding with no attempts to obtain additional funding
c. failing to provide a supportive environment and adequate supervision for trainees, or
d. display substantiated deceptive or unethical practices or academic misconduct

IV. Guidelines for Appointment and Promotion in Specific Tracks/Pathways and Ranks

Overview

The Department of Radiation Oncology has a multidisciplinary faculty covering a wide range of professions and expertise, including several clinical sciences, physical sciences, biological sciences, chemistry, and radiation sciences. There are several faculty tracks and pathways available in the Department of Radiation Oncology including:
a. Regular Track
    i. Clinician Educator Pathway
    ii. Clinician Scientist Pathway
b. Research Track
c. Salaried Clinical Faculty (Annual Appointments)

The criterion for appointment and promotion of faculty within each of these tracks/pathways is described below. When a specific Department Policy is not documented the University Policy is the sole criteria.

A. Regular Track –

These are the general guidelines for the ranks within the Regular track. Appointment to and promotion within the Regular Track requires an MD, DO, and/or PhD degree. Following this section, more specific guidelines will be listed for the two pathways within this track. The candidate must meet the requirements in both this overview section and the section specific to their pathway for appointment and promotion. Evidence of published scholarly activity is an essential component for all pathways within the Regular track.

1. Assistant Professor

University Policy: At the time of appointment, an Assistant Professor is expected to have demonstrated ability in research and teaching

Department Policy: Appointment to the rank of Assistant Professor requires completion of a doctoral degree (i.e., MD, DO, PhD, MD/PhD, or an equivalent degree). Those involved in patient care are expected to have successfully completed residency training and to be certified by or eligible for certification prior to appointment. Any physician faculty member with a clinical practice or involved in clinical care must become appropriately board certified within 3 years of his/her initial appointment unless this requirement is waived by the Department Chair due to specific and unusual circumstances.

2. Associate Professor

University Policy: At the time of appointment, an Associate Professor must show evidence of substantial record of success in research and teaching.

Department Policy: To be appointed or promoted to the rank of Associate Professor the candidate must meet the requirements of Assistant Professor. Appointment or promotion to the rank of Associate Professor requires regional/national recognition and a record of substantial success in effective teaching and research, except that in individual cases a superior record in one of these activities may be considered sufficient achievement with satisfactory performance in the other area. Teaching and research must demonstrate creativity and scholarship as defined under the general criteria presented on page one.

In addition, the provision of clinical care and administrative leadership are important missions of the School of Medicine and therefore excellence in these areas will be given consideration. Regardless of an individual's balance between teaching, research and service, evidence of scholarly contributions might include research published in refereed journals; texts, chapter and review articles; prepared written or audiovisual materials; or other types of educational or program development. Success in clinical teaching and patient care will be measured by resident, student, staff, and peer evaluation to document good to excellent performance. Quantity and quality of achievements in all of these areas will be considered, but excellence in clinical care, clinical teaching or administrative function alone will not suffice.

Regional/national recognition may be documented by peer evaluation, by such things as participation on editorial boards, study sections, invitations to speak at meetings, symposia and other institutions, or by special honors, awards, or other recognitions. National recognition for other than scholarly contributions will not in itself substitute for this requirement.

3. Professor

University Policy: Appointment to the rank of Professor requires outstanding mature scholarship as evidenced by accomplishments in teaching and in research, as evaluated in terms of national recognition.

Department Policy: The successful candidate for promotion will be expected to have established an international reputation in his or her field of interest, to be deeply engaged in scholarly work, and to have shown him or herself to be an effective teacher. These are the main criteria. However, either superior teaching or superior scholarship, sustained over many years, and satisfactory performance in the other area could also in itself justify eventual promotion to the rank of Professor. Administrative or other service to the University and related activities will be taken into account in assessing candidates for promotion, but given less weight than the main criteria; promotion will not be based primarily on such service. Promotion to Professor is not automatic, but it is expected that the majority of full-time tenured or without tenure due to funding faculty will eventually attain this rank.

Building upon the requirements for Associate Professor, appointment or promotion to the rank of Professor requires outstanding, mature scholarship as evidenced by national and international recognition. National and international recognition may be documented by peer evaluation, by such things as participation on editorial boards, study sections, invitations to speak at meetings, symposia and other institutions, or by special honors, awards, or other recognitions. National or international recognition for other than scholarly contributions will not in itself substitute for this requirement.

A Professor is expected to maintain high quality and substantial contributions to teaching, research, and service upon which promotion to this rank are based in the department.

Listed below are more specific departmental criteria for the specific ranks within the Regular faculty Track.

A.1 Clinician Educator Pathway

Overview

The Clinician Educator Pathway has been developed to provide clinicians, including, but not limited to Physicians and Medical Physicists committed to clinical service and teaching an opportunity to successfully pursue full-time academic careers as members of the faculty of the University of Washington School of Medicine. Evidence of scholarship is required for promotion contributing to medical education through peer review articles, development of teaching materials such as evidenced-based clinical guidelines, teaching program curricula and methodology to evaluate success of educational programs and the progress of trainees if appropriate. Evidence of scholarship may also include contributions to research.

Individuals in the pathway should devote the majority of his/her time to clinical practice and clinical teaching at one of the University's major affiliated clinical sites. Individuals on this pathway will have an MD, DO, PhD or equivalent.

Promotion within the Clinical Educator Pathway requires superior clinical performance. This should be demonstrated by fund of knowledge, problem solving skills, management of complex patients, and overall clinical skills. Humanistic qualities such as integrity, compassion, professional behavior and attitudes, interpersonal skills, and effectiveness in working in multidisciplinary settings are also required.

      1. Assistant Professor

An individual who is a physician and practicing radiation oncologist appointed to this rank must be Board-eligible or Board-certified in Radiation Oncology or appropriate field, have advanced clinical credentials and hold at least an advanced degree. If Board-eligible, the practicing radiation oncologist must become Board-certified within 3 years of their initial appointment. If foreign trained, equivalent international qualifications will be accepted. This requirement can be waived by the Department Chair due to specific and unusual circumstances. The individual must have a valid appropriate State license to practice medicine, if appropriate for field, be able to practice in an independent manner, if appropriate, and participate in the teaching, research, and administrative functions of the Department.

A non-physician appointed to this rank must have a PhD or equivalent from a recognized graduate program. If required for their profession, they must possess a valid appropriate State license. The individual must be able to and actively participate in the teaching, research, and administrative functions of the Department.

The mandatory promotion clock begins with the appointment to Assistant Professor.

2. Associate Professor

To be appointed or promoted to the rank of Associate Professor the candidate must meet the requirements of Assistant Professor. Appointment or promotion to the rank of Associate Professor requires a record of substantial demonstrated success and exemplary commitment to teaching and creative professional activity over a period of time as an Assistant Professor. In addition, the individual must have demonstrated excellent clinical care and administrative leadership. Regardless of the individual's balance between teaching, research, and service, evidence of sufficient scholarly contributions is important.

Such contributions may include refereed journal articles, texts, chapters, and review articles, audiovisual materials, and/or other educational program development. Contributions may also include mentorship programs for undergraduate students, medical students, residents, or peers within and outside the UW community. Quality of teaching will be measured by student, resident, and peer evaluation. It is expected that the individual will have demonstrated high productivity as a clinician with regional/national recognition as a clinician, administrator, or medical educator.

3. Professor

To be appointed or promoted to the rank of Professor the candidate must meet the requirements of Associate Professor. They must also have high ranking as a teacher and clinician, evidence of mature scholarship, and national/international recognition as a clinician, teacher, or medical educator.

The successful candidate for promotion will be expected to have established a wide reputation in his or her field of interest, to be deeply engaged in scholarly work, and show him or herself to be an effective teacher. There must be evidence that the activity has changed policy-making, organizational decision-making, or clinical practice beyond the candidate's own institution or practice setting, including when the target audience is the general public.

A.2 Clinician Scientist Pathway

Overview

Individuals on the Clinician Scientist Pathway are expected to be involved in research that generates "new knowledge". They will also participate in the clinical, educational, and administrative missions of the Department. Scholarship is evaluated by quality and quantity of published work, range and variety of intellectual interest, grant and fellowship awards, and success in training graduate and professional students. The regional/national/international scientific reputation of the faculty member will be considered in promotion decisions. It is expected that during his/her career the faculty member will obtain independent grant funding although it is not necessary that currently funded grants be in place at the time or promotion. In general, individuals on this pathway will be Board-certified in Radiation Oncology or Medical Physics unless the individual's contributions in non-clinical areas are such that this may be waved.

1. Assistant Professor

Individuals must have an MD, DO, PhD or equivalent. At the time of appointment the Assistant Professor is expected to have demonstrated activity in research and teaching. If clinically active and a physician, the individual is expected to have successfully completed resident training in Radiation Oncology and be Board-certified or Board-eligible prior to appointment. If Board-eligible, the practicing radiation oncologist is expected to become Board-certified within 3 years of the initial appointment. If foreign trained, equivalent international qualifications will be accepted. This requirement can be waived by the Department Chair due to specific and unusual circumstances. The physician must have a valid unrestricted State license to practice medicine.

A non-physician appointed to this rank must have a Ph.D. or equivalent from a recognized graduate program. If required for their profession, they must possess a valid appropriate State license. The individual must be able to and actively participate in the teaching, research, and administrative functions of the Department.

The mandatory promotion clock begins with the appointment or promotion to Assistant Professor.

2. Associate Professor

To be appointed or promoted to the rank of Associate Professor the candidate must meet the requirements of Assistant Professor. Appointment or promotion to the rank of Associate Professor requires a record of demonstrated substantial success in research, teaching, excellent clinical care, and administrative leadership. Regardless of an individual's balance between teaching, research, and service, evidence of published scholarly contributions is essential.

Such contributions may include refereed journal articles, text, chapters and review articles, audiovisual materials and/or other types of educational program development. Quality of teaching will be measured by resident, student, and peer evaluation. In rare circumstances, an individual with an outstanding record in one or two of these areas with satisfactory accomplishments in the other areas would be considered for promotion. It is expected that the individual will have a demonstrated record of grant funding although, it is not necessary that the individual have active grant funding at the time of promotion or appointment.

3. Professor

The candidate must meet the requirements of Associate Professor. Additionally, individuals promoted to the rank of Professor must have demonstrated outstanding mature scholarship as evaluated by national and international reputation in research and/or teaching. This may be documented by peer evaluation, participation on editorial boards of appropriate journals, invitations to speak at national/international meetings, symposiums, and visiting professorships at other institutions. The individual should also have contributed to the educational mission of the Department and be a respected mentor as evidenced by his/her teaching evaluation.

B. Research Track

Overview

Research faculty will be permitted and generally expected to conduct independent research programs. Research professional track appointments will be distinguished from regular track appointments by the absence of expected teaching or clinical responsibility although research faculty will be permitted to contribute to teaching activities to the extent that time and interest permit. Appointment to one of the ranks within the Research track requires qualifications corresponding to those prescribed for that rank, with primary emphasis upon research.

Research professor and research associate professor appointments are term appointments for a period not to exceed five academic years. The question of their renewal shall be considered by the voting faculty who are superior in academic rank to the person being considered and are faculty of the department in which the appointments are held. An exception is that the voting faculty at rank of professor shall consider whether to recommend renewal or non-renewal of the appointment of a research professor.

Research assistant professor appointments are for a term not to exceed three years with renewals and extensions to a maximum of eight years.

1. Research Assistant Professor

Appointment to the rank of Research Assistant Professor requires a doctoral degree (MD, PhD, MD/PhD or equivalent) and the individual is expected to have demonstrated activity in research, such as a postdoctoral research experience with publications in relevant journals.

2. Research Associate Professor

The candidate must meet the requirements of Research Assistant Professor. Additionally, appointment or promotion to the rank of Research Associate Professor requires a record of demonstrated significant success in research as measured by the development of new knowledge and its publication in refereed journals. Other scholarly contributions such as texts, chapters, and reviews and any teaching, administrative or other service junctions may contribute to qualification but will not replace publications in referred journals as the primary criterion.

3. Research Professor

The candidate must meet the requirements of Research Associate Professor. Additionally, appointment or promotion to the rank of Research Professor requires an outstanding and currently active mature scholarship sufficient to command a (national and international reputation in research and related scholarly contributions. National and international recognition may be documented by peer evaluation, such as participation on editorial boards, study sections, invitations to speak at meetings, symposia and other institutions, or by special honors, awards or other recognitions. National and international recognition for other than scholarly contributions will not substitute for research as the primary criterion.

C. Clinical Faculty Track (Annual Appointment) – Salaried and Non-salaried Appointments

Overview

A clinical appointment in the appropriate rank is usually made to a person who holds a primary appointment with an outside agency or non-academic unit of the University, or is in private practice. However, it may also be given to individuals providing full or part-time clinical service at one of the academic units. Clinical faculty members make substantial contributions to University programs through their expertise, interest and motivation to work with the faculty in preparing and assisting with the instruction of students in practicum settings. Clinical appointments are annual; the question of their renewal shall be considered each year by the faculty of the department in which they are held. Clinical faculty members are not eligible to vote on faculty appointments or promotions.

The salaried full-time clinical faculty appointment has been developed to provide individuals devoted primarily to patient care who practice in affiliate institutions a vehicle for a career as a full-time faculty member of the University of Washington, School of Medicine. For the purposes of this document, an "affiliate institution" is one that has a relationship with the School of Medicine via a professional services agreement with the Department of Radiation Oncology through the University of Washington physicians practice plan.

This recognizes the need for the University to provide decentralized specialty medical services at locations that are often some distance from the main campus where opportunities in research and teaching may be more limited than at UWMC or the SCCA or one of the major affiliated research and/or teaching sites such as HMC, VAPSHCS, NWH, or VMC. These appointments are for physicians supported through practice income flowing through UWP. This appointment also may be offered at one or more of the major teaching sites, for example, UWMC or SCCA.

Individuals in the salaried full-time clinical faculty pathway will carry the titles of Clinical Instructor, Clinical Assistant Professor, Clinical Associate Professor, or Clinical Professor. To be eligible for these appointments as a physician, individuals must be eligible for full-time appointment at the hospital or medical center where UWP has a site-of-practice agreement for Radiation Oncology Services. Both physicians and non-physicians shall have demonstrated a level of clinical competence appropriate for the appointment rank. Participation in appropriate clinical research protocols is expected and encouraged. If assigned to a site with resident teaching, participation in a UW resident training program will be identified in the individual's job description.

Faculty appointed to this track shall be expected to generate sufficient salary via their clinical activities to financially support their level of appointment.

Promotion Criteria

Criteria for evaluation of clinical faculty focuses on clinical activity. Teaching and research activities are clearly secondary and if expected, will be identified in the individual's job description. The individual must demonstrate excellence in patient care, be able to work well with referring physicians and support staff, and adhere to the general treatment policies of the Department of Radiation Oncology.

1. Clinical Instructor

An individual appointed to this rank must at a minimum be Board eligible in their discipline. Physicians must have a valid and appropriate State license to practice medicine and able to practice radiation oncology with only limited supervision. Non-physicians must have a valid and appropriate State license to practice in their discipline when legally required. A faculty member will serve at least 2 years at this rank before being eligible for promotion.

2. Clinical Assistant Professor

An individual appointed to this rank must be Board eligible or Board certified in Radiation Oncology or Radiation Oncology Physics. If Board eligible, the individual must become Board certified within 3 years of the initial appointment. If foreign trained, equivalent international qualifications will be accepted. Physicians must have a valid and unrestricted State license to practice medicine and be able to practice radiation oncology independently. Non-physicians must have a valid and appropriate State license to practice in their discipline when legally required. Appointment to the rank of Clinical Assistant Professor as a physician requires a doctoral degree (MD, DO, or equivalent degree) and the potential to actively participate in developing the cancer program at their assigned center. Appointment to the rank of Clinical Assistant Professor as a non-physician requires a doctoral degree (Ph.D. or equivalent doctoral degree) and the potential to actively participate in developing technological or scientific aspects of cancer treatment programs at their assigned center

An individual will normally serve six (6) years at this rank before being eligible for promotion. Promotion requires superior clinical performance. This should be demonstrated by fund of knowledge, problem solving skills, management of complex patients, and overall clinical skills. Humanistic qualities such as integrity, compassion, professional behavior and attitudes, interpersonal skills, and effectiveness in working in multidisciplinary settings are also required. Outstanding individuals may be considered for earlier promotion.

3. Clinical Associate Professor

The individual must meet the requirements of Clinical Assistant Professor. Additionally, appointment or promotion to the rank of Clinical Associate Professor requires a successful leadership role in developing and guiding discipline relevant aspects of the cancer program at their affiliate center. This may be demonstrated through service on cancer-related committees, new program development, and administrative duties. Being recognized for community service in relation to the affiliate center's cancer program will be viewed positively. Participation in the Department's clinical research program, such as enrolling patients in clinical trials or assisting in their development will also be viewed positively The individual is expected to occasionally lecture on Radiation oncology topics to residents in training. An individual will normally serve six (6) years at this rank before being eligible for promotion. Success in patient care will be measured by resident, student, staff, and peer evaluation to document good to excellent performance. Outstanding individuals may be considered for earlier promotion.

4. Clinical Professor

The individual must meet the requirements of Clinical Associate Professor. Additionally, appointment or promotion to the rank of Clinical Professor requires demonstrated success and productive mentoring (serve as mentor) of junior Radiation Oncology faculty at the center to which the individual seeking promotion is assigned. The individual must be recognized by peers for skill and knowledge of Radiation Oncology or Radiation Oncology Physics and its role in the treatment of the cancer patient. The individual must have a senior-level role in developing and guiding the cancer program at their assigned center/site of practice specific to their discipline. This may be demonstrated through having served as Chair on cancer-related committees, new program development, and senior administrative duties.
The individual is expected to be recognized for outstanding community service in relation to the assigned center's cancer program.

D. Other Faculty titles

D. 1. Teaching Associate

Teaching Associate is the appointment title of non-physicians such as nurse practitioners, physician assistants, social workers, and others practicing in UW Medicine clinical settings. Appointment with the title of teaching associate is made to a non-student with credentials more limited than those required of an instructor. Teaching associate appointments are annual, or shorter; the question of their renewal shall be considered each year by the faculty of the department in which they are held.

D.2. Lecturer

Lecturer is an instructional title that may be conferred on persons who have special instructional roles and who have extensive training, competence, and experience in their discipline. Full-Time Lecturers appointed through a competitive recruitment may be either on an annual or a multiple-year contract (up to 5 years) and may be considered for promotion in the last academic year of the appointment term. Full-time lecturer appointments are considered annual if a competitive search is not conducted.

Full-time lecturer appointments not made through a competitive search are not eligible for promotion. Lecturers may be reappointed indefinitely.

D.3. Adjunct:
Adjunct appointments are made to faculty already holding a regular or research appointment in another department. This title recognizes the contributions of a faculty member to a secondary department.

D.4. Affiliate:
Affiliate appointments recognize the professional contribution of an individual whose principal employment responsibilities lie outside the colleges or schools of the University. Appointment or promotion requires qualifications comparable to those required for appointment to the corresponding faculty rank in the Department of Radiation Oncology.

D.5. Emeritus
The emeritus appointment must at minimum meet the requirements specified in Section 24-34. B13 of the University faculty code. Appointment is recommended by departmental action for a faculty member whose scholarly, teaching, or service record has been meritorious. It requires holders to have provided at least ten years of prior service as a member of the faculty and to have achieved the rank of professor or associate professor. Non-paid faculty can be considered for emeritus status. If being paid as an emeritus faculty member, the individual is eligible to vote on appointments and promotions. Appointees must have served the department with distinction beyond that typically achieved by an average faculty member in any one of the categories of scholarship, teaching or service. Examples of meritorious service include;

> i). Previous service as chair of the department or high office at the university or state or national level.
> ii). Recognition by external national and professional bodies in their discipline.
> iii). National and international awards and prizes related to their discipline.
> iv). Creation of large clinical programs ab initio and leading clinical trials.
> v). Post-retirement ongoing contributions to the educational, research, or clinical missions of the department.

V. Faculty Performance and Time Allocation

Promotions will be based on a faculty member's overall performance and quantity of achievements in the areas of teaching, administrative service, clinical practice, research and professionalism. To attain promotion a faculty member must have an overall superior performance and a number of documented achievements in their areas of activity. Faculty members have the responsibility to keep records of his/her achievements, and to make sure necessary supportive documents are obtained for the promotion packet. It is important that appropriate documents be obtained whenever possible. One document that provides a measure of performance is the review of the faculty performance given by the department chair (e.g. annually for Assistant Professor level). It is an expectation that faculty members will operate at a high level of professionalism at all time, so the level of *professionalism will always be appropriate*. An unacceptable professionalism rating will have disciplinary consequences. A level of unacceptable professionalism negates any superior or satisfactory performance ratings given in a review.

The different levels of appointment on the Regular, Research and Clinical Faculty tracks have performance expectations commensurate with that rank (e.g. Lecturer, Assistant Professor, Associate Professor or Professor), as outlined in section III. For promotion consideration, the expectation is that faculty appointees at the Assistant Professor level might have ratings of satisfactory performance in the first few years, while learning and developing their skills in the new position. However, ratings should become superior in focus areas during subsequent years. For the Associate Professor level, superior performance must be demonstrated in his/her focus area over a several year period. It is an expectation that once the level of Professor is obtained, the faculty member will continue operate at the superior performance level.

On initial appointment and at annual performance reviews, or sooner if appropriate, faculty members will negotiate with the department chair the percentage effort to be spent in teaching, administrative service, clinical practice, and research, such that the interests of the faculty member and the needs of the department are met. The percentage effort in the different areas can change, and will be reassessed at each faculty performance review with the department chair. As stated previously, there is a requirement that a minimum of 5% effort be conducted in both administrative service and teaching. The only exception for this is that the Research Professor track does not have a requirement for teaching. The expectation is that it will be more difficult to attain a high number of achievements in those areas that have a low percentage of effort, but the performance might still be superior. Thus, the level of performance will be gauged annually on expectations of achievement based on the percent effort in a particular area set for the previous year.

VI. Faculty Advisory Committee

Overview

It is the goal of the Department of Radiation Oncology that junior faculty will be given every opportunity to qualify for and obtain promotions in rank. Preparation for and progress towards promotion is the responsibility of each individual faculty member. To assist faculty below the rank of Associate Professor, Research Associate Professor and Clinical Associate Professor, a Faculty Advisory Committee will be established. The Faculty Advisory Committee will be made available to individual faculty to provide annual, timely, constructive feedback to the junior faculty on his/her progress towards meeting departmental expectations for promotion. It is expected that the Faculty Advisory Committee will be a resource to junior faculty as they work towards their own promotions. The different aspects of the Faculty Advisor Program are outlined below.

Role

The role of the Committee is to serve as a resource to help the junior faculty meet and exceed the expectations of the department for promotion to the next rank. To assist in this process, the Faculty Advisory Committee will help the junior faculty members identify/contact one or two other investigators, not necessarily from within the department, who can act as mentors. In the role of mentor the other investigators can help to determine what might be expected in the junior faculty's discipline so that "reasonable" goals can be set and help judge the progress toward those goals. The Faculty Advisory Committee will be available to meet with the junior faculty member a minimum of twice a year (more often is recommended) to review the junior faculty member's progress. The Committee functions as a peer review for promotion and provides advice and guidance to junior faculty. The Committee may also identify resources and methods for junior faculty to enhance their scholarly effort. It is expected that the individual faculty member actively take advantage of the Faculty Advisory Committee's guidance, as the faculty member hold ultimate responsibility for his or her progress towards promotion. In the event a Faculty Advisory Committee is unable to perform its duties in any given year, then the department Appointments and Promotions Committee may temporarily serve as its substitute.

Evaluation

The junior faculty will provide a self-evaluation report to the Faculty Advisory Committee prior to his/her departmental annual review. The report will include a summary of the past year's activities in the areas of research/scholarly activities, teaching and service as is appropriate (and agreed upon) in their original appointment and most recent annual review, as appropriate. The report will be discussed by the junior faculty and Faculty Advisory Committee, and may be revised as warranted. The report will be sent to the Chair prior to his/her annual review meeting with the junior faculty.

Expectations for Promotion

The Faculty member should take steps to become familiar with the expectations for promotion to the next rank and continuously work towards exceeding those expectations as their careers advance. The Faculty member should consult with the Faculty Advisory Committee for help in defining some minimum expectations and setting goals to exceed those expectations. The Committee will help set goals for junior faculty both as a group. The expectations and goals set for the junior faculty should be discussed and agreed upon between the faculty, Faculty Advisory Chair and the Department Chair.

The various parameters evaluated in considering promotions in the Department of Radiation Oncology are provided with each of the professional pathways listed in this document. As a general rule, promotion to a higher rank requires that a faculty member make significant contributions to his/her field and be recognized for those contributions by peers in the field. It is recognized that different disciplines often have different peer-reviewed publications. It is also recognized that some faculty positions have significantly higher service roles for the department, and those circumstances will be factored in when evaluating productivity.

It is the responsibility of faculty members to take steps to document their contributions in the area of research/scholarship, teaching and service. This is usually done by maintaining a current Curriculum Vitae and gathering copies of materials such as publications, abstracts, and student evaluations of instruction. . Those reviews must be sent directly to the department administrative office and not received by the faculty member performing the instruction.

References

1. AAUP 1949 statement of principles on academic freedom and tenure. https://www.aaup.org/report/1940-statement-principles-academic-freedom-and-tenure.
2. Walling A. Understanding tenure. Soc Teach Fam Med. 2015;47(1):43–7. https://www.stfm.org/FamilyMedicine/Vol147Issue1/Walling43.
3. Golden DW, Ingledew PA. Radiation oncology education. In: Halperin EC, Brady LW, Perez CA, Wazer DE, editors. Perez & Brady's principles and practice of radiation oncology. 7th ed. Philadelphia: LWW, https://www.ovid.com/product-details.12608.html.
4. Simpson D, Fincher RM, Hafler JP, et al. Advancing educators and education: defining the components and evidence of educational scholarship. Med Educ. 2007;41(10):1002–9, https://pubmed.ncbi.nlm.nih.gov/17822412/.
5. Disis ML, Slattery JT. The road we must take: multidisciplinary team science. Sci Transl Med. 2020;2(22):22cm9, https://stm.sciencemag.org/content/2/22/22cm9.full.
6. University of Washington department of radiation oncology criteria for promotion and tenure.

Maintenance and Assessment of Skills and Knowledge Over the Career Continuum

Paul E. Wallner, Lisa A. Kachnic, and Kaled M. Alektiar

Past

The American Board of Radiology (ABR) was established in 1934. Between 1934 and 1986, 2024 certificates were awarded in therapeutic radiology.[1] In 1986, the designation of the specialty was changed to radiation oncology. Between 1986 and 1995, an additional 1295 certificates were awarded to radiation oncology diplomates [1]. All certificates bore the initial date of the award, but no expiration dates were memorialized. In the absence of an expiration date on the certificate, it was inferred, but never actually stated, that the credential would be in force for the individual's entire career, that is, "lifetime" or "non-time-limited" certificates. A similar situation existed for all Member Boards of the American Board of Medical Specialties (ABMS), the umbrella organization for 24 independent specialty certification organizations, except for the American Board of Family Medicine, which from the time of its founding in 1969 awarded only time-limited certificates [2].

---

[1] Additional certificates were awarded in disciplines termed roentgen therapy, radium therapy, and general radiology, which were discontinued in 1954, 1960, and 1989, respectively.

P. E. Wallner
GenesisCare USA, Fort Myers, FL, USA

American Board of Radiology, Tucson, AZ, USA

L. A. Kachnic (✉)
Department of Radiation Oncology, Columbia University Irving Medical Center,
Herbert Irving Comprehensive Cancer Center, New York, NY, USA
e-mail: lak2187@cumc.columbia.edu

K. M. Alektiar
Department of Radiation Oncology, Memorial Sloan Kettering Cancer Center,
New York, NY, USA

© Springer Nature Switzerland AG 2021
R. A. Chandra et al. (eds.), *Career Development in Academic Radiation Oncology*, https://doi.org/10.1007/978-3-030-71855-8_19

From the early years of the medical specialty board certification movement through 1945, progress in clinical medicine was slow, with only a modest number of new drugs, techniques, and discoveries [3]. After World War II, however, the pace of innovation changed dramatically, such that leaders within the medical specialty boards began to question the validity of lifetime certificates. Candidates for initial certification were examined during and immediately following completion of residency training but then never again during careers that might span 4 or more decades. State medical licensing boards and facilities routinely required that physicians provide proof of a current medical license and that they earn a predetermined number of continuing medical education (CME) credits, but the content of these credits was typically self-selected and often unrelated to the individual's actual medical practice. Skills and/or knowledge attained from the CME content were rarely assessed. ABMS Member Boards were routinely called upon by credentialing entities to "certify" that diplomates had maintained the necessary knowledge and skills for the benefit of the public, but aside from publicly available records of state or federally based disciplinary actions, the boards lacked current data regarding diplomates, including such basic information as whether the individual even remained in practice. Initial certification by an ABMS member board is considered by the public, credentialing entities, regulators, and legislators as the sine qua non measure of clinical quality. Careers in academia and often in private practice are effectively impossible absent board certification. That being the case, the regimen of a single, early career assessment was problematic.

The ability of organized medicine to self-regulate as a profession is deeply engrained, highly valued, and scrupulously guarded. Concerns about the weaknesses of the existing certification system intensified in the 1950s and 1960s, and as early as 1971, senior ABR leaders began to raise the idea of initiating time-limited certificates [1]. Potential legislative and regulatory limitations of professional self-regulation coupled with previously unimagined advances in clinical practice in the 1980s and early 1990s amplified concerns about shortcomings in a regimen of initial certification that assessed knowledge and skills only at the outset of practice. Certification by a Member Board of the ABMS had been considered the primary acceptable and reliable metric of physician quality by other professionals and the public for more than half a century but was increasingly questioned under this "once and done" process [4–6]. Continuation of the status quo, absent some type of diplomate requirements and evaluations following initial certification, was deemed to be inconsistent with the rigorous process of initial certification. In the early 1990s, to maintain the public trust and hard-fought elements of professional self-regulation, leaders of the medical certification board movement determined that the regimen of initial certification should be transitioned into awards with specified time limitations, that is, time-limited certificates. All ABMS Member Boards committed to making this complete transition by 2020. Several of the Member Boards had either unilaterally determined to end non-time-limited certification or anticipated the ABMS decision and moved into their time-limited certificate programs immediately [7]. A majority of the remaining boards made the transition during the 1990s. The ABR awarded its last non-time-limited certificate in radiation oncology in 1994, and beginning in 1995, all certificates awarded in the discipline were limited to 10 years [1].

As part of this process, the ABMS Member Boards collectively developed and agreed to adhere to basic elements of continuous certification collectively referred to as the new Maintenance of Certification (MOC) program. The foundation of MOC was based on continuous reinforcement and assessment of six essential competencies that had been developed conjointly by the Accreditation Council for Graduate Medical Education (ACGME) and the ABMS [8], and included:

- *Medical knowledge*, including knowledge of established and evolving biomedical, clinical, epidemiological, and social behavioral sciences, as well as the application of this knowledge to patient care.
- *Patient care and procedural skills*, including attributes such as provision of patient care that is compassionate, appropriate, and effective for the treatment of health problems and the promotion of health, and demonstration of competence in all current modalities and procedures appropriate to the specialty.
- *Interpersonal and communication skills*, including attributes such as competence in communicating effectively with patients, families, and the public, as appropriate, across a broad range of socioeconomic and cultural backgrounds, and communicating effectively with physicians, other health professionals, and health-related agencies.
- *Professionalism*, including attributes such as compassion, integrity, respect for others, and responsiveness to patient needs that supersedes self-interest.
- *Practice-based learning and improvement*, including attributes such the ability to investigate and evaluate care of patients, to appraise and assimilate scientific evidence, and to continuously improve patient care based on constant self-evaluation and lifelong learning.
- *Systems-based practice*, including attributes such as an awareness of and responsiveness to the larger context and system of health care, including the social determinants of health, and the ability to call effectively on other resources to provide optimal health care.

Individual ABMS Member Boards were provided some flexibility in the interpretation and implementation of how ongoing education and assessment of those competencies would be incorporated into their emerging MOC initiatives. Four framework elements (parts) were required of all programs (described below and in Table 1). Some Member Boards initially opted for a 5- to 6-year cycle of program components to be completed, while the ABR selected a cycle of 10 years.

- *Part 1: Evidence of Professional Standing* – Diplomates were required to provide primary documentation of medical licensure and state- and/or institution-based disciplinary actions.
- *Part 2: Lifelong Learning and Self-Assessment* – Diplomates were required to provide primary documentation of a predetermined number of CME and self-assessment-CME (SA-CME) credits of relevant content.
- *Part 3: Cognitive Examination* – Diplomates were required to pass a computer-based examination once during each 10-year MOC cycle.
- *Part 4: Evidence of Evaluation and Improvement of Performance in Practice* – Diplomates were required to perform at least one Practice Quality Improvement project every 3 years.

Table 1 MOC elements and requirements (1/1/2020)

Element	Descriptor	Requirements
Part 1	Professionalism and professional standing	Throughout the Maintenance of Certification (MOC) process, the physician must hold a current, full, and unrestricted license to practice medicine in all states in which the physician currently practices in the United States, its territories, or Canada
Part 2	Lifelong learning and self-assessment	To satisfy Maintenance of Certification (MOC) Part 2, the ABR requires diplomates to attain 75 CME credits every 3 years, at least 25 of which must be credits from Self-Assessment CME (SA-CME) activities
Part 3	Assessment of knowledge, judgment, and skills	Part 3 requires passing the most recent summative decision for the Online Longitudinal Assessment (OLA) or having passed a traditional exam in the previous 5 years. In May 2016, the ABR announced its plans to move away from the 10-year exam to OLA
Part 4	Improvement in medical practice	With the implementation of Continuous Certification, diplomates must have completed at least one Practice Quality Improvement (PQI) Project or Participatory Quality Improvement Activity in the previous 3 years at each MOC annual review. A PQI Project or Activity may be conducted repeatedly or continuously to meet PQI requirements

Note: Full and timely details of requirements for each element are available on the ABR website: https://www.theabr.org/radiation-oncology/maintenance-of-certification#moc Printed with permission of the American Board of Radiology

The requirements initially established for Parts 1 and 2 were similar to those that already existed for most state agencies, provider facilities, and many specialty societies, except for the need to provide primary documentation. Parts 3 and 4 were new and believed to be important for maintaining continued clinical proficiency.

At the outset of the MOC program, Part 4 participation was interpreted by the ABMS Member Boards as consisting of Practice Quality Improvement (PQI) projects that demonstrated positive impact on patient care, conceived and implemented by the diplomate. Subsequent guidelines were modified to include projects designed by specialty societies for use by their members (template projects), as well as those developed and implemented by practice groups and/or their institutions, often with incorporation of data sets embedded in existing health records.

As initially conceived and implemented, the MOC programs represented a radical departure from previous Member Board programming, and there was always an anticipation that elements of the programs would evolve over time, both at the national ABMS level and within individual Member Boards. The ABMS and its Member Boards remained fully committed to continuing the programs and to making periodic appropriate changes to provide activities that were clinically relevant to physicians [5, 9].

The ABR has carried out periodic radiation oncology Clinical Practice Analysis (CPA) surveys to evaluate what diplomates are actually doing in the field. The 2013 survey revealed that many diplomates limited their practice to one or several disease or system sites. To reduce some of the stress related to the cognitive exam, in 2015 the ABR introduced a modular MOC exam format [3, 10]. The exam remained unchanged in length, with 200 questions, but was divided into modules of varying lengths. All diplomates were required to complete a general radiation oncology module of 120 scorable units, but the remainder of the exam could be populated by modules selected by the individual diplomate based on areas of interest and/or preference. A compulsory general radiation oncology module was necessary because all radiation oncology certificates are for the general discipline, rather than for a specific site or modality.

In 2015, the Part 4 guidelines were also modified to include "activities" as well as projects. The definition of activities then included almost all institutional and/or peer review programs, as well as participation in clinical trials and registries [11–13].

Present[2, 3]

The initial enrolled and progressively increasing number of diplomates involved in the emerging MOC programs, the variety of their practice settings, and the complexity and novel nature of the programs themselves assured that progressive changes in implementation would be anticipated and essential. For the most part, individual member boards determined the pace of these changes based on feedback from their own diplomates and stakeholder organizations. Some modifications were small and evolutionary, while others were more rapid and significant [9]. The level of concern raised by diplomates of the American Board of Internal Medicine was unique among the Member Boards, including issues related to the cost of the programs, perceived high Part 3 exam failure rates, and a requirement for broad cross-subspecialty assessment regardless of the diplomate-specific practice pattern. These concerns were not generally raised by diplomates of other Member Boards, but program modifications to improve the diplomate experience were enacted throughout the ABMS board movement in general and by the ABR specifically [11–14].

For ABR diplomates, primary documentation is no longer required for Part 1: when accessing their personal ABR website profile, diplomates are simply prompted to attest to meeting the current requirements. Primary documentation is required only in the event of a random and infrequent MOC audit. Diplomates must report any state or federal disciplinary action within 60 days of that action.

Part 2 documentation has been similarly changed to require only attestation of CME and SA-CME credit rather than requiring primary documentation, which would be requested only in the event of an audit. Diplomates have significantly greater flexibility in determining the relevance of program content for their own

---

[2] Specific requirements of the various parts have changed periodically following initial adoption. Details current as of this writing are provided in Table 1.

[3] As with any active ABMS or ABR program, determination of current policies, procedures, and requirements should be based on the details available on the ABMS and/or ABR websites at the time of the query.

benefit. A minimum of 75 AMA Category 1 CME credits are required every 3 years, of which 25 credits must be SA-CME. Significantly greater flexibility has been provided regarding the types of SA-CME permitted. Additional documentation for Parts 1 and 2 is also provided to the ABR from the Federation of State Medical Boards and the American Society for Radiation Oncology, further simplifying documentation requirements for diplomates.

The most significant MOC programmatic changes have been implemented for Parts 3 and 4 [11–13]. Administration of the Part 3 modular exam was discontinued in 2017 and in January 2020, the once-every-10-years multiple-choice cognitive exam was replaced for radiation oncology by the ABR Online Longitudinal Assessment (ABR OLA) instrument. Unlike the previous Part 3 modular exam that was administered only at commercial test centers, ABR OLA is a web-based platform that can be accessed from any desktop or mobile device. In addition to eliminating the need for travel to a test center, the ABR OLA instrument differs significantly from the previous Part 3 exam. Each week, participating diplomates receive an email reminder of question availability, with a link to their ABR homepage. The homepage report provides an update to their MOC and Part 3 status and a portal to the OLA platform where they are provided with an opportunity to answer one of two available questions. On average, only one question per week must be answered, for a total of 52 questions each year. There is no requirement that questions must be answered weekly, and up to eight questions can be stored for later access. Individual questions are available for 4 weeks, after which time they expire. Diplomates may elect to answer more than one question per week to accelerate completion of their annual requirement. Diplomates can decline up to 10 questions each year without penalty at the discretion of the individual. ABR OLA items will be distributed to individual diplomates and the entire diplomate population on a random basis, with the total number of items distributed annually based on the blueprint developed from the Clinical Practice Analysis and other practice sources. The ABR OLA instrument has a summative evaluation that will be completed after each diplomate completes 200 individual questions, which for most will not occur until almost 4 full years after initial participation in the instrument. Diplomates will receive feedback regarding their performance on an ongoing basis, but a critical element of the ABR OLA platform is also immediate, dynamic feedback. After completing a question, diplomates immediately receive confirmation of the correct answer, a brief rationale in support of that answer, and a reference for the appropriate information source. If the question is answered incorrectly, a similar question, essentially querying the same topic, will be directed to the diplomate within 3–6 weeks as one of their weekly options, to determine if they have learned from their initial incorrect response. Diplomates will receive updated performance data on a regular basis and are always able to review previously answered questions.

A critical difference between the ABR OLA instrument and the previous Part 3 exam is the level of knowledge required and the perceived need for preparation. Questions in the ABR OLA inventory are developed by volunteers who are overwhelmingly in private general radiation oncology practices, rather than by site-specific content experts. These individuals, as do all ABR private and academic practice volunteers, contribute their time and expertise to serve the profession and public, and for many, to enhance career opportunities and personal satisfaction. The target for the required level of knowledge is "walking-around knowledge," that is, basic material that should be known to all practicing radiation oncologists without a need for further investigation. Any physics or biology material will be directly related to current clinical practice. Upon completion of each question, diplomates will have an immediate and optional opportunity to rate the question on its relevance to their own practice and its difficulty level. This aspect of the ABR OLA instrument is a significant difference from the standard setting of initial certification exams, in which the Angoff technique is carried out by a small sample group. Standard setting for the ABR OLA questions will be carried out dynamically, by the entire pool of diplomates, at the time they complete the response. Analysis of this diplomate feedback will inform future question development.

The ABR OLA instrument effectively addresses other concerns raised by diplomates regarding the previous Part 3 exam. Travel to a commercial site, with associated expenses and lost office time, is no longer required. ABR OLA questions are timed to allow either 1 minute or 3 minutes to complete, based on their length and complexity, so they can be answered any time a diplomate has a brief amount of free time. Diplomates will also have the option of saving and batching items, if they choose to do so. The perceived concern regarding a high-stakes, single-sitting exam has been eliminated with an instrument for which the summative evaluation will be almost 4 years in development and for which there is continuous feedback.

Part 4 participation has been significantly simplified and opportunities for completion, greatly expanded. Individual, group, institutional, or national organization projects remain encouraged but are no longer required. Instead, a broad range of Practice Quality Improvement and peer review activities are now included in the menu of options available to MOC participants [11–13] (Table 2). For many

Table 2 Available part 4 participatory activities (1/1/2020)

Participatory quality improvement activities	Acceptable documentation of active individual participation (retain for use if audited)
Participation as a member of an institutional/departmental clinical quality and/or safety review committee Examples include meaningful participation as a member responsible for creating, reviewing, and/or implementing clinical quality improvement safety activities; service as a radiation safety officer (RSO)	One of the following bulleted options: Institution/department documentation of attendance at committee meetings (such as minutes, if available), OR Submission of completed and signed MOC Part 4 Participatory Quality Improvement Activity
Active participation in a departmental or institutional peer-review process, including participation in data entry/ evaluation and a peer-review meeting process or Ongoing Professional Practice Evaluation (OPPE)	One of the following bulleted options: Minutes, with peer-protected information redacted, showing attendance at peer-review meetings, or other forms of participant feedback, OR Logs showing active participation in submitting and reviewing cases as well as having your own individual work reviewed in the course of daily workflow, OR Submission of completed and signed MOC Part 4 Participatory Quality Improvement Activity

(continued)

Table 2 (continued)

Participatory quality improvement activities	Acceptable documentation of active individual participation (retain for use if audited)
Participation as a member of a root cause analysis (RCA) team evaluating a sentinel or other quality- or safety-related event	One of the following bulleted options: Minutes or other institutional/ departmental documentation showing attendance at RCA meetings, OR Submission of completed and signed MOC Part 4 Participatory Quality Improvement Activity
Participation in at least 25 prospective chart rounds every year (peer review of the radiation delivery plans for new cases – radiation oncology and medical physics only)	One of the following bulleted options: Conference attendance sheets, OR CME credit logs (if appropriate), OR Submission of completed and signed MOC Part 4 Participatory Quality Improvement Activity
Active participation in submitting data to a national registry	One of the following bulleted options: Log of cases/data submitted to organization, OR Letter from registry stating participation (including dates of participation)
Publication of a peer-reviewed journal article related to quality improvement or improved safety of the diplomate's practice content area	Copy of journal article
Invited presentation or exhibition of a peer-reviewed poster at a national meeting related to quality improvement or improved safety of the diplomate's practice content area	Copy of the meeting program showing that the poster was presented/exhibited and listing the diplomate as an author
Regular participation (at least 10/year) in departmental or group conferences focused on patient safety Examples include regular attendance at tumor boards, morbidity and mortality conferences, diagnostic/therapeutic errors conferences, interprofessional conferences, surgical/pathology correlation conferences, etc.	One of the following bulleted options: Conference attendance sheets, OR CME credit logs (if appropriate), OR Submission of completed and signed MOC Part 4 Participatory Quality Improvement Activity
Creation or active management of, or participation in, one of the elements of a quality or safety program Examples include a department dashboard or scorecard, a daily management system to ensure quality and safety, a daily readiness assessment using a huddle system	One of the following bulleted options: Other documents describing and documenting work, (e.g., copies of scorecards created, minutes from daily readiness huddles, etc.), OR Submission of completed and signed MOC Part 4 Participatory Quality Improvement Activity
Local or national leadership role in a national/international quality improvement program, such as Image Gently, Image Wisely, Choosing Wisely, or other similar campaign Local participation roles include implementation and/or maintenance of, or adherence to, program goals and/or requirements	Submission of completed and signed MOC Part 4 Participatory Quality Improvement Activity

Table 2 (continued)

Participatory quality improvement activities	Acceptable documentation of active individual participation (retain for use if audited)
Completion of a Peer Survey (quality or patient safety-focused) and resulting action plan. Survey should contain at least five quality or patient safety-related questions and have a minimum of five survey responses	Summary of process, including a copy of the survey administered, results, and action plans taken
Completion of a Patient Experience-of-Care (PEC) survey with individual patient feedback. Survey should contain at least five quality/patient safety-related questions and have a minimum of 30 survey responses	Summary of process, including a copy of the survey administered, results, and action plans taken
Active participation in applying for or maintaining accreditation by specialty accreditation programs such as those offered by ACR, ACRO, or ASTRO	Submission of completed and signed MOC Part 4 Participatory Quality Improvement Activity
Annual participation in the required Mammography Quality Standards Act (MQSA) medical audit or ACR Mammography Accreditation Program (MAP)	Submission of completed and signed MOC Part 4 Participatory Quality Improvement Activity
Completion of a Self-directed Educational Project (SDEP) on a quality or patient safety-related topic (medical physics only)	Submission of completed and signed MOC Part 4 Participatory Quality Improvement Activity
Active participation in a National Cancer Institute cooperative group clinical trial (for diagnostic radiologists, radiation oncologists, and interventional radiologists, entry of five or more patients in a year; for medical physicists, active participation in the credentialing activities)	One of the following bulleted options: Log of cases submitted, OR Letter from registry stating participation (including dates of participation), OR Other documents showing individual participation

Printed with permission of the American Board of Radiology

diplomates, these available activities will represent opportunities in which they already participate on a routine basis.

Early in implementation of the national ABMS-conceptualized MOC programs, questions arose regarding the efficacy and sustainability of a rolling MOC cycle that encompassed a full decade. Could episodic CME and SA-CME activities and a cognitive exam administered only once every 10 years appropriately fulfill the implied contract with the public regarding medical self-regulation and professional oversight? Equally important was an emerging legislative concern regarding a lack of appropriate continuous participation in regular MOC activities. With passage of Public Law 111–148, the Patient Protection and Affordable Care Act of 2010 (ACA), Congress codified ABMS Member Board MOC participation as part of Title III,

Improving the Quality and Efficiency of Health Care, as an amendment to the Social Security Act (Section 1848) [15, 16]. This amendment effectively embedded MOC participation into the physician incentive reimbursement schema that was part of the Physician Quality Reporting System. The Act further defined the MOC programs as "continuous," and the Medicare Physician Fee Schedule for calendar year 2011 applied a "more frequent" participation qualifier to its description of the MOC incentives within its Value-based Purchasing initiatives. In a significant effort that included ABMS and Member Board leaders, the Centers for Medicare and Medicaid Services (CMS) were encouraged to allow the ABMS and Members Boards to determine the meaning and implementation of "continuous" and "more frequent" participation.

To meet the requirements placed on the ABMS and Member Boards by agreement with CMS, and with their own concerns regarding the then-active programs, in 2012 the ABR amended its MOC interval from the previous 10-year cycle to what was effectively a continuous regimen of participation [12, 13]. On January 1 of the year following attainment of initial certification, each ABR diplomate is automatically enrolled in the MOC program. CME, SA-CME, and Practice Quality Improvement activities completed during the period between the award of initial certification and entry into MOC are counted toward MOC credit. All diplomates participating in MOC receive a status report on March 2 each year. This report includes the individual's status on each of the four parts of MOC, enables updating of the Parts 1, 2, and 4 attestations, and is available only to the individual diplomate. Payment for annual participation may also be made at this time.

In parallel with annual reporting to individual diplomates, the ABR is required to report the certification status of each diplomate to the ABMS for updating its public Certification Matters™ website [17]. In addition to displaying the initial certification status of the diplomate, the site also reports whether the individual is participating in MOC. For diplomates holding non-time-limited certificates and participating voluntarily in MOC, that participation is noted. If the individual has elected not to participate in MOC, the site will indicate nonparticipation but will also provide a qualifying statement that MOC participation is not a requirement for the practitioner. The ABR website provides similar information. ABR diplomates who elect to participate voluntarily in MOC can never lose their non-time-limited initial certification. Although no diplomate is required to participate in MOC, those with time-limited certificates who do not participate will have their initial certification lapse on the date indicated on the certificate. Subsequent to that date, they are no longer permitted to use the designation "board certified." Return to certification later is possible and is defined on the ABR website [13].

Future

The ABR OLA instrument will provide invaluable and previously unavailable data to educational content developers and individual diplomates regarding gaps in knowledge for which a variety of educational programming can be developed. Approximately 3600 radiation oncology diplomates will answer a random distribution of 104 question opportunities each year. Most diplomates will likely elect to answer 52 questions each year. Thus, after completion of a single year of implementation, this participation will generate over 187,000 data points of information for analysis of areas of strengths and weaknesses. The ABR will share this information with stakeholder organizations and use the data to inform additional modifications of its MOC program.

All aspects of the US health care delivery system, including education and assessment, continuously evolve. The ABMS and its Member Boards recognize that frequent MOC program amendments produce concern and confusion within the diplomate community, and they have committed to reducing the frequency of significant programmatic changes. This commitment has been made with an understanding that the significant programmatic changes already adopted were necessary to meet the needs of diplomates and fulfill the board movement's mission to the public. As changes are considered and implemented, they will be sensitive to the needs of diplomates to better integrate the MOC processes into routine clinical practice while adhering to the missions and intentions of the ABMS and its Member Boards. As objective evidence of its long-term commitment to continuation of the MOC programs, with modifications as appropriate, in early 2018 the ABMS empaneled a Continuing Board Certification: Vision for the Future Commission. The Commission consisted of 27 members from diverse backgrounds representing a variety of stakeholder interests, including educational, professional, and health advocacy sectors. The Commission was charged with reviewing how all aspects of continuing certification impact not only diplomates, but also healthcare institutions, member boards, and especially, patients, their caregivers, and the public at large. Overarching topics of interest to the Commission were the purpose of continuing certification, the value of continuing certification to diplomates, and the value of continuing certification to the public. The final report of the Commission, released in February 2019, addressed each of these issues with supporting documentation and recommendations [18]. The recommendations specifically considered concerns previously raised by diplomates, many of which had already been addressed in programmatic modifications [9].

One often mentioned issue of diplomate concern has been the belief that continuing certification lacks proof of value, despite an intuitive notion that career-long education, assessment of that education, and participation in peer evaluations are beneficial, and indeed, essential. At the time of conceptualization and implementation of the programs in the 1990s as new and unique initiatives, objective proof of value remained to be demonstrated. In a scientific milieu that recognized randomized controlled clinical trials as the highest level of evidence, this criterion could likely never be met for MOC. The population of non-time-limited certificate holders was continuously diminishing, and that cohort had no incentive to participate in any type of evidence development that would match their performance or knowledge with time-limited certificate holders. Despite these obstacles, and with almost 3 decades of experience with MOC by early-initiator member boards, a significant body of literature now exists regarding the value of the MOC programs to many studied disciplines and stakeholders [19, 20].

The current iteration of MOC programming and the intent for any future modifications are and will be intended to fulfill limited specific goals: meaningful and

nonintrusive educational, assessment, and practice improvement elements for diplomates; sensitivity to the concerns of credentialing, regulatory, and legislative entities; and, most importantly, adherence to the ABMS and Member Board mission of
assuring the public that certified diplomates represent the best providers of health
care in their disciplines.

Summary/Bullets

- The concept of "lifetime certification" in medical specialties existed for over 6
  decades, despite the fact that the notion of a "once and done" assessment of skills
  and knowledge for medical professionals defied a basic understanding of continuous and dynamic scientific advances and clinical practice changes.
- Increasing concerns from within and outside of organized medicine recognized
  that some form of continuous assessment of provider maintenance of skills and
  knowledge was essential to maintain high-quality patient care, public trust in the
  value of specialty certification, and the high level of self-regulation currently
  enjoyed.
- To meet these challenges, the American Board of Medical Specialties (ABMS)
  developed a framework for its 24 member specialty boards to implement similar
  maintenance of certification (MOC) programming across their disciplines.
- Individual medical specialty boards were allowed a degree of flexibility in development of discipline-specific maintenance of certification programs within the
  constraints of adherence to the six core concepts of quality practice and four
  foundational parts of MOC.

For Discussion with a Mentor or Colleague

- Why was the previous policy of "lifetime certification" changed to continuous
  certification to be maintained throughout the diplomates career?
- What are suitable activities for PQI (MOC Part IV)?
- What are some appropriate self-assessment continuing medical education
  activities?
- Why is professional self-regulation an appropriate goal?

References

1. Linton OW. The American Board of Radiology, 75 years of serving the public. Tucson: The
   American Board of Radiology; 2009.
2. The American Board of Family Medicine Certification Process. https://www.theabfm.org/
   continue-certification/how-do-i-remain-certified. Availability verified 2 Jan 2020.

3. Wallner PE, Shrieve DC, Kachnic LA, et al. American Board of radiology maintenance of certification program: evolution to better serve stakeholders. Int J Radiat Oncol Biol Phys. 2016;94(1):16–8.
4. American Board of Medical Specialties History of Certification Development. https://www.abms.org/about-abms/history/. Availability verified 4 Nov 2019.
5. American Board of Medical Specialties Statement on Commitment to Board Certification and Maintenance of Certification (MOC), March 2, 2015. https://www.abms.org/news-events/abms-commitment-to-board-certification-and-maintenance-of-certification-moc/. Availability verified 4 Nov 2019.
6. American Board of Medical Specialties Maintenance of Certification. https://en.wikipedia.org/wiki/American_Board_of_Medical_Specialties#Maintenance_of_certification. Availability verified 4 Nov 2019.
7. MOC Overview and History, the American Board of Dermatology, https://www.abderm.org/about-moc/moc-overview-and-history.aspx. Availability verified 31 Oct 2019.
8. Accreditation Council for Graduate Medical Education Milestone Guidebook. https://www.acgme.org/Portals/0/MilestonesGuidebook.pdf. Availability verified 7 Nov 2019.
9. Cook DA, Holmbee ES, Sorenson KJ, et al. Getting maintenance of certification to work. JAMA Intern Med. 2015;175(1):35–42.
10. Wallner PE, Gerdeman A, Willis JM, et al. The American Board of Radiology radiation oncology maintenance od=f certification part 3 modular examination: evaluation of the first administration. Pract Radiat Oncol. 2016;6:436–8.
11. American Board of Radiology Maintenance of Certification Frequently Asked Questions. https://www.theabr.org/radiation-oncology/maintenance-of-certification/moc-faqs. Availability verified 6 Nov 2019: 56–64.
12. American Board of Radiology Maintenance of Certification Brochure. https://www.theabr.org/wp-content/uploads/2019/01/MOC_Brochure_DR_IR-DR_RO_2019.pdf. Availability verified 7 Nov 2019.
13. American Board of Radiology Maintenance of Certification Program. https://www.theabr.org/radiation-oncology/maintenance-of-certification#moc. Availability verified 5 Nov 2019.
14. American Board of Internal Medicine Announcement, February 3, 2015. https://www.abim.org/media-center/press-releases/abim-announces-immediate-changes-to-moc-program.aspx. Availability verified 4 Nov 2019.
15. PL 111, the Patient Protection and Affordable Care Act of 2010. https://www.govinfo.gov/content/pkg/PLAW-111publ148/pdf/PLAW-111publ148.pdf. Availability verified 21 Nov 2019.
16. American College of Radiation Oncology Maintenance of Certification Report. https://www.acro.org/washington/Maintenance%20of%20Certification.pdf. Availability verified 20 Nov 2019.
17. American Board of Medical Specialties Certification Matters TM Website. https://www.abms.org/verify-certification/certification-matters-service-for-patients-and-families/. Availability verified 21 Nov 2019.
18. American Board of Medical Specialties Continuing Board Certification Vision for the Future report. https://www.abms.org/media/194956/commission_final_report_20190212.pdf. Availability verified Nov. 13, 2019.
19. American Board of Medical Specialties Value of Board Certification https://www.abms.org/board-certification/value-of-board-certification-to-health-care/. Availability verified 6 Nov 2019.
20. American Board of Medical Specialties Research and Education Foundation Reference Library. https://www.abms.org/about-abms/research-and-education-foundation/abms-continuing-certification-reference-center/. Availability verified 7 Nov 2019.

Networking

Mutlay Sayan and Bruce G. Haffty

Introduction

Networking is a process undertaken with the intent of developing and sustaining relationships with those who have the prospective ability to assist in one's career or personal goals [1, 2]. It requires active behavior, which often includes the nurturing of networks both inside and outside one's home institution. While the concept of networking originated in the business world, its benefits extend well beyond it. Indeed, companies in the technological and research fields have come increasingly to rely on networking to find success in today's world [3, 4].

There are many benefits to engaging in effective networking. Much of the literature suggests that networking activity is indispensable to a successful career [5], and scholarly research has reinforced the reality that networking is positively related to objective and subjective measures of career success [6, 7]. Most crucially, one will often see the creation of new projects, find a mentor, and gain access to career advancement [6–11]. Indeed, the task of networking can be a key overall to raising one's career prospects [11–16]. It is clear that people are more likely to recommend, employ, and support projects of people with whom they are personally familiar [14, 16, 17].

One hypothesis has been devised that identifies three skills as being predictors of career advancement: "knowing why," "knowing whom," and "knowing how" [18]. The skill most relevant and directly related to networking is the "Knowing whom." Under this hypothesis, there are two crucial types of networks that will improve one's career development: one's developmental network (including mentoring), and the extensiveness of one's network both internal and external to an institution. The key advantages that come from "knowing whom" is that the sources you cultivate

M. Sayan · B. G. Haffty (✉)
Radiation Oncology, Rutgers Cancer Institute of New Jersey, New Brunswick, NJ, USA
e-mail: hafftybg@cinj.rutgers.edu

© Springer Nature Switzerland AG 2021   289
R. A. Chandra et al. (eds.), *Career Development in Academic Radiation Oncology*, https://doi.org/10.1007/978-3-030-71855-8_20

will provide wisdom, guidance, reputation, advancement, and knowledge. "Knowing whom" also grants important access to additional contacts and potentially career opportunities.

Some benefits of networking can seem less tangible but are no less important. For instance, networking can lead to new acquaintances and friends who will provide valuable sources of emotional support. According to the longitudinal social network analysis over 20 years in the Framingham Heart Study, happiness is very often found through support networks, especially as one's network extends out through a variety of social areas [19]. Put simply, "people's happiness depends on the happiness of others with whom they are connected." These kinds of connections are very often found through networking.

While the practice of networking is most heavily emphasized and relied upon when one is looking for employment opportunities, it is no less important as a method for continued success and advancement in one's current position. Networking involves making meaningful contacts that are enduring, and such contacts can be found in almost any context that provides interaction with colleagues.

Types of Networks

There are several different types of networks, each of which offers various opportunities to individuals. The type of network to pursue, develop, and sustain will depend heavily on one's goals.

Personal Networks

In the first instance, a great place to start with networking is through one's personal community. This includes members of one's family, friends, and other people within the immediate local community. Such contacts are often a primary tool in enhancing one's career prospects and are the starting point for forming a larger network [2, 20]. While people have very different levels of access to influential contacts, for many people it is true that those already within their circle can be extremely helpful in searching for new opportunities [21].

Academic Networks

While not everyone has access to high-powered or influential connections in their personal lives, such contacts can often be found in one's academic career. Relationships are usually formed upon entering a university community, where both undergraduate and postgraduate students can find new contacts within their fields of interest. This continues into residency, where trainees have the opportunity to connect with others from different specialties. By the end of one's educational experience, a network can be built of friends, peers, and colleagues who either become powerful connectors themselves or sources of information on where to locate such connections. Additionally, organizations such as alumni groups can offer networks of former students who are inclined to offer career help [22].

Transient Networks

Temporary communities are those that are encountered when we take part in events. Examples of this include conferences, seminars, and multidisciplinary tumor boards. Annual meetings organized by the American Society for Radiation Oncology (ASTRO), American College of Radiation Oncology (ACRO), and American Radium Society (ARS) are all examples of such events. Encounters like these can provide small windows of opportunity to form bonds with other participants. Often by their nature, they demand quite vigorous networking activities. A proactive, curious, and energetic attitude is essential when approaching activities in these setting [14].

Online Networks

Social media is universally used in today's world. Digital media allows communication between people with minimal effort. Such networks are widely relied upon by patients, healthcare workers, hospitals, and businesses, and they have helped both to better inform patients and to encourage innovation in the practice of healthcare. Social media enables communication instantly without regard to the barriers of geography, resources, or even language (thanks to translation software in many applications.) Clinical educators on social media, through rich peer-to-peer discussions, share the newest research advancements to enhance the practice of evidence-based medicine.

As one example of these social media platforms, LinkedIn is a site used by more than 500 million professionals to grow and interact with their professional network. Many physicians have LinkedIn accounts to promote their academic standing, network with colleagues around the world, and find possible career opportunities [23]. Indeed, even when one is not seeking employment, social media platforms such as LinkedIn, Twitter, and ResearchGate, when used judiciously, can be quite valuable as a networking opportunity, as they can help to find new connections, probe additional knowledge, and raise one's own profile.

Strategies to Improve Networking Opportunities

Included here are some useful insights when it comes to improving and developing networking skills. The strategies below were drawn from sources such as business literature, medical education literature, and personal experiences.

Start with an Existing Network

To varying extents, everyone has some personal network on which to rely. This would often include mentors, colleagues, medical school classmates, and friends in other fields, both medical and nonmedical. This is often the most fertile place to begin. Friends and acquaintances can assist in connecting you with someone from their own circle and coordinate an introduction process [4, 5, 7, 10, 24]. If you know that someone in your own inner circle has a connection with a contact of interest to you, it is usually worth asking whether he or she would be willing to get in touch with them on your behalf.

Committees offer another promising opportunity to expand one's network. The work of such groups – regular attendance at meetings and collaboration on various projects – offers invaluable chances to interact with new people, both within your hospital and within the field. Indeed, finding and sustaining connections with one's own peers can be especially worthwhile, because such people will be the cohort of colleagues with whom you will ultimately spend the most time.

Use Conferences Wisely

National conferences are golden opportunities for networking. Such events are filled to the brim with fellow practitioners, future colleagues, and leaders in the field. Other than conferences, it is rare to find situations in which sizable numbers of people from across the country, and the world, are all under the same roof at the same time. This can be taken advantage of, as opportunities to network abound [15, 24]. This might involve attending an abstract presentation and speaking with the presenter, serving as a resident representative to a committee, or even simply attending preplanned events geared toward networking.

Planning ahead is a key component of conference networking. Generally, a conference's website will provide a list of attendees and presenters. One could easily review this information and make a personal list of speakers and possible attendees he/she would be interested in getting to know. This could be followed by contacting such people via email before the conference and requesting a meeting [16, 24].

Just as one would prepare for a committee meeting with clear goals in mind, so too should one have explicit desired outcomes for networking interactions. Before the meeting, it is a good practice to take the time to figure out what can be ideally achieved from meeting a new contact. The goals don't need be complex: learning more about an aspect of the field, brainstorming a new research idea or potential collaboration, or establishing a new mentor are all realistic and worthy goals for a meeting. Flexibility is essential too [25]. Keep in mind that the conversation may go down a path very different from the one originally intended. Your contact may have his or her own intentions with the meeting, and this can be beneficial. Both personally and professionally, the most powerful relationships are built on shared goals [12].

Don't Forget to Follow Up

As simple as it sounds, the step of following up after each interaction is often forgotten but quite critical [16, 24]. Strong networking skills require following up and maintaining contacts. This can be as quick as a short email thanking the contact for taking time to meet with you and reiterating your shared interest or articulating the next steps that might be involved in a project. After the initial interaction, in order to maintain the new connection, regular contact is essential. The simplest way to keep in touch is by email.

Conclusion

Networking is a series of behaviors which one can employ toward the goal of developing and sustaining relationships with those who have the potential ability to help with one's goals both in one's career and in one's personal life. There are several types of networks, each of which offers various opportunities to individuals. The type of network to pursue, develop, and sustain will depend heavily on one's goals. It requires an active effort to seek out and harvest such connections through the networking process, and several strategies exist for doing so. By knowing the type of networking necessary, and by pursuing connections in a consistent, strategic manner, a diligent professional can turn many potential contacts into lasting friendships and academic partnerships.

Key Points

- Networking is an active process of developing and sustaining relationships with those who have the potential to assist in one's career or personal goals.
- There are several different types of networks, including personal, academic, transient, and online networks.
- Many strategies can be employed to improve and develop networking skills, such as starting with one's home network, using contact opportunities like national conferences, and remembering to follow up.

For Discussion with a Mentor or Colleague

- Which kinds of networks are best for personal goals, and which are best for professional goals?
- Do the opportunities for networking provided in a university setting help to equalize the playing field for those without extensive personal networks?
- Aside from job opportunities, what are some other specific benefits that come with having an extensive network of contacts?

References

1. Quinlan KM. Enhancing mentoring and networking of junior academic women: what, why, and how? J High Educ Policy Manag. 1999;21:31–42.
2. Wolff HG, Moser K. Effects of networking on career success: a longitudinal study. J Appl Psychol. 2009;94:196–206.
3. Baum JAC, Calabrese T, Silverman BS. Don't go it alone: alliance network composition and startups' performance in Canadian biotechnology. Strateg Manag J. 2000;21:267–94.
4. Bougrain F, Haudeville B. Innovation, collaboration and SMEs internal research capacities. Res Policy. 2002;31:735–47.
5. Nierenberg AR. Nonstop networking: how to improve your life, luck, and career. Sterling: Capital Books; 2002.
6. Monica LF, Dougherty TW. Networking behaviors and career outcomes: differences for men and women? J Organ Behav. 2004;25:419–37.
7. Michael J, Yukl G. Managerial level and subunit function as determinants of networking behavior in organizations. Group Org Manag. 1993;18:328–51.
8. Orpen C. Dependency as a moderator of the effects of networking behavior on managerial career success. J Psychol. 1996;130:245–8.
9. Jack SL. The role, use and activation of strong and weak network ties: a qualitative analysis*. J Manag Stud. 2005;42:1233–59.
10. Thompson JA. Proactive personality and job performance: a social capital perspective. J Appl Psychol. 2005;90:1011–7.
11. Emmerik IH, Euwema M, Geschiere M, et al. Networking your way through the organization: gender differences in the relationship between network participation and career satisfaction. Women Manag Rev. 2006;21:56–64.
12. Jackson VA, Palepu A, Szalacha L, et al. "Having the right chemistry": a qualitative study of mentoring in academic medicine. Acad Med. 2003;78:328–34.
13. Ismail M, Rasdi RM. Impact of networking on career development: experience of high-flying women academics in Malaysia. Hum Resour Dev Int. 2007;10:153–68.
14. Haynes L, Adams SL, Boss JM. Mentoring and networking: how to make it work. Nat Immunol. 2008;9:3–5.
15. Warren OJ, Carnall R. Medical leadership: why it's important, what is required, and how we develop it. Postgrad Med J. 2011;87:27–32.
16. Streeter J. Networking in academia. EMBO Rep. 2014;15:1109–12.
17. Higgins MC, Kram KE. Reconceptualizing mentoring at work: a developmental network perspective. Acad Manag Rev. 2001;26:264–88.
18. Eby LT, Butts M, Lockwood A. Predictors of success in the era of the boundaryless career. J Organ Behav. 2003;24:689–708.

19. Fowler JH, Christakis NA. Dynamic spread of happiness in a large social network: longitudinal analysis over 20 years in the Framingham heart study. BMJ. 2008;337:a2338.
20. Arthur M, Khapova S, Wilderom C. Career success in a boundaryless career world. J Organ Behav. 2005;26:177–202.
21. Silliker SA. The role of social contacts in the successful job search. J Employ Couns. 1993;30:25–34.
22. Blackford S. Harnessing the power of communities: career networking strategies for bioscience PhD students and postdoctoral researchers. FEMS Microbiol Lett. 2018;365:1–8.
23. Huang J. Promote education, research, and networking in cardiac anesthesia with journal of cardiothoracic and vascular anesthesia social media. J Cardiothorac Vasc Anesth. 2020;34:315–7.
24. Gottlieb M, Sheehy M, Chan T. Number needed to meet: ten strategies for improving resident networking opportunities. Ann Emerg Med. 2016;68:740–3.
25. Cristancho S, Varpio L. Twelve tips for early career medical educators. Med Teach. 2016;38:358–63.

Leadership Versus Service: What's the Difference? Is There a Difference?

Sue S. Yom and Iris C. Gibbs

The Evolution of Physician Leadership in the Modern Era

The traditional hierarchical view of the physician's role is that of an individual practitioner coordinating and managing a patient's care. In this view, the physician is assisted by a team that may include a number of nonphysician providers and staff, but in the end, the physician makes most of the decisions which are then executed, with the goal of providing the best care for an individual patient. The physician is personally responsible for the outcomes of the plan of care as well as any logistical failures associated to that plan.

However, this view of the physician is increasingly becoming outmoded. Team-based medicine that diffuses decision-making and provision of care across multiple providers has increasingly emerged as the dominant model over the past decades [1]. This model relies heavily on administrative protocols and clinical guidelines and has largely replaced traditional hierarchical models. Similarly, the work environment has also evolved, placing a greater emphasis on enabling and optimizing teamwork for the betterment of the healthcare system [2].

In the modern era, it is increasingly realized that physicians now most commonly work in interdisciplinary teams which may change and evolve in cohesion, size, and complexity over time [3]. The goals of these teams not only include excellence in caring for the individual patient but also work together on process improvement metrics such as communication, efficiency, and quality improvement [4]. Furthermore, the rise of the healthcare triple aim has brought specific emphasis to patient satisfaction metrics, the health of populations, and reducing costs [5].

S. S. Yom (✉)
University of California San Francisco, San Francisco, CA, USA
e-mail: Sue.Yom@ucsf.edu

I. C. Gibbs
Stanford University, Stanford, CA, USA

© Springer Nature Switzerland AG 2021
R. A. Chandra et al. (eds.), *Career Development in Academic Radiation Oncology*, https://doi.org/10.1007/978-3-030-71855-8_21

Medicine will be defined by an increasing focus on population- and value-based care which cannot be carried out by focusing only on the individual level [6].

Rather than focusing exclusively on direct patient care, the physician is now expected to demonstrate managerial acumen. The unique knowledge and management skills needed to navigate these complex sets of responsibilities are domains of leadership that are not emphasized in most medical school curricula [7]. In the current era, most physicians in training will graduate without formal instruction in leadership or management, and due to the pressing demands of standard medical school requirements, they cannot be expected to have the time or resources to seek out these opportunities on their own [8].

Unfortunately, a gap in these skills is likely to lead to a dearth of physicians who are prepared to take on leadership roles and assist in the effective advancement of medical practice. It is commonly recognized that few physicians have the ability to be truly effective at the highest levels of institutional or national service [9]. Moreover, this may become a self-reinforcing phenomenon, as physicians who are unable to gain the skills needed to advance in leadership and service are likely to become discouraged and withdraw from engagement in these types of activities which are increasingly needed by the medical profession.

"Service Work" as Negatively Defined and Perceived

It is not uncommon to hear the term "service" being mentioned in a negative manner [10]. In fact, many institutions actively discourage younger or mid-level faculty from taking on a large amount of service, as it is frequently viewed as noncontributory to the common benchmarks needed for academic advancement [11]. In this view, service is typically portrayed as an obligation to be met at the minimum level required and ideally without any great amount of investment of energy or time. Furthermore, service may be considered a potential distraction from the core elements of clinical, teaching, and research productivity which will be judged in academic assessments [12]. Because of these perceptions, many faculty may conclude that service is relatively unimportant to their careers and become disinterested in it.

There are numerous burdens and pitfalls associated with service. For instance, there is a very real concern that service can be disproportionately leveraged on underrepresented groups who, for various reasons, may take on more service than others. It has been documented, for example, that women spend more time on service assignments that do not lead to direct personal gain, learning, or promotion [13]. In this study, despite both working about 64 hours per week, male associate professors spent 37% of their time on research, while females spent 25% of their time on research. Female associate professors spent 27% of their time on service, while males spent 20% of their time on service. In science, technology, engineering, and medical (STEM) fields, these differences were more pronounced, with associate STEM men spending 42% of their time on research compared to 27% of STEM women's time. Associate STEM women spent 21% of their time mentoring and 25% on service compared to 15% and 20%, respectively, for STEM men [14].

In another survey study of academic faculty, these service-related differential efforts were driven by a greater number of internal rather than external assignments accepted by women, and with regards to the external assignments, women performed more community and national service as opposed to higher profile and more visible service to professional organizations or the international community [15]. In this type of scenario, providing labor- or time-intensive service to one's department or institution without obvious recognition or reward could add to a faculty member's feelings of discouragement, alienation, and underappreciation.

Furthermore, institutions often rely upon physicians from racial and ethnic groups underrepresented in medicine to promote diversity initiatives. These physicians can in turn incur a "minority tax," [16] which can be colloquially defined as the collection of additional responsibilities that institutions place on minority faculty in their efforts to display diversity. An example of this might be excessive service on numerous search committees to ensure an emphasis on diversity as part of these search processes. Despite providing these important institutional contributions, underrepresented faculty may not be afforded additional access to mentorship or opportunities for promotion as result of these activities [17]. Thus, many such faculty report social isolation, racism, and bias as part of their experiences in academic medicine [18, 19]. While provision of extra service may be only one factor in this complex issue, it adds to the stress and separation that a faculty member may feel.

Also, these factors may have a tendency to become dangerously self-reinforcing. For example, women and minority physicians may resign themselves to the reality of reduced power or powerlessness which leads to acceptance of less desirable assignments. Specific cultural factors may be operative in women who may face consequences from not being seen as a "team player" or have an inability to say no [20]. Culturally conditioned factors may also lead some women or minorities to accept demotion of their personal interests for the benefit of the institution in a form of self-sacrifice that they hope will be recognized. Alternatively, there may be a personal interest or commitment which drives women or minorities to allocate larger amounts of time to service that may not be recognized as prestigious or important. This is a particular influence in the area of community service.

For these reasons, it is important to define one's service carefully and to understand fully the scope and nature of the work. It is also important to analyze one's reasons for taking on service commitments and what that means in the context of one's professional and personal life. This requires a strategic and intentional formulation of one's service agenda, which ideally should be coherent with the parts related to each other and the whole [21].

This process should be regularly revisited and evaluated as one's career evolves over time [22]. There can be extremely valid reasons for engaging in service that may not be assessed by others as significant or impactful, but this should be managed in the context of all of one's other competing academic responsibilities. This can be a complex calculus as most universities do not define clearly what the expectations for service are or under what conditions service, even if outstanding or exceptional, may factor into one's academic evaluations [23].

The Varieties of "Service" and Their Relationship to Professional Values

Despite these valid multiple concerns, it is extremely important not to dismiss the meaning of service. Service may represent an important source of personal value and fulfillment and may even contribute to finding deeper meaning within a professional career. Service is also valuable from a civic and public standpoint, as organizations clearly cannot function without engagement and participation from their members [24]. Most importantly, we believe that service and leadership are inextricably intertwined. From this perspective, we propose that service is a source and avenue for developing leadership skills and opportunities, and conversely, service is a necessity and functional component of leadership.

Traditionally, service in the context of academia has meant membership on committees formed for the purposes of program review, grant/funding awards or review, academic programming, academic search/promotion, or operations/governance. These memberships can vary in the level of time and attention required. Their value to one's career can vary widely, but in some cases can potentially offset some of the perils of the "minority tax." Aligning one's service with an area of passion can be mutually beneficial by providing unique insights into organizational structure and the inner workings of the institution. However, it is important to acknowledge that various types of service are not regarded as equally significant and some types of service may require much greater amounts of time and effort than others. Furthermore, different types of service may result in different benefits in terms of the knowledge that is acquired or the networking and personal connections that may be developed (Table 1).

A newer development over the past couple of decades is that many institutions are increasingly recognizing public or community service as valid forms of service [25]. Uniquely for academic physicians who are interested in community-based research, it is possible for these activities in some cases to tie closely to one's research or teaching, or for these engagements to lead to new ideas or funding opportunities. The emerging fields of dissemination and implementation research increasingly require expertise and real-world knowledge of community organizations.

General Benefits of Service Work

While specific benefits of different types of service may result (Table 1), there are also general benefits of service which are important to describe.

Table 1 Types and benefits of service

Type of service	Benefits of service
Departmental committees	Learn about department decisions Contribute to forming department policies and processes Demonstrate your abilities to your colleagues and chair
Medical school committees	Make connections to other departments Learn about other departments Better understand educational or faculty development processes Show value as a representative of your department
Medical center committees	Make connections to other departments Learn about other departments Better understand operational and organizational processes Show value as a representative of your department
Community organizations	Learn about the challenges, needs, and priorities of the organization Gain expertise in community–academia relationship building Learn about nonprofit and organizational management Potential for collaboration with the organization or support from the organization
Professional organizations	Make connections to other institutions Learn about other institutions' strategies and processes Preview emerging trends and issues within and affecting the profession Build external professional reputation

Networking and Support

An important part of academic success and promotion is recognition by one's peers, both within the institution and around the country and world. Service can be an important way to establish one's reputation [26]. A real and tangible benefit of service commitment is identifying people who may be able to write letters of recommendation or write in support of one's promotion. In particular, junior faculty may benefit from making the acquaintance of senior faculty who are in a position to assist and advise.

Furthermore, service can be a means to connect personally with researchers and educators in other departments and/or institutions. This can lead to learning more about new advances in one's research area, collaborations to investigate areas of common interest, and friendships that may be a source of valuable support over the course of a career [27]. When evaluating whether to take on a new service commitment of this nature, it may be useful to spend considerable time learning about it first, specifically considering its potential alignment to one's academic interests and priorities. Particularly in the case of membership in a professional organization, these commitments should be evaluated for the likelihood of a long-term commitment.

Ability to Make an Impact

Many who enter academia wish to enact change and contribute to progress, and some forms of service can yield meaningful impact. Usually, the ability to have an impact will come after a period of sustained and consistent service in one particular direction. At that point, there will often be opportunities or projects that may fall to those who show genuine interest and competence in the work. It is thus important to engage in service commitments that are personally meaningful, as enthusiasm and commitment are valued when persons are selected for these types of opportunities and cannot easily be feigned.

Finding meaning in one's work should also be a priority. This consideration is easily dismissed, but fulfillment and enjoyment are very important to the long-term sustainability of a faculty member's academic effort [28]. Certain forms of service may provide a personal satisfaction that justifies the effort. It can be extremely gratifying to contribute knowledge and skills to a service work that has a high level of particular personal meaning.

Soft Skills and Leadership Development

There are definable skills which are needed to function effectively in groups, and service work can be a very important training ground for the development of complex skills such as negotiation, time management, prioritization, and conflict resolution. Working in groups provides training in interpersonal skills that may benefit many aspects of one's academic interactions in the future [29].

In addition, observing and working with a talented leader provides an up-close case study in learning how to manage effectively. With sustained and visible commitment, there may also be leadership opportunities that become available. There may be the opportunity to obtain valuable mentoring from other leaders within the group. Leadership development includes consensus-building, change management skills, and skills in managing group meeting and agendas effectively.

Developing a Service Agenda and Portfolio

For junior faculty, service commitments will likely be mostly time-limited, involving short-term assignments to reviews, courses, or group projects. For these types of work, it is important to estimate the amount of time and energy that will be needed. Junior faculty should ask what the usual time commitment and meeting schedule is that should be expected for each project. Our strong suggestion is that this should be planned and/or calendared just like any other form of work commitment. It can be helpful for junior faculty to consult with a senior advisor within their department to discuss their service commitment portfolio.

It is very reasonable for a starting faculty member to choose to be significantly involved in at least one departmental or institutional committee and one professional society. As the faculty member progresses in their career, additional committees and societies may be added but these should be strategically selected for their value to the faculty's career interests and promotion. This might include activities that have a possibility to help in improving their scholarship or teaching, for example.

As seniority increases, service commitments tend to involve more ongoing and sustained involvement and perhaps leadership. For instance, in one's fourth year as faculty, it would be reasonable to consider initiating a community engagement activity. There might also be opportunities to expand one's role into leadership of a section or committee.

It is important to manage one's service portfolio actively, both to allocate time and effort in reasoned manner and to assure receipt of appropriate credit for these activities. To this end, organized documentation of one's service should be maintained. It is best to keep a spreadsheet listing each service commitments with its associated working groups, subcommittees, or project assignments. Under these sub-assignments, the dates of service, the role taken in the group (member, chair, lead), and the specific contribution that was made (voting, research, writing, review) should all be documented.

Flexible Leadership for the Twenty-First Century

We believe that it is not possible to develop a rich and meaningful academic career in the total absence of service. Service offers the opportunity to share knowledge and expertise with others, which is one of the foundations of academic life. We also believe that a carefully curated program of service leads naturally to leadership development and leadership opportunities. To lead effectively, it is important to understand all aspects of service and vice versa.

Here it may be helpful as one framework to introduce the concept of the servant-leader. Traditional leadership theory focused on the performance of the organization, and the main goal of leadership was to enhance one's own performance, influence, and visibility. The alternative concept of the servant-leader emerged in 1970 with the publication of a foundational essay introducing this concept [30]. A servant-leader's main focus is to serve, putting others' needs first and helping others to develop and perform as well as possible. Instead of "I lead" the concept is that "I serve."

The servant-leader formulation resonates well with physicians because the practice of medicine is ultimately about helping others. This model has become a highly influential and guiding principle for numerous large organizations [31]. To act as a servant-leader requires maturity, a desire to understand others' needs, a background in the organization and institution to enable others, and a practice of selfless concern for the well-being of others. While no clear consensus exists on the exact criteria or standards for judging this style of leadership, research efforts have focused on altruism, self-sacrifice, and leader-member exchange. Other emphases include charismatic, transforming, authentic, spiritual, and transformational leadership [32]. Leadership can exist at many levels and in many contexts, but the fundamental construct of servant-leader defines a large part of modern leadership and is helpful in conceptualizing the complex connection between service work and leadership.

The modern management concept of the servant-leader puts the emphasis back on service to others and fundamentally links the concept of service and leadership in a revolving and renewing cycle. This would seem to be one appropriate conceptualization of the interdisciplinary and fluid nature of teams in contemporary medicine and medical administration. Service work is hence the training ground and fundamental bedrock that underlies leadership. Leaders in medicine today do not exist to lead alone; they need to be able to draw the best out of the persons around them and motivate those persons to excel; they exist to provide service and mentorship to others.

Unfortunately, in ineffective or poorly functioning teams, the potential perils of the servant-leader model are similar to the traditional hierarchical leadership model in that the overwhelming sense of personal responsibility can lead to burnout. The self-sacrificing emphasis and excessive subjugation of ego can lead to distress and fatigue in both leaders and followers. Also, in some organizations, the servant-leader structure may also result in overreliance on the leader with disconnection and loss of motivation by other team members, with resultant downstream negative effects on interpersonal relationships.

Thus an ideal leader should be aware of the advantages as well as pitfalls of various forms of leadership and demonstrate flexibility in their application. Every leader must be proficient in multiple styles and skills of leadership which may require formal study. As engagement at higher levels progresses or becomes more complex, senior faculty may need deeper engagement in studying models of leadership formally. To study leadership more, there are many good books on various aspects and other valuable experiences are to take a course or seminar or engage a private coach.

If truly abiding by the concept of servant-leadership, leadership is strictly defined as a self-sacrificing activity, not ever being about obtaining a title or advancement. In reality, however, from a practical perspective, leadership roles should be recognized and compensated appropriately, whether through financial compensation or formal recognition. An overly self-sacrificing adherence to the servant-leader approach could be detrimental to further advancement in leadership, particularly for women and minorities.

Whether for themselves or others, academic leaders must be adept at negotiation, decision-making, equitable resource allocation, and collaboration [33]. As a new leader, it is important to form alliances with persons within the organization who can help you learn about effective means of leadership and help you to contribute meaningfully. Mentorship, just as it was an important part of service learning, is also important in leadership development, and new leaders should seek out persons who are willing to serve in that role.

Service and Leadership: Personal Experiences from the Authors

Sue Yom

I tend to see any committee or leadership role I go into as an opportunity to serve something, whether that's the organization or a cause that I care about, or whether it's the people involved in that initiative whom I want to do right by. I don't know if some part of that comes necessarily from one of my minority identities, but it might. Certainly, I've felt what it's like when structures aren't working for me or other people, and I've always hoped there might be ways to help set them right so that they do work for more people.

I usually notice when people seem unhappy or upset and it deeply bothers me. I still have a lot of faith that a listening, collaborative dialogue between groups and leadership can fix at least some if not all of those problems. I have strong convictions about certain basic principles, and I see my involvement in any group or leadership role as an opportunity to follow through on those. I also know I'm not perfect and that probably no one is, so I perceive leadership skills as something everyone including me can continue to work on. One of the biggest lessons in my life has been to try to really listen to others' feedback and be open to it, even if it is painful or doesn't make sense to you at the time, because you can always learn something from the experience. I believe this is true in all aspects of academic life, even research collaborations.

When I was very early on in my career, I personally really enjoyed being on committees, because I thought of them as opportunities to shape the dialogue or process. I never was careful about limiting my commitments and probably should have managed my time better in retrospect. I gradually learned to set limits and say no but that honestly came with age and more self-confidence. I probably sacrificed research time in favor of committees and organizational opportunities - and I happened to be in a flexible career track that for better or worse, allowed me to make these kinds of choices.

The best situation is when you're on a committee or in a group possibly leading something that really excites you and that makes you want to look at it all the time and do work on it and do extra. The very best, of course, is if there is some learning in it, either that contributes directly to your research or your career, or that deeply influences you or changes you in some way. I regard all the service work and leadership I've done so far in my career as having contributed to developing my personal style and thus I do think it's all been valuable in some way in the end. I strongly advise people to follow their passions in life and not be afraid to be involved in things that mean a lot to you, because that is how you will discover your own uniqueness and enrich your professional life.

Iris Gibbs

I have not always viewed myself as a leader. However, as I have traversed my journey through training and academic medicine, increasingly it has become evident that people who share my background and who look like me are scarce. Hence, my journey to leadership has caused me to venture out of my own comfort zone and to speak more vociferously than I would otherwise. I have always walked a tightrope, and while I do not think consciously about it, I know that I shoulder the responsibility of representing more than myself—whether I intend to or not. My choices and responses will invariably open or close opportunities for other minorities. This is the fact of my underrepresentation. Because I so abhor tokenism, I have made sure to offer my unique perspectives to committees and become the voice of the voiceless. Being in this position has given me the opportunity to learn several lessons: (1) If not me then who? (2) If you are not at the table, you may very well be on the menu. (3) To define for myself what opportunity looks like—not every lemon is suitable for lemonade, but often through innovation, untoward service can be turned into opportunities. (4) While no one is indispensable, potential leaders need to nurture a skill that is unique and valuable. (5) Seize the moment, as not all opportunities will come again.

During my early training, I learned an adage, "If there's a chair sit in it; if there is food, eat it; if they tell you to go home, go home because the longer you stay the longer you stay." I have taken these lessons with me, though they have evolved. I have learned the value of having a seat at the table—and, yes, I literally will almost never sit along the chairs aligning the walls of a boardroom if there are seats at the table. Sometimes this garners me strange looks about my place, but I persevere. I understand that issues of great importance and livelihood are made at these tables, resources are allocated at these tables, and I insist on being in the room at the table when I can. I do not want to be on the menu—my fate or resources being determined without my input. Despite these efforts, sadly most minorities have not been afforded the opportunity to serve at the most powerful tables at my institution.

Mentorship and sponsorship of others while taxing are also incredibly rewarding. As an individual who is underrepresented in medicine, mentorship is a powerful leadership skill that ensures legacy. Mentorship is mutually beneficial to the mentor and mentee, renewing one's sense of purpose. Mentorship is almost always "good" service.

Summary

Service is essential to the trajectory along the journey to leadership. While some types of service may not be personally beneficial to career advancement, other services can open up to opportunities for meaningful impact. Understanding how best to devote one's academic time and energy toward service can be challenging and can be particularly so for women and minorities, owing to the "minority tax." It is important to balance one's service with other competing priorities and account for the time and effort spent, with consideration as to whether there is appropriate compensation either professionally or personally for these activities. The prevailing concept of the servant-leader is a popular and suitable style of leadership in team-based medicine, but must be balanced with other styles of leadership in order to be most effective for the leader and to permit continued upward mobility. Leadership is a process of personal development that requires time and attention.

Take Home Messages

- While not all service will lead to career advancement, service to others is required to become a good leader.
- Mentorship is good service.
- Persons underrepresented in medicine have a unique vantage point that can be leveraged for mutual benefit of the individual and the institution but needs to be carefully managed to avoid a "minority tax."
- Service obligations should be actively evaluated and managed for their relevance to personal and professional goals.
- Nurturing leadership skills lays the groundwork for academic advancement.

For Discussion with a Mentor or Colleague

- I am most passionate about …. How can I best channel these passions into my work as a physician?
- Could you help me with balancing service that energizes me the most and what feels draining or forced or inauthentic?
- Do you have suggestions about which committees or organizations would benefit me the most personally or professionally?
- How do you see me developing as a leader? What aspects of my personal leadership style should I improve or develop further?
- Could you review my 5-year plan for academic, personal, and community success?

References

1. Gawande A. Cowboys and pit crews. The New Yorker. 26 May 2011.
2. Mitchell PH, Institute of Medicine (U.S.), Institute of Medicine (U.S.). Roundtable on Value & Science-Driven Health Care. Best Practices Innovation Collaborative. Core principles & values of effective team-based health care. Discussion paper. Washington, DC: Institute of Medicine; 2012.

3. Salas E, Wilson KA, Murphy CE, King H, Salisbury M. Communicating, coordinating, and cooperating when lives depend on it: tips for teamwork. Jt Comm J Qual Patient Saf. 2008;34(6):333–41. https://doi.org/10.1016/s1553-7250(08)34042-2.
4. Shea CM, Turner K, Albritton J, Reiter KL. Contextual factors that influence quality improvement implementation in primary care: the role of organizations, teams, and individuals. Health Care Manag Rev. 2018;43(3):261–9. https://doi.org/10.1097/HMR.0000000000000194.
5. Kirch DG, Ast C. Interprofessionalism: educating to meet patient needs. Anat Sci Educ. 2015;8(4):296–8. https://doi.org/10.1002/ase.1504.
6. Gourevitch MN. Population health and the academic medical center: the time is right. Acad Med. 2014;89(4):544–9. https://doi.org/10.1097/ACM.0000000000000171.
7. Dine CJ, Kahn JM, Abella BS, Asch DA, Shea JA. Key elements of clinical physician leadership at an academic medical center. J Grad Med Educ. 2011;3(1):31–6. https://doi.org/10.4300/JGME-D-10-00017.1.
8. Myers CG, Pronovost PJ. Making management skills a core component of medical education. Acad Med. 2017;92(5):582–4. https://doi.org/10.1097/ACM.0000000000001627.
9. Gabel S. Expanding the scope of leadership training in medicine. Acad Med. 2014;89(6):848–52. https://doi.org/10.1097/ACM.0000000000000236.
10. Group SSFNRI. The burden of invisible work in academia: social inequalities and time use in five university departments. Humboldt J Soc Relations. 2017;39:228–45.
11. Lampe C. Why I love academic service. Medium. 12 July 2016.
12. Macfarlane B. Defining and Rewarding Academic Citizenship: the implications for university promotions policy. J High Educ Policy Manag. 2007;29(3):261–73. https://doi.org/10.1080/13600800701457863.
13. Misra J, Lundquist JH, Templer A. Gender, work time, and care responsibilities among faculty. Sociol Forum. 2012;27(2):300–23. https://doi.org/10.1111/j.1573-7861.2012.01319.x.
14. Misra J, Lundquist JH, Holmes E, Agiomavritis S. The ivory ceiling of service work academe. Washington, DC: American Association of University Professors; 2011. p. 22–6.
15. Guarino CM, Borden VMH. Faculty service loads and gender: are women taking care of the academic family? Res High Educ. 2017;58(6):672–94. https://doi.org/10.1007/s11162-017-9454-2.
16. Rodriguez JE, Campbell KM, Pololi LH. Addressing disparities in academic medicine: what of the minority tax? BMC Med Educ. 2015;15:6. https://doi.org/10.1186/s12909-015-0290-9.
17. Bergeron D, Ostroff C, Schroeder T, Block C. The dual effects of organizational citizenship behavior: relationships to research productivity and career outcomes in academe. Hum Perform. 2014;27(2):99–128. https://doi.org/10.1080/08959285.2014.882925.
18. Mahoney MR, Wilson E, Odom KL, Flowers L, Adler SR. Minority faculty voices on diversity in academic medicine: perspectives from one school. Acad Med. 2008;83(8):781–6. https://doi.org/10.1097/ACM.0b013e31817ec002.
19. Campbell KM, Rodriguez JE. Addressing the minority tax: perspectives from two diversity leaders on building minority faculty success in academic medicine. Acad Med. 2019;94(12):1854–7. https://doi.org/10.1097/Acm.0000000000002839.
20. Cardel MI, Dhurandhar E, Yarar-Fisher C, Foster M, Hidalgo B, McClure LA, et al. Turning chutes into ladders for women faculty: a review and roadmap for equity in academia. J Women's Health. 2020;29(5):721–33. https://doi.org/10.1089/jwh.2019.8027.
21. Pfeifer HL. How to be a good academic citizen: the role and importance of service in academia. J Crim Justice Educ. 2016;27(2):238–54. https://doi.org/10.1080/10511253.2015.1128706.
22. Neumann A, Terosky AL. To give and to receive: recently tenured professors' experiences of service in major research universities. J High Educ-UK. 2007;78(3):282−+. https://doi.org/10.1353/jhe.2007.0018.
23. Filetti JS. Assessing service in faculty reviews: mentoring faculty and developing transparency. Mentor Tutor. 2009;17(4):343–52. https://doi.org/10.1080/13611260903284416.
24. Lynton EA. Making the case for professional service. Washington, DC: American Association for Higher Education; 1995.

25. Driscoll A, Lynton EA, Lynton EA, Forum on Faculty Roles & Rewards (American Association for Higher Education). Making outreach visible : a guide to documenting professional service and outreach. Washington, DC: American Association for Higher Education; 1999.
26. Porter CM, Woo SE. Untangling the networking phenomenon: a dynamic psychological perspective on how and Why people network. J Manage. 2015;41(5):1477–500. https://doi.org/10.1177/0149206315582247.
27. Wolff HG, Moser K. Effects of networking on career success: a longitudinal study (vol 94, pg 196, 2009). J Appl Psychol. 2017;102(2):150. https://doi.org/10.1037/apl0000199.
28. Brown S, Gunderman RB. Viewpoint: enhancing the professional fulfillment of physicians. Acad Med. 2006;81(6):577–82. https://doi.org/10.1097/01.ACM.0000225224.27776.0d.
29. Martin GP, McKee L, Dixon-Woods M. Beyond metrics? Utilizing 'soft intelligence' for healthcare quality and safety. Soc Sci Med. 2015;142:19–26. https://doi.org/10.1016/j.socscimed.2015.07.027.
30. Greenleaf RK. Servant leadership : a journey into the nature of legitimate power and greatness. New York: Paulist Press; 1977.
31. Bujak JS. Approaches to influencing physician behavior. Seek to be a servant leader when building partnerships with your physicians. Healthc Exec. 2009;24(1):68–9.
32. Eva N, Robin M, Sendjaya S, van Dierendonck D, Liden RC. Servant leadership: a systematic review and call for future research. Leadersh Q. 2019;30(1):111–32. https://doi.org/10.1016/j.leaqua.2018.07.004.
33. Grant A. Give and take: a revolutionary approach to success. New York: Viking; 2013.

Disease Site Leadership

Salma K. Jabbour and Sue S. Yom

Introduction

Achieving disease site leadership functions as a mechanism for personal growth and fulfillment, by mastering a topic and serving as an expert in a particular subspecialty. To develop an expertise may require patience, concentrated study, pursuit of research and quality improvement, and other collaborations and networking. Identifying stakeholders and opportunities for cooperation can provide career enrichment and building of new endeavors and initiatives. Persistence, resilience, and adaptability are key characteristics to reach a desired outcome.

Working with Colleagues to Build Expertise

In radiation oncology, it is common for physicians to associate themselves with a particular topic or an interest for which they may garner a local, national, and/or international reputation. Most often we think of this topic or interest as relating to a particular cancer subtopic (i.e., management of early-stage non-small cell lung cancer) or a topic related to the discipline of radiation oncology (i.e., negotiating a contract or job offer in radiation oncology), and in either instance, this subspecialty within radiation oncology is based on a particular dedication to the topic, either in the form of lectures, publications, or advocacy. These subspecializations may occur

S. K. Jabbour (✉)
Rutgers Cancer Institute of New Jersey, Rutgers University, New Brunswick, NJ, USA
e-mail: jabbousk@cinj.rutgers.edu

S. S. Yom
University of California San Francisco, San Francisco, CA, USA

© Springer Nature Switzerland AG 2021
R. A. Chandra et al. (eds.), *Career Development in Academic Radiation Oncology*, https://doi.org/10.1007/978-3-030-71855-8_22

naturally from an affinity or passion about the topic and accrete over time by virtue of increasing familiarity and expertise on a topic, or because of the patient volume and/or clinical or administrative responsibilities assigned within a department. Subspecialized interests are not only applicable to those working in academic practices, although these associations may occur more frequently as many academicians focus on one or two disease areas of interest; in any case, specialized interests are often taken up by experts working in private settings who develop a commitment to a specific topic or area. In either situation, the individual spends time and effort to promote and develop this interest by educating others through research, education, improvements in care or workflow, or advocacy.

When faced with a topic about which one is expected to become an expert, one may gather this wealth of information over time and/or may delve deeply into a thorough understanding of the topic over a condensed time course. The necessity or urgency to learn a topic may result from the environment (i.e., a case presentation at tumor board in the upcoming week for which one is the only radiation oncologist) or the nature of the need (i.e., composing a review article over many months about a topic). Regardless of the reason for learning about a topic, the importance of this knowledge lies in its dissemination to colleagues in a clear and consistent manner, often with the need to be convincing (Table 1). One concrete example might be in the debate at an institutional tumor board about the utility of a particular preoperative therapy in which surgery provides the curative intent. It might be important to provide detailed, succinct information by citing the data about the pathological complete response rates or notable local control benefits that can be achieved with preoperative chemoradiation compared to chemotherapy alone, perhaps using the format of brief presentation with a slide deck or printed bullet-point summary sheet. In the absence of presenting supporting information, the physician may face difficulties in persuading colleagues from other disciplines about the utility of chemoradiation for this case or similar, future cases. Although it may take extra effort to prepare for sharing knowledge which seems obvious to another radiation oncologist, providing multidisciplinary education based on the expertise of the radiation oncologist is central to acquiring the support of colleagues for a recommendation

Table 1 Potential obstacles to disease site leadership and potential approaches

Obstacle	Potential approach
Lack of consensus on patient care discussion	Education of colleagues through brief presentations or circulation of brief summaries of the literature
Unreceptive colleagues in areas of interest	Diplomatic and amicable demeanor; consider tweaking area of interest if unable to overcome differences
Difficulty managing collaborator's participation in a project	Arrange deadlines and routine meetings to track of progress; if unable to resolve, then consider open and honest discussion to optimize/reduce colleague commitment
Key stakeholder unaware of progress in subspecialty	Schedule regular meetings to provide updates and ask for advising and connection to opportunities
Unable to garner strong outside networking	Approach outside collaborators with forethought having a clear vision and goals that align multiple interests

involving patient care and can improve patient care outcomes [1, 2]. One could think of similar instances in trying to persuade one's leadership about a process to benefit the department, or discussing with the hospital CEO the importance of a technology. Being prepared with data is pivotal to developing expertise and one's reputation as an authority, and these points may require many repetitions to involved stakeholders before they materialize into a desired outcome.

Continuing to demonstrate a depth of knowledge about a topic over repeated instances may allow others to look to this individual as someone who will emerge as a leader. Leadership does not occur overnight, and in the rare circumstances it does, this is because a predecessor has laid the groundwork for this path or there are colleagues who are usually receptive to this development. It is perhaps more often the case than not, particularly when trying to sway those in your group who may be less familiar with your perspective, that developing into an expert could take months or years. At the heart of this discussion about developing into an authority, we must understand that that resilience and persistence are required. It may take repeated discussions about the same topic to influence others or to appreciate other points of view or to derive a consensus. Why do the opinions or beliefs of others not change immediately? The answer to this question may be multifactorial and could include long-held biases, lack of familiarity with the topic, and the need to build a level of trust and respect within the group. All of these belief systems as well as others may be truly ingrained and may take time to change. During this period of relationship building, the radiation oncologist should be consistent in presenting the data, must remain patient and diplomatic, must continue to provide timely and thoughtful involvement, and should try to engage colleagues through collaborative efforts if possible (Table 1). Collaborative efforts may include working together in presenting a lecture or performing a retrospective review on a mutual topic of interest or holding informal group meetings to encourage more candid interpersonal dialogue.

The take-home messages are that knowledge, partnership, patience, resilience, and often time will achieve the desired results of building expertise. Regardless of the topic at hand, following a passion or topic of vested interest will make this work more satisfying by building on a baseline level of enthusiasm and relevance to one's personal development.

Tumor Boards/Cancer Center Initiatives

Circumstances may permit for establishment of a new subspecialty tumor board or committee, but for this group to take hold and become a consistent force, a core constituency with the same or greater vested interest as the original visionary must be present. Otherwise, the group will lack roots and regularity. Three to four committed individuals can form a vision into a continuing reality, but with only one to two individuals, there will likely be an insufficiency of ideas and energy. Within this core group of individuals, we will likely harness the capital of the visionary, formal and informal leaders, and several committed members. Roles can include publicizing the group, organizing the logistics and mission, and following through with the mission of providing increased knowledge and fulfillment to the members.

Developing such a committee can lead to other desirable endpoints. For example, initiation of a liver tumor board can lead to the growth in the fund of knowledge about liver cancers, followed by increased expertise, then a research endeavor, or perhaps a potential set of new patient referrals for radiation therapy. Also, as an integral part of the early discussion and as an early adapter, the radiation oncologist may help to develop treatment paradigms and work with colleagues to provide evidence-based care. Having a seat at the table, and getting there early, can build experience and shape the role of radiotherapy within the group.

Continuing to be responsible for incorporating modern techniques and philosophies can allow the radiation oncologist to grow as a central part of the tumor board working group. The radiation oncologist may contribute meaningfully by bringing important initiatives to the group, by using novel techniques, being up-to-date and educating colleagues about newly released data, and facilitating the care of patients efficiently. The radiation oncologist may be a front-runner in arranging collaborations with different specialties, such as interventional radiology, or arranging clinical trial protocols that draw on the expertise of multiple disciplines within the group. Close collaborations with colleagues can make the tumor board experience rewarding and stimulating.

Cancer center initiatives focusing on a particular research or quality improvement endeavor may allow for sources of funding, access to certain key thought leaders within the institution, and opportunities to work on a timely project in an expedited manner. The collaborative nature of these multiple-principal investigator projects may propel the project forward due to its strong base of participants. In sum, getting involved, even if outside of one's comfort zone, can build relationships and provide access to knowledge and involvement that would have not been otherwise possible.

Building Expertise Within the Division and Institution

As one's particular expertise grows, sharing this interest with immediate colleagues will become routine, but keeping a supervisor aware of this growth remains an essential consideration. The supervisor may not be fully aware of the details of growth, and providing updates and communication to leaders in the department can help keep them abreast of the ongoing advances in an area of expertise. This communication remains relevant as there is progression in career growth where advice and guidance may be needed. There are many instances in which a chair or leader has a lack of overlap in subspecialization or daily practice that would keep them fully apprised. Providing updates about the continued development of expertise may aid them in connecting the faculty member with networking inside and outside of the institution or other opportunities. If nothing else, this communication will aid the leader to understand the strides that have been accomplished and ways to support one's continued progress in a subspecialty. Although periodic meetings may be mandatory, one can demonstrate initiative by proactively arranging meetings to explicitly discuss achievements and future goals. Other casual communication can foster this relationship as well.

Other important stakeholders within the institution can include those from the discipline with whom there is a shared common interest with regard to the specialty (i.e., thoracic cancers). These relationships may be initiated in tumor boards but may continue to develop outside of tumor boards through continued collaboration in research or quality endeavors or patient care. To this end, one may develop a mentor in medical or surgical oncology based on common interests or possible partnerships. Other stakeholders may include senior leaders in the cancer center, including the cancer center director or executive committee members. Opportunities to be involved in cancer center grants can also foster important friendships and chances to extend horizons of the radiation oncologist. For example, a grant that incorporates early-phase clinical trials with novel agents may present opportunities to use these agents preclinically as radiosensitizers or in phase I clinical trials. Involvement in community-based initiatives at the cancer center level may lead to opportunities for the radiation oncologist to extend their network of services and education. Interaction with other individuals may lead to opportunities or resources that may align with the topic or work and can result in networking opportunities that allow for continued development of expertise.

Managing Others

When embarking on a research endeavor or building a programmatic initiative, one cannot go at it alone. Although a radiation oncologist may have physician collaborators from within radiation oncology, it is likely that many needed collaborators will be located outside of the department; to manage their involvement requires a foundation of trust and strong communication built up from previous interactions. It may be necessary to manage a team of physician colleagues, residents, and students to complete a deadline or direct an administrative assistant who may help with the submission of an application or manuscript. At the heart of management is creating a dialogue of information exchange including clear expectations for deadlines and the quality of the work (Table 1). To propel a project to the finish line, a critical component is frequent communication through periodic meetings where future goals are set for the next meeting (serving as an interim deadline), and this step can be repeated until a desired outcome is achieved, or until there is confidence that another colleague or trainee can complete the work at hand based on the initial guidance and feedback. Also in dealing with nonmedical staff, key pieces of delegation may include direction, follow-up on progress, and personal involvement until a certain task has become familiar and can be fulfilled independently. These processes can seem repetitive at first, but once the radiation oncologist has sculpted these elements, it will prove easier to carry out a similar project or task in the future requiring less oversight and with outcomes mirroring those of close involvement. In some instances, it will be important to work with colleagues who concur with the goal at hand or your leadership role (Table 1). In these scenarios, maintaining a positive and amicable disposition as well as focusing on the relevance of the common goal can aid in the inception and completion of a project.

How to Develop and Realize Research Goals

Often research goals morph from the specific experiences of a seasoned radiation oncologist and are based on a new connection or sudden attentiveness to a topic. Availability for implementation and maintenance of a particular technology, with the aid of one or more dedicated physicists, may lead to an expertise in this technology in the setting of a disease subspecialty (i.e., proton therapy (technology) for pancreatic cancers (subspecialty)). Alternatively, as noted above, a cancer center with strong programs of excellence may lead to radiation oncologists having access to novel phase I agents or clinical or community initiatives that could incorporate radiation therapy. Frequently there are prospects that are readily accessible within the department or cancer center which will most easily lend themselves to development into a focused interest, and for early-career radiation oncologists, leveraging pre-existing strengths of the institution will be viewed as most feasible and supported by colleagues and leadership. It is also feasible for the radiation oncologist to build on a topic where there has not been a prior infrastructure, but this may require at least one other committed and established stakeholder in order to form a partnership. For example, to start a radioembolization program could require working closely with an interventional radiologist, and such an enterprise could flourish with a committed partnership and loyalty. Building up a new interest is only likely to succeed in a context of personal accessibility, mutual interest, and high initiative.

It is also possible to pursue a new interest by collaborating with stakeholders outside of the institution; however, it will be important for one to be able to contribute meaningfully to this collaboration by providing a large patient population or a developed preclinical research expertise (Table 1). Should there not be access to the patient population or a relevant technology, it may be difficult to develop a two-way street and be able to contribute significantly to the endeavor. Strong, mutually beneficial collaborations can result in lifelong friendships and shared accomplishments. Therefore, the development of new interests is most likely dependent on the commitment of the one's institution and the available resources at hand which can be deployed. Similar to other pursuits, one should expect hindrances at times, and rejections at first, but continued persistence, authenticity, and strong personal interest – with perhaps some needed fine-tuning to develop a less resistance-prone path – are the avenues to eventual success.

Networking, Cooperative Groups, and Clinical Trials

Forming connections with colleagues outside of one's department or institution often leads to abundant personal fulfillment and stimulating collaborations. Such connections are usually based on common interests and result in noteworthy discussions and work that can advance a particular topic of interest (Table 1). Networking can occur at institutional, local, or national conferences and also through the use of social media. Committee meetings organized by professional organizations (ASTRO, ARS, ASCO) or of groups located within the National Clinical Trials Network (NTCTN) (NRG Oncology, ECOG, SWOG, Alliance) present opportunities to become involved with other experts sharing similar interests, and frequently the most meaningful collaborations will gain additional strength from these in-person meetings. Finding a committed collaborator from another discipline or institution can result in fruitful endeavors, such as shared work on clinical practice statements or outcome reviews, development of quality or technology metrics, or initiation of joint prospective clinical trials. Networking is not a quick process and may take multiple meetings and interactions to emerge as well as a shared vision and often friendship. Opportunities may exist to network through visiting professorships occurring within the institution where it may be feasible to meet with additional uninvolved persons for lunch or discussion. Building such networks in the best-case scenario will augment career satisfaction and prosperity on the part of all parties.

Summary Points

- Building expertise may take time, patience, and persistence in addition to gaining knowledge. Following a passion about a specific interest will help in maintaining enthusiasm for the topic.
- Growing a particular expertise outside of one's comfort zone can lead to new collaborations, patient referrals, and achievements which can spawn new areas of growth and personal fulfillment.
- Connecting with committed stakeholders can lead to unrecognized opportunities, and keeping various persons in leadership informed of your progress may help connect to new partners.
- The success of new developmental goals may be predicated on available resources of institutional strengths, and latching onto these opportunities may provide a source of patients and/or technologies to gain expertise. These prospects may allow for networking with experts outside of the department or institution with similar interests.
- Networking is a source of satisfaction and growth that stems from enhanced achievements, expertise, and friendships.

For Discussion with a Mentor or Colleague

- What are the main strategies to make an interaction with a colleague at an outside institution successful?
- What areas of strength or reputation are available at our center in which I could be involved?
- What are the best techniques for managing others at this institution? How do you manage others who have a different viewpoint than yourself?
- Who are some key stakeholders at our institution or other institutions with whom you recommend to connect?

References

1. Specchia ML, Frisicale EM, Carini E, et al. The impact of tumor board on cancer care: evidence from an umbrella review. BMC Health Serv Res. 2020;20(1):73. Published 2020 Jan 31. https://doi.org/10.1186/s12913-020-4930-3.
2. Liu JC, Kaplon A, Blackman E, Miyamoto C, Savior D, Ragin C. The impact of the multidisciplinary tumor board on head and neck cancer outcomes. Laryngoscope. 2020;130(4):946–50. https://doi.org/10.1002/lary.28066.

Additional Reading/Resources

Long JC, Cunningham FC, Wiley J, Carswell P, Braithwaite J. Leadership in complex networks: the importance of network position and strategic action in a translational cancer research network. Implement Sci. 2013;8:122. Published 2013 Oct 11. https://doi.org/10.1186/1748-5908-8-122.
Long JC, Cunningham FC, Carswell P, Braithwaite J. Patterns of collaboration in complex networks: the example of a translational research network. BMC Health Serv Res. 2014;14:225. Published 20 May 2014. https://doi.org/10.1186/1472-6963-14-225.
Sangaleti C, Schveitzer MC, Peduzzi M, Zoboli ELCP, Soares CB. Experiences and shared meaning of teamwork and interprofessional collaboration among health care professionals in primary health care settings: a systematic review. JBI Database System Rev Implement Rep. 2017;15(11):2723–88. https://doi.org/10.11124/JBISRIR-2016-003016.

The Role of Department Chair

Christopher G. Willett and Quynh-Thu Le

This chapter is based on a commentary by one of the authors (CGW)

Reflections from a chair: leadership of a Clinical Department at an Academic Medical Center. Cancer 2015;121:3795–8.

Introduction

The responsibilities of a chair of a clinical department at an academic medical center (AMC) include the leadership and oversight of the care of oncology patients; supervising and mentoring of faculty, trainees, and staff; as well as guiding the research and educational missions of the department. In addition, there is intensive interaction with other elements of an AMC, including the school of medicine (SOM), the university hospital, the health system, other departments, a physician's organization, other affiliated hospitals, and the cancer center or institute (Figs. 1 and 2). These interactions are often complex, and involve understanding and balancing diverse viewpoints with different goals and interests. The search for common ground is both challenging and rewarding. Thoughtful navigation of these group discussions is required in achieving the short-term and long-term goals of a department.

A chair needs to recognize that success is measured by the accomplishments of the faculty and the department as a whole, leading to growth, prosperity, and well-being. Importantly, one's honesty and professional conduct in all interactions are

C. G. Willett (✉)
Department of Radiation Oncology, Duke University, Durham, NC, USA
e-mail: christopher.willett@duke.edu

Q.-T. Le
Department of Radiation Oncology, Stanford University, Palo Alto, CA, USA
e-mail: qle@stanford.edu

© Springer Nature Switzerland AG 2021   319
R. A. Chandra et al. (eds.), *Career Development in Academic Radiation Oncology*, https://doi.org/10.1007/978-3-030-71855-8_23

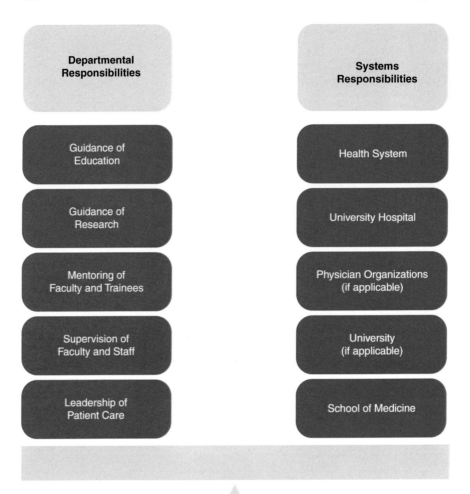

Fig. 1 The chair's balance

critical. The development of trust among colleagues and leadership are of paramount importance to the long-term success and credibility of a chair and department. The objective of this chapter is to provide the readership a better understanding of the multifaceted elements of a chair's position.

With the COVID-19 pandemic, the leadership of a chair has become even more important in advancing the critical needs of patients, faculty, staff, and learners. In addition to local leadership, effective collaboration with the AMC, the university, and local, regional, and national agencies is crucial in navigating this unprecedented challenge.

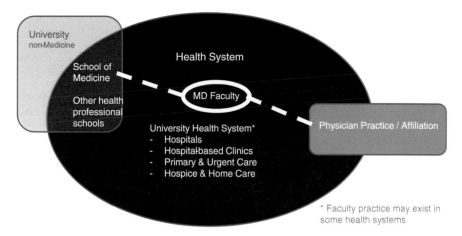

Fig. 2 Components of an academic medical center

The Department

A clinical department at most AMC has three missions: clinical, research, and education. The primary clinical mission is to provide outstanding care of patients. It is critical that the chair instill and support a culture of patient-centric care and safety throughout the department by example and actions. In oncology, the leadership of a chair can have a profound impact on the care of patients with cancer. Ideally, the chair should be actively engaged in the clinic: caring for patients and working in the same environment in which patients and providers coexist to fully understand and appreciate the day-to-day experiences of patients and caregivers. For oncology patients receiving specialized treatment such as radiotherapy, there is an interwoven stream of interaction with staff and faculty including receptionists, physicians, physicists, nurses, dosimetrists, radiation therapists, and others. It is critical that the functions of all providers are aligned and communication is optimized to ensure that the path of caregiving is seamless and transparent. Given the increasing complexity of oncology and radiotherapy, the establishment of robust quality assurance is mandatory, including all elements of the patient's management. These include checklists, time-outs, and other processes during treatment evaluation and planning, before treatment, at the time of first and subsequent treatments and during follow-up. Redundancy in systems of care affecting a patient is important to ensure safe and effective treatment. All members of the department must work as a collaborative team to achieve clinical excellence.

Departments are comprised of faculty, including clinicians, scientists, physician-scientists, educators, clinical investigators, and physicists. Mentorship and guidance of faculty is a very important charge of a chair. The recruitment and retention of talented faculty are critical to the success of a department. The interests, skills, and goals of individual faculty member vary greatly, and the chair must seek to understand an individual's strengths, passions, and limitations to define strategies to aid and enhance their performance. There is no substitute for one-on-one time and discussion to achieve this understanding. Ultimately, the chair serves as an advocate of the faculty in their professional development. The department must provide faculty with resources, time, and opportunities to pursue scholarly activities. Pilot research funds and the provision of core resources such as space, clerical, statistical, and clinical trial research support are tools that can aid faculty in the conduct of their scholarly activities. With the increasing demands of clinical activity and decreasing reimbursement for clinical care, it is imperative to ensure protected time for the faculty to undertake the academic mission. Faculty members working as collaborative teams may facilitate this goal. Personnel support to assist with clinical care such as advance practice providers, nurse coordinators, patient flow coordinators, and/or scribes is an invaluable help to our faculty, residents, and importantly patients. This has been a key strategy to mitigate physician burnout [1, 2]. Physician-scientists are instrumental in bridging translational and basic science research to the clinic and vice versa. Significant and sustained investment of protected time, resources, and culture is required to optimize their success, and the rewards may be profound with creative and practice-changing discoveries. Many departments also have basic scientists in the biological sciences in the department. Their collaborations with physician-scientists, clinicians, and clinical physicists can lead to transformative science and help to foster both basic and translational research in the department. This type of collaboration is also important for the education and training of students and other learners in the sciences. Last but not least are clinical physics faculty members who are involved with not only the day-to-day machine maintenance and patient treatment but also translating new radiation treatment plans or algorithms to patients. The professional success of all faculty members, regardless of line or function, is a critical commitment of a chair and is key in achieving the academic missions of a department. This is further strengthened by increasing the diversity of a department balancing gender, race, ethnicity, and other factors. True excellence is achieved by the innovations created by faculty. It is one of the major rewards of a chair to contribute to the success of a faculty member or faculty team.

In contrast, the oversight of problematic faculty can be vexing and time-consuming. Establishing objective and transparent expectations of a faculty's professional activity and conduct is required. If basic standards are not met, remedial steps should be initiated promptly. Ultimately, formal and even legal steps of recourse may be required to achieve resolution of a faculty member's conduct and performance. The potentially corrosive effects of one individual's actions on colleagues and the department must never be underestimated. One important lesson in conflict resolution is to address issues timely, directly, dispassionately, and objectively within the context of what is best overall for patients, faculty, and the department.

Given the scope and breadth of activities within a department, it is typical for a chair to involve additional leaders within the department to oversee all its diverse undertakings. Delegation of responsibilities to talented faculty greatly enriches the department, creates a cohesive leadership team, and fosters leadership skills in other faculty members. Many departments have several leadership positions such as vice-chair of clinical operations, vice-chair of translational and basic science research, division head (if a department has multiple divisions), director of residency training, directors of affiliated departments in other hospitals, and subspecialty directors. Other emerging leadership areas include those in education of medical students, graduate students, and fellows, safety and quality, network growth, and physician wellness. These faculty teams are not only necessary but enhance the department by including individuals with leadership in different areas. Importantly, the relationship between the chair and faculty must be based on mutual trust and recognition of talents as the ultimate accountability resides with the chair.

Participation of all faculty in the education of students, residents, and other trainees within a department is a key mission of a department. The impact of this education is profound in shaping the next generation of clinical practitioners, scientists, and leaders. The members of a department must support and respect the educational process to ensure that residents and other trainees are able to fully participate in teaching conferences, didactic sessions, multidisciplinary conferences, and other valuable educational opportunities. There is little substitute for instructive learning through the experience of working closely with faculty in patient care or hands-on research. Residency program directors are crucial for the advocacy of both didactic and practical learning experiences for residents, which may conflict with departmental clinical demands. The scope and breadth of knowledge to be mastered by physician trainees is rapidly expanding. Innovative tools are required to facilitate the acquisition of knowledge as well as creating and supporting new experiences in global medicine, clinical trials, and basic science. Of all the missions of a department, education is the most vulnerable to the changing economics of an AMC. Philanthropy has been invaluable in the support and enhancement of our educational mission.

School of Medicine

In most AMC, the dean of the SOM administratively oversees many departments (basic science and clinical), as well as centers, institutes, and programs. Although a given chair may envision the faculty and the activities of their department as central and all-important to the SOM, the reality is that the SOM has many important constituencies and executes multiple agendas. The SOM's mission is the advancement of scholarly activities, specifically research and education. In addition, it oversees and implements an increasingly complex regulatory environment that faculty and departments must observe. It is ideal for all chairs to have collegial and constructive relationships with the dean of the SOM and with other chairs to advance the goals and missions of each department within the context of the SOM's agenda. Access to funds, resources, research space, program development, and collaborations are typically adjudicated and facilitated by the dean. As the start-up package for a chair wears thin over time, the ability of a chair and department to recruit talented new faculty and initiate new programs requires continued support from the SOM and other sources, such as philanthropy and clinical revenue. Departments require renewal to ensure the vitality of their missions. All organizations need new ideas, and these often come from new faculty. Major research agendas of the past should be reevaluated. New core resources need to be developed. New directions should be initiated (e.g., initiatives in quality and safety over the past decade) and the ability to change research directions quickly.

The Hospital and Health System

Although the SOM and the hospital and health system (H/HS) may exist within the same organization, their missions are not the same, even with the same leader at the top. The bonds with a chair and department are fundamentally different between these constituencies. In contrast to the SOM, the relationship of a chair and department to the H/HS is aimed at an effective partnership in the care of patients. Typically, the hospital provides equipment, clinical space, nursing, and staffing support to plan treatment and deliver care to patients. Departmental faculty work closely with nurses, therapists, and other hospital staff involved in patient care. Although the head nurse, radiation therapist, and other staff may not report directly to the chair, it is invaluable for the chair to meet regularly and maintain a strong working relationship with key personnel individually. Similarly, group meetings with the chair often optimize and ensure the productive functioning of the clinic. The H/HS is a healthcare network with clear goals of growth, productivity, accountability, and expense management. Consequently, the chair and the department's business team directly manage professional revenue generated by clinical services. There is inevitably a close yin and yang with the revenue elements of the H/HS. The interactions and experience of the chair with the H/HS are a contractual business-like relationship. Metrics are increasingly used by H/HS administration to assess the performance of a department and faculty. External consultants can provide counsel to the H/HS with regard to the staffing, operations, and productivity of the department and its performance. An increasing administrative burden addressing these requests is a facet of a chair's position. As long as revenues are robust, the collaboration of a department with the H/HS is straightforward. In times of challenging revenues, efforts at expense reduction, searching for novel revenue streams, enhancing the clinical productivity of faculty, philanthropy, and other steps should be pursued, lest academic missions become compromised leading to declining education and research activities.

Other Departments, Centers, and Institutes

Relationships with other clinical and basic science departments, centers, and institutes of an AMC vary greatly with regard to activity and significance. Oncology as an entity thrives on the strengths of the departments of medicine and surgery (with subspecialty divisions), radiation oncology, radiology, pathology, and the overarching cancer center or institute. The orchestration of all these facets is critical in providing the highest-quality clinical services to oncology patients and growing a multidepartmental collaborative research enterprise. Given the multidisciplinary nature of oncology, faculty from multiple departments work closely in both clinically and scholarly activities. These collaborations should be strongly encouraged and supported. At the level of leadership, the alignment of missions across departments is ideal, but fiscal realities may be challenging. Competing services provided by different departments may arise in the care of patients. For example, a patient with prostate cancer could be an appropriate candidate for either surgery or radiotherapy. Many patients would be best managed in multidisciplinary clinics with thoughtful attention by an experienced team. However, open discussions may not always occur. Effective collaboration and the pooling of resources across departments, centers, and institutes are important methods of recruitment of talented research-oriented faculty as well as new program implementation.

Physician Organizations

At some AMC, physician organizations can serve as an umbrella providing representation for the clinical faculty. In addition, these organizations may manage an array of services in the support of the physicians and their practices, including healthcare benefits, professional billing management, malpractice plans, legal services, retirement plans, and others. Increasingly, these organizations advocate for the clinical faculty in growth and development independently or together with the H/HS. At some institutions, the leadership of physician organizations represents departments and faculty in discussions and decision-making with the dean of the SOM and leadership of the H/HS.

Conclusions

The leadership position of a departmental chair can be a positive and rewarding opportunity. These rewards principally stem from the success of the faculty, trainees, staff, and everyone supporting the department. With healthcare reform and the constraints of the federal budget, increasing attention and time has become directed toward administrative management. Formal courses and training in executive leadership and business management may be helpful in enhancing knowledge and skills in these disciplines. There are multiple and often competing constituencies and agendas requiring thoughtful strategies to achieve departmental goals. The objectives of the chair are advancing patient care, education, and research as well as a continual presence and visibility in the department. The true excellence of a department is achieved by the innovation of its faculty and trainees.

For Discussion with a Mentor or Colleague

- At my institution, what are the formal courses and training in executive leadership and business management that may be helpful in enhancing knowledge and skills in these disciplines?
- How can I best prepare for the promotion process at my institution?

References

1. Dyrbye LN, Shanafelt TD, et al. Burnout among health care professionals: a call to explore and address this underrecognized threat to safe, high-quality care. NAM Perspectives. Discussion Paper, Natinal Academy of Medicine, Washington: 2007. https://nam.edu/burnout-among-health-care-professionals-a-call-to-explore-and-address-this-underrecognized-threat-to-safe-high-quality-care.
2. West CP, Dyrbye LN, Shanafelt TD. Physician burnout: contributors, consequences and solutions. J Intern Med. 2018;283:516–29. https://doi.org/10.1111/joim.12752.

Successful Strategies to Exploit the Intersection Between the Radiation Oncology Department and the Cancer Center

Nancy P. Mendenhall, Kathryn E. Hitchcock, and Jonathan D. Licht

Introduction

It is possible that our true purpose in life is to make it better for someone else.

As radiation oncologists, we can make life better for someone else through practicing excellent patient care; but, as academic radiation oncologists, we are charged to also find and teach ways of making life better for all patients, not just those we treat, through making radiation oncology better.

So how can we make radiation therapy better? We have partnered with physics to better understand radiation dose delivery and create better treatment machines, customized dose modification devices, and dose calculation programs, and we have partnered with biology to better understand the relationship between radiation fractional and total dose effects, hypoxia, and tumor kinetics. We have partnered with surgery and medical oncology to optimize the roles of local therapies in each clinical situation and to best combine systemic and local therapy to balance the competing risks of local and distant tumor control and normal tissue injury. But the world of oncology has evolved, and there are new partners who have much to offer, many of whom can be found in or through the cancer center. Figure 1 shows potential new partnerships facilitated through a cancer center to improve radiation oncology.

N. P. Mendenhall (✉)
Department of Radiation Oncology, University of Florida College of Medicine, Gainesville, FL, USA

University of Florida Health Proton Therapy Institute, Jacksonville, FL, USA
e-mail: menden@shands.ufl.edu

K. E. Hitchcock
Department of Radiation Oncology, University of Florida College of Medicine, Gainesville, FL, USA

J. D. Licht
University of Florida Health Cancer Center, Gainesville, FL, USA

© Springer Nature Switzerland AG 2021
R. A. Chandra et al. (eds.), *Career Development in Academic Radiation Oncology*, https://doi.org/10.1007/978-3-030-71855-8_24

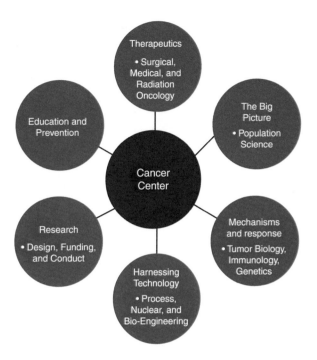

Fig. 1 Potential new partnerships facilitated through a cancer center to improve radiation oncology

As we consider how to improve radiation oncology, we may think about harnessing technology through creating better radiation modalities and delivery methods with the help from process, nuclear, and bioengineering as well as medical physics. We may think about strategies that focus on the nature of cancer, the mechanism of action and effects of radiation, and the body's response to both with the help from tumor biologists, molecular geneticists, and immunologists. We think creatively about the most effective and efficient clinical research methods to test our hypotheses with the help from biostatistics and experts in clinical trial design, grant acquisitions and administration, and trial management and monitoring. We may think broadly about the social impact of our work with the help from population scientists who understand how to analyze and link large data sets that provide us with the big picture.

Many options exist for the success in academic radiation oncology. In medical school and university-based health-care systems, success on an academic track is measured by achievements such as publications, grants, patents, and leadership roles, and milestones such as tenure and promotion. Academic tracks generally require accomplishments in teaching, research, and service for promotion. While historical intradepartmental approaches to these areas may be successful, new opportunities have arisen from team-based activities that intersect multiple disciplines, apply new technologies, and use sophisticated research and data analysis techniques that are promising but require extradepartmental mentorship and collaboration typically available in cancer centers.

Although some radiation oncology departments provide support for clinical research coordination, regulatory paperwork, grant writing, and manuscript preparation, few have intradepartmental resources to support the varied academic career paths that are now possible for academically oriented radiation oncologists at the start of their careers, such as support for biostatistics, clinical trial design, grant applications and administration, laboratory management, bioengineering and nuclear engineering collaboration, eHealth, and deployment of new oncologic tools such as gene sequencing and immunotherapy. Without access to the experts and resources, intradepartmental teaching opportunities may be limited to traditional didactic presentations, and research opportunities may be limited to retrospective disease-site outcome studies and dosimetry projects, which are typically nonfundable and increasingly difficult to publish.

Cancer centers, particularly those associated with large medical schools, universities, and hospital systems, tend to be comprised of members from multiple disciplines, have an extensive repertoire of resources and expertise, and welcome involvement from all clinical disciplines. They often share resources with or have affiliations with other university or health science centers or institutes focused on genetics, bioengineering, drug design, immunotherapy, nanoparticle, aging, emerging pathogens, brain, clinical and translational science, and more, which further extend the possibilities for unique and creative academic contributions. Cancer centers typically have the broad missions of patient care, service, education, and research across the spectrum of cancer interests from mechanisms of origin, prevention, early detection, and optimal therapies. Although radiation oncology is the only traditional medical college department solely focused on cancer, it is often underrepresented in cancer center activities, and so radiation oncology involvement may be viewed by a cancer center as particularly valuable.

The sections below cover a sample of the kinds of resources that may be available in your cancer center, describe a method for accessing the resources, and offer some examples of hypothetical academic career pathways enriched by integration into cancer center resources.

Typical Cancer Center Resources

Clinical Research Office

Most cancer centers will have an office to facilitate clinical research. The functions and resources in this office may be shared with or overlap with services provided by other university entities such as a clinical and translational science institute or core program described below. A major goal will be to help develop and conduct investigator-initiated clinical research. Typically, support will be provided for developing research projects, assuring compliance with pertinent regulatory bodies, and securing necessary funding. Specific services may include assistance with protocol and informed consent writing; feasibility assessments and budget development; regulatory management including submission to institutional review boards (IRBs), the Food and Drug Administration, and study sponsors; clinical trial coordination including recruitment, data management and monitoring, ClinicalTrials.gov management, and laboratory processing; financial management including budget development and contract negotiations, study invoicing and payments, and billing compliance; and oversight activities including a scientific review and monitoring committee, data integrity and safety committee, and quality management and audit services. The clinical research office may also monitor and maintain membership with regional or national cooperative groups and support participation in extramurally initiated clinical research.

Funding

Most cancer centers will provide a listing of external research funding sources and templated language to assist with applications. In addition, most will have a listing of internal funding opportunities available that may include pilot project awards, early and established investigator awards for high-scoring studies that just missed the pay-line, and specific funding opportunities through philanthropic foundations or state-supported grants. Often, there are special seed monies to aid young investigators in preparing for major awards.

In addition, some of the following special resources may reside within the cancer center or be shared with other university entities.

Biostatistics and Quantitative Sciences

Increasingly, a strong statistical study design and analysis are required for grant funding for and publication of clinical studies. Most major journals have a statistics section and engage statisticians as one of the peer reviewers. Essentially, all clinical research funding agencies require thorough statistical design and analysis plans. Some funding agencies may even publish extensive and detailed statistical methodology that would be incomprehensible to most clinical scientists. Ultimate success in obtaining a grant or in publishing a manuscript may rest on the statistical validity of the study design and analysis, so a core resource in biostatistics can be invaluable.

Most cancer centers will have or share a core resource that provides biostatistical and quantitative support for clinical, translational, population, and bench research. Expertise in this core will include at least one experienced biostatistician and possibly a whole biostatistics team. This core will have access to a variety of software tools and statistical codes for standard biostatistical and bioinformatical analyses such as SAS Macros, Demograph Table, Frequency_t, TTest_FDR, SAS Code, as well as data cleaning instructions.

Such a group may also aid in developing statistically viable research questions and hypotheses; developing a study design with sample size justifications, power analyses, and analysis planning; developing the study database, data quality monitoring procedures, and data management plan; statistical analyses and interpretation of results; grant writing; manuscript writing; and education in basic biostatistics for cancer researchers.

Population Science

There is a growing awareness that historically popular randomized controlled trials (RCTs) may not provide the best answers to all questions. Only 2–3% of adults with cancer participate on clinical trials, so the generalizability of clinical trials may be in question, particularly for certain segments of the population who are particularly disinclined to participate in historically typical RCTs. The expense and outcome maturation time also make some prospective randomized controlled clinical trials unfeasible. Thus, there is a growing interest in mining large existing databases to gain broad brushstroke answers to important clinical questions. The data may not be sufficiently granular to answer certain questions, but will be inherently generalizable and possess validity because of its volume; as such, this kind of data-driven research may be hypothesis generating, providing excellent background for a prospective clinical study, if not conclusive in itself. It can provide critically important context, in essence, the big picture. Large databases can be linked to provide broad brushstroke impressions on relationships, e.g., diagnostic codes from a registry can be linked to claims codes to estimate costs of care. Skill and experience are required in linking and using surrogate data effectively. Some large academic programs have clinical research networks and access to large databases, and are focused on mining existing national databases. Mentors and tools in this area of investigation can stage-set a clinical research career, providing an excellent foundation for grants for prospective trials.

The expertise in such a core may include epidemiologists, health outcomes researchers, statisticians, and researchers with expertise in designing, linking, or analyzing large electronic databases. It may also include behavioral scientists and health disparity researchers who are interested in subpopulations and can aid in patient engagement and recruitment.

Informatics and eHealth

As the sheer volume of data bearing on patient care has mandated the move to electronic medical records, similarly in research the myriad of data elements that must be considered in clinical research has mandated web-based systems for data management. Some cancer centers will have or share a core for informatics and "eHealth." These resources may aid in the design, development, and implementation of novel informatics methods, tools, and systems for archiving, mining, and integrating research data with other relevant sources such as electronic medical records; provide tools for engaging communities and key stakeholders in clinical research; and assure compliance with privacy standards.

Cellular, Molecular, Immunologic, and Genetic Analytics

Cellular, molecular, immunologic, and genetic analytics resources may reside within the cancer center or as a shared resource with another university entity. The investigators may include pathologists, tumor and molecular biologists, and genetics researchers, and the services may include flow cytometry, confocal microscopy, gene sequencing, and tools for functional annotation of sequence data, multomics data integration, and statistical analysis of gene expression data. Increasingly, therapeutic development and outcomes assessment is informed by knowledge of cellular, molecular, and genetic characterization, so access to such resources can provide an opportunity to develop cutting-edge treatment approaches or to understand heterogeneous treatment effects.

Process, Nuclear, and Bioengineering

Radiation oncology is technology intense. Optimal radiation therapy requires meticulous quality control with the development of predictable technology and fail-safe processes, an in-depth understanding of radiation dosimetry and effects, and the development of both class solutions and customized design to best serve patients. Access to process engineering may help in the onboarding of a new technology to assure accuracy and efficiency. Access to nuclear engineering may enable sophisticated Monte Carlo dose calculations to better understand the effects of very low radiation doses as well as high and moderate radiation doses in or near the treatment field. Such knowledge can be used to develop predictive models for outcomes and late effects. Access to bioengineering may provide the creativity and skill to solve challenging clinical problems particularly in the domain of normal tissue protection. Access to process, nuclear, and bioengineering directly or through cancer center affiliations can enrich research programs designed around quality and safety or prediction of radiation effects, both areas of growing scientific interest.

In addition to cancer center-specific and shared resources, the cancer center will include a broad range of research programs and investigators that may be open to collaboration.

Basic Laboratories with Interest in Cancer Biology, Radiation Effects, and Immunology

There is increasing interest in understanding radiation effects at the molecular level, the impact of the microenvironment on both tumor response and radiation effects, and interactions between the immune system and tumors and radiation. Many basic scientists benefit from understanding clinical priorities, may be interested in obtaining clinical specimens for analysis, and may be willing to collaborate on clinical/translational projects. Having access through the cancer center to researchers in these areas may facilitate unique opportunities for clinical, translational, and basic research.

The overall success of the cancer center depends on the number and success of investigators and programs it supports, so it is likely that the cancer center will prioritize the development of young investigators setting out on a fresh career path.

Strategies for Accessing Cancer Center Resources

Website Review

A first step in understanding what resources and expertise might be available to you would be a perusal of your cancer center's website. The website will likely list core resources, featured and developing programs, recent publications and grants, educational opportunities, and connections to other university or health science centers. It may list openings in labs and invitations to join developing research or educational teams. It may provide an announcement of visiting professor lectures and seminars. It may list community outreach activities and opportunities for volunteers. The website will likely include a mission statement. While most cancer centers will have patient care, community service, education, and research included in this mission statement, there may be specific descriptors in that indicate some of the particular strengths and more focused goals of the cancer center. Subscribing to a cancer center listserve can also provide useful and timely information.

Educational Programs

The cancer center will be involved in the education of medical students, residents and fellows, graduate students, postdoctoral graduates, faculty, and the community it serves. Most student education will be through laboratory apprenticeships, but there will be a host of seminars and lectures given by students, professors, and visiting scholars. The cancer center may identify its service area as a city, a state, or region, and may emphasize certain community subsets of particular interest. There may be novel educational programs focused on these special groups that represent a strategic cancer center goal. For example, in an effort to increase young students in the STEM pipeline, a program might aim at inspiring high school science teachers by exposing them through a 2-day seminar to exciting research presentations from a broad range of disciplines. Another example might be a novel summer program for promising students from historically black universities and colleges to attract minorities to careers in STEM; they might live in dormitories on the university campus; attend daily lectures on cancer etiology, epidemiology, natural history, therapeutic options, and ongoing research; and work on a specific clinical, translational, or basic research project with an assigned mentor.

Community Outreach Programs

An important function of the cancer center will be service through community outreach. The primary goals of these programs are often to provide education and access to the community for the purpose of cancer prevention and early detection of cancer. These activities may be in concert with other cancer advocacy groups. In addition to education, these events and programs may offer windows into research opportunities, for example, the creation of a stakeholder group or study population for a particular research project or funding opportunities from cancer advocacy foundations.

   If you know your career path, getting involved in the cancer center education and community outreach programs can introduce you to specific projects or laboratories you may wish to join, mentors or collaborators you may wish to work with, stakeholders and study populations you may wish to engage. If you do not know your career path, getting involved in the cancer center education and community outreach programs will expose you to a broad range of possibilities, including structured programs, resources, and expertise that may help you focus your interests and build a unique career path.

Hypothetical Examples of How a Cancer Center Might Enrich a Radiation Oncology Career

Example 1
- A radiation oncology resident with a bioengineering background assigned to a service dealing with skin cancer learns the treatment technique for using orthovoltage with customized lead face shields to protect nontargeted adjacent and underlying tissues. She notes the multistep manual process involved in creating the shield and realizes that she could work with *bioengineering* colleagues asso-

ciated with the cancer center to develop a much more efficient process using a three-dimensional printer. As a resident, she obtains a small intramural grant from the cancer center to create a new process for creating customized lead shielding. This leads to a first-authored technical publication in a radiotherapy journal.

- After joining the faculty, she joins a medical school teaching team and uses this clinical experience as a team project in a problem-based medical student course she co-teaches. She involves multiple members of the cancer center including a *pathologist* interested in skin cancer pathology, an *epidemiologist* studying geographic distribution of skin cancers, a Mohs *surgeon* who discusses the potential morbidity of resection of advanced skin cancers around the nose, and a *medical physicist* who explains the dose distribution advantages of orthovoltage compared with conventional electron beam treatment and the adequacy of lead sheet shielding with orthovoltage. She wins a creative teaching award from the medical school.

- She decides to review the departmental experience with radiation for advanced skin cancer. With assistance from the cancer center clinical research office, she obtains IRB permission for a longitudinal outcomes project and finds that patients with advanced disease, particularly those with perineural spread, have both a poor prognosis and significant treatment-related morbidity. This finding results in another publication in a radiation therapy journal detailing the disease control and morbidity rates of high-dose radiation for advanced skin cancer.

- The outcomes for advanced skin cancer treated with radiation therapy make clear the benefits of skin cancer prevention and/or early detection. She searches the cancer center website for programs and individuals with interests in skin cancer prevention and connects with an *oncologic research nurse* interested in skin cancer prevention and *a health outcomes researcher* interested in engagement and clinical trial participation. Discussions ensue on the best approach for engaging people in their teenage years and early 20s in skin cancer prevention. They decide the best strategy to engage young people is through other young people who are already in recognized leadership roles. They identify more senior male and female university service club members willing to distribute sunscreen samples and short bullet-point pamphlets at fall football games. She participates in gaining industrial donations for sunscreen samples and an intramural cancer center grant to distribute educational pamphlets and sunscreen samples at football games to teenage and young adults as a preventive intervention.

- As the project evolves, she and her colleagues realize this activity also has research potential and could provide an opportunity to build a large cohort of subjects at risk for skin cancer who could be followed over time to (1) evaluate the efficacy of the engagement approach and (2) evaluate the long-term efficacy of the sunscreen and education intervention, but funding would be needed. With a concept for a significant research project built around the community skin cancer prevention project, they go back to the cancer center to search for potential funding agencies and assistance in grant and protocol preparation. As part of this overall research program strategy, the young radiation oncology attending applies for and receives (1) an American Cancer Society career development award to provide time over the next 3 years to develop a skin cancer-preventative medicine program.

- With knowledge and experience gained in the early prevention project, she creates a stakeholder group that includes skin cancer patients, recipients of the football game sunscreen samples, and an industrial partner who makes sunscreen; she also creates a research group that includes the Mohs *surgeon, pathologist,* cancer center *ARNP,* and *health outcomes researcher.* With the help from the cancer center research office and clinical and translational science institute, they obtain a grant to supply sunscreen samples from an industrial entity for the next 2 years.
- With the clear demonstration of the ability to engage a community of stakeholders including patients and industry, she applies for and obtains a PCORI award to cover the cost of building the patient cohort through the initial mechanism of sunscreen samples and an educational brochure handed out at football games along with an invitation and incentive to join the study.
- After 12 home football games, she has distributed sunscreen samples to 24,000 students between the ages of 18 and 25, and 12,000 have agreed to be part of the outcome study, completing data forms once a year on their use of sunscreen for a $50 gift certificate to a coffee shop.
- With her success in building the cohort, she obtains funding through a foundation for extending follow-up for her cohort to 10 years.
- With 10-year follow-up assured, she works with collaborating investigators in the cancer center who have identified gene signatures that are associated with increased skin cancer development to secure funding to gene sequence all 12,000 in the study who agreed to complete baseline and follow-up data forms that include family history and lifestyle data.
- With correlative family history data and gene sequence data, she develops a high-risk surveillance program that involves routine dermatology screening which is adopted into national practice guidelines.

Example 2

- A young physician-investigator's institution recently acquired a new proton therapy machine. His area of assigned clinical activity is prostate cancer. Because of the prevalence of the disease and the utility of radiation, a large number of patients are treated in the new proton center for prostate cancer, creating an opportunity for clinical research into the comparative effectiveness of proton therapy in prostate cancer and the less expensive and more commonly available sophisticated photon-based radiation therapy techniques such as intensity-modulated radiotherapy (IMRT) and volumetric-modulated arc therapy (VMAT). He designs and conducts a series of pilot studies to establish benchmark outcomes using statistical expertise, assistance with IRB submission and regulatory activities, and data management, analysis, and monitoring provided by the cancer center clinical research office. These studies lead to a series of outcome publications in a variety of radiation oncology and urological oncology journals.

- A *disparity researcher* in the cancer center who has teamed up with a historically black college to identify promising undergraduates for a summer research program to expose them to ongoing bench, translational, and clinical research activities is aware of his work and invites him to serve as a mentor for one of the students over the summer and to deliver a lecture to the student group on prostate cancer.

- In an effort to make his lecture meaningful to the young students, he decides to include in his presentation information on prostate cancer in African Americans. He realizes that not only is the incidence of prostate cancer higher in African Americans, but the prognosis is worse as well. In his literature search, he finds theories as to why—limited access to health-care versus biology—but little convincing data exist to confirm a cause. As he digs further, he discovers that only 2–3% of adults with cancer go onto clinical trials in the USA and that African Americans are particularly underrepresented, suggesting the possibility that available clinical trial data guiding common therapeutic practice may not be generalizable to the African-American population.

- This research leads him to a review of the proton experience in prostate cancer including a subset analysis of African-American outcomes, which prove to be identical to the outcomes of white patients. This leads to a publication in an oncology journal. He wonders if the previous discrepancy in outcomes was indeed related to access or whether the finding could also be explained with a different theory: differential molecular effects of proton therapy relative to photon therapy that could potentially overcome the underlying genetic heterogeneity accounting for worse outcomes in African-American men treated with photons.

- Based on his benchmark data and a growing body of molecular data suggesting differential molecular effects between protons and photons, he plans to conduct a comparative trial of proton and photon therapy in men with prostate cancer. He is aware of the probable need for a large study population and a study design that would be attractive to men, and particularly African-American men. He teams up with a cancer center *health outcomes researcher* to determine what kind of trial design might be attractive to men with prostate cancer. He also engages a *disparity researcher* to determine how best to attract African-American men to the trial.

- With intradepartmental seed monies, the *health outcomes researcher* conducts a series of focus groups to identify the main priorities of men with lived experience of prostate cancer and what their attitudes are toward research. The findings result in a survey sent to men over 50 years old across the country, and the responses validate the focus group's recommendations on what cancer control and treatment toxicity outcomes matter most to men, what endpoints of a study would be meaningful, what trial design men would accept, and what demographic factors might be associated with particular responses. The survey leads to a presentation at a national meeting and a publication in a clinical trial journal.

- His *disparity research collaborator* advises the creation of culturally specific recruitment materials and strategy to be administered by trusted members of the African-American community and a minority engagement group within an overall patient-stakeholder group to guide the study.

- He also engages through the cancer center an established well-funded *clinical researcher* with extensive experience on research funding agency study sections, a *bioethicist*, and a *business ethics professor* from the university's law and business schools to discuss a potential trial design from the perspectives of scientific validity, feasibility, and human subject research ethical principles.
- With cancer center statistical assistance, he develops the hypotheses, endpoints, assessment tools and times, and a statistical analysis plan for a multi-institutional clinical trial involving 45 US sites and 3000 patients.
- The cancer center research office assists with budgeting—work time for key personnel, site payments for the cost of study activation, site payments for the incremental costs of patient enrollment and follow-up data gathering and submission, consulting costs for creation of a web-based data archiving and mining system, treatment plan collection in DICOM format and processing for quality assurance assessment, and patient stipends for data form completion. After gaining letters of support from multiple prospective site principal investigators, he applies for and receives an award from the Patient-Centered Outcomes Research Institute (PCORI) to conduct the proposed trial.
- To accept the award, he must have an institutional contract between his institution and PCORI, so he engages the contracts and grants office of the university's clinical and translational science institute as well as university *attorneys* to aid in executing the contract. He engages the cancer center in streamlining the institutional study process approval, which includes review by the scientific review committee, the institutional resource allocation committee, the radiation safety committee, and the institutional review board. Once the study is activated at his site, he engages the cancer center in helping to secure IRB approval at other sites, either through new regulatory mechanisms for institutional ceding of IRB responsibilities or sharing of regulatory documentation and processes through Smart IRB. Once the study is activated, he also engages the cancer center data integrity and safety committee to monitor the study.
- This study becomes the backbone and inspiration for numerous other studies that require him to engage other cancer center resources and members.
- After obtaining permission from the patients, the pertinent IRBs, and the funding agencies, he works with the cancer center population science core to retrospectively compare the cost-effectiveness of protons and photons in prostate cancer using the patient cohort and data linkage with claims databases.
- After obtaining permission from the patients, the pertinent IRBs, and the funding agencies, he works with the cancer center genetics researchers and an industry partner to correlate prostate cancer outcomes in the proton and photon cohorts with other prognostic factors and genetic signatures.
- At a cancer center-sponsored educational program to inspire high school science teachers, the investigator-physician becomes aware of a collaboration between a tumor *biologist* studying the impact of abnormal vasculature on the tumor microenvironment and an exercise *physiologist* who hypothesizes that abnormal vasculature around tumors may lead to preferential blood flow to tumors during exercise, alleviating tumor hypoxia and making tumors more responsive to

radiation. He begins discussions with the tumor *biologist* and the *physiologist* that lead to pilot studies demonstrating imaging markers of hypoxia visible in prostate cancer magnetic resonances images that correlate with tumor hypoxia markers in prostate cancer biopsies and with circulating tumor cells in prostate cancer patients. With feasibility demonstrated by the pilot studies and the success in building the patient cohorts as background, he enlists the cancer center to aid in identifying funding agencies interested in healthy lifestyle research. His team receives funding to conduct a prospective controlled study assessing the impact of vigorous pretreatment exercise immediately before proton therapy on tumor control as estimated by prostate-specific antigen progression-free survival.

Example 3
- With IRB approval and assistance from *biostatisticians* in study design, a radiation oncology resident conducts a retrospective longitudinal outcomes assessment in a large institutional Hodgkin lymphoma population treated with radiation and discovers late effects in survivors, including several types of heart disease and second malignancies that begin at 10 years but appear to increase in incidence at least 40 years after treatment. The study results in a publication in a radiation oncology journal.
- He engages the cancer center clinical research office, biostatistics, and population science to help in mining the Surveillance, Epidemiology, and End Results (SEER) database to determine whether the longitudinal department experience of increasing incidence of second malignancies and cardiac morbidity appears significantly increased in comparison with age- and gender-matched patients with no history of Hodgkin lymphoma or radiation therapy. The increased incidence is confirmed, and this study results in a publication in a high-impact general medicine journal.
- Because radiation continues to be a valuable tool in the therapeutic armamentarium of Hodgkin lymphoma, he decides to determine whether these late effects are correlated with parameters describing dose and volume of irradiated tissue which could be modified with new radiation therapy techniques. He decides on a two-pronged approach. In a backward-looking approach, he plans to collaborate with *nuclear engineers* and *medical physicists* to mine radiation records to determine what dose-volume histogram (DVH) parameters were associated with events that occurred 5–40 years after treatment. In a forward-looking approach, he plans to collaborate with *nuclear engineers, and medical physicists*, and *biostatisticians*, to assess comparative proton and photon treatment plans to model comparative risks for late effects with the two approaches.
- Since many of the late effects occurred in patients treated 20–45 years earlier, radiation equipment, treatment planning, and diagnostic procedures have changed. Cobalt machines are largely eliminated from US radiation oncology practices. The radiation output was related to the machine design and age of the cobalt source. Treatment planning was based on two-dimensional kilovoltage simulation films and image guidance, and verification was based on kilovoltage port films. Dose calculations were based on simple cobalt and X-ray depth dose

tables by Clarkson calculations for points in the target volume located according to assumed target depths relative to a wire surface contour and caliper-measured patient thickness at those points. There was no three-dimensional imaging available for three-dimensional target contouring or three-dimensional treatment planning or daily image-guided radiation dose delivery.

- Therefore, in a multistep process, nuclear engineering researchers are engaged to reconstruct historical radiation dose distributions. First, the nuclear engineering team creates a virtual cobalt machine based on historic specifications and tests the validity of its predicted output using with one of the few existing extant cobalt machines left in the USA. Second, they use a series of anthropomorphic three-dimensional phantoms matched to patient histories based on gender, age, height, and weight and apply the historic cobalt prescription and field design to the phantom to determine dose distribution to a variety of organs. Third, the locations of the late events are determined through a review of medical records and ascribed a radiation dose based on the patient's individual phantom dose distribution by the radiation oncology team. These activities result in three publications in nuclear engineering, medical physics, and radiation oncology journals.
- Next, the cancer center biostatistics team is engaged to aid in creating a predictive model for second malignancy events and specific cardiac events based on knowledge of the actual late effects and estimation of the associated radiation dose distribution. The model could be used to predict probabilities of late events with different radiation strategies, e.g., simple three-dimensional conformal photon-based radiation, intensity-modulated photon radiotherapy, and intensity-modulated proton radiotherapy. With the help from the cancer center clinical research office, a grant is obtained from the National Institutes of Health for the predictive model study. The model is published in a high-impact oncology journal.
- Finally, cancer center cost-effectiveness researchers aid in correlating predicted differential outcomes with differential overall health-care costs, and another publication results in impacting practice patterns across the USA.

Summary

- Cancer centers offer expanded opportunities for unique academic radiation oncology careers.
- They will vary in what resources and expertise they offer, but each will have unique strengths and present unique opportunities.
- Website review and participation in cancer center service and educational activities are good ways to assess cancer center resources and refine your career path.
- The cancer center can provide resources for the design, funding, and conduct of your clinical research as well as novel opportunities for translational and basic research and context through population science.

For Discussion with a Mentor or Colleague

- Based on its website, mission statement, research, educational opportunities, and activities, what are the strengths of my cancer center?
- Given my own interests and the resources and potential collaborators within my department and my cancer center, what are potential career paths I might take?
- How could I enrich this path by enlisting resources from the cancer center?

Conflicts of Interest   None

Funding   None

Business Development from Research, Entrepreneurship Within Academic Medicine

Sara T. Rosenthal and Joanne B. Weidhaas

Background

Joanne Weidhaas grew up in an affluent suburb of Detroit, Michigan, where her father worked as a high-level executive at Ford. Scientific minds ran in her family—her uncle, Roy Vagelos, trained as a cardiologist and biochemist, and went on to build a career in life sciences, serving as the CEO of Merck starting in the mid-1980s. Weidhaas herself first planned to study biochemistry, but changed course after some genetics classes and her time volunteering at a hospital in New Haven, Connecticut, while earning her undergraduate bachelor of science degree at Yale. Having decided to pursue a career in medicine, but still having a passion for science, she enrolled in Tufts University's MD/PhD program, where she obtained her PhD in the lab of one of the world's foremost scholars in the field of retroviruses, Dr. John Coffin. In the end she was drawn to oncology, both because she was fascinated by the science and also because she felt drawn to the patients who showed such courage and determination to beat their disease in partnership with their physicians.

Weidhaas completed her radiation oncology residency at Memorial Sloan Kettering Cancer Center in New York City before taking an academic position at Yale in 2004. While at MSKCC she was a Holman Fellow, allowing her to pursue postdoctoral work in genetics, where she developed a genetic model of radiation resistance. She loved her training, appreciating each patient she met along the way, and became extremely well-versed in cancer of all types by the end of her time there. At Yale, Weidhaas intended to split her time between clinical work and research focused on *RAS* genes, an interest which developed during her PhD in the

S. T. Rosenthal
MiraKind, Los Angeles, CA, USA

J. B. Weidhaas (✉)
University of California Los Angeles, Los Angeles, CA, USA
e-mail: jweidhaas@mednet.ucla.edu

© Springer Nature Switzerland AG 2021
R. A. Chandra et al. (eds.), *Career Development in Academic Radiation Oncology*, https://doi.org/10.1007/978-3-030-71855-8_25

343

Coffin laboratory and continued during her postdoc. *RAS* genes, and one known as *KRAS*,[1] are part of a class of genes known as proto-oncogenes, which share the common property of being involved in normal cell growth, but have the ability to cause cancer if not appropriately controlled.

At Yale, Weidhaas continued her research on *KRAS* while simultaneously overseeing the Yale Cancer Center's Radiation Oncology breast cancer program. Her days included time in the clinic seeing breast cancer patients, as well as applying for grant funding to build a group to pursue her scientific interests. During a weekly "Worm meeting" (so named because the researchers who attended were all studying a primitive wormlike organism called *C. elegans*, a nematode that was a common focus of study for developmental biologists), Weidhaas sat in on a presentation that caught her attention. Frank Slack, also on faculty at Yale, was presenting his findings on an entirely new area of genetic discovery—microRNAs, small RNA molecules shown to work as master gene controllers.

In 1999, during his postdoc, Slack discovered the second-known microRNA and first human microRNA, called *let-7*. Whereas DNA, deoxyribonucleic acid, contains the genetic instructions for how organisms develop and function, RNA, or ribonucleic acid, is responsible for helping carry out those instructions by activating gene regulation, gene expression, and the coding and decoding of genes. Slack's presentation at the Worm meeting detailed his findings on how *let-7* played an integral role in controlling *KRAS*. Further, he had shown that without *let-7*, there was excess *KRAS* protein production, and thus cell division could proceed unfettered, very similar to what was seen in cancer.

Coincidentally, Weidhaas knew Slack when they were both graduate students at Tufts, and she thus reintroduced herself to him after his talk. She was intrigued by his work, and, as he was very interested in moving his research on *let-7* and microRNAs into cancer, he asked if she would join him on a grant he was resubmitting about *let-7*, *KRAS*, and lung cancer. This conversation was the beginning of an extremely productive partnership and friendship between Weidhaas and Slack. They submitted numerous grants together, and worked extremely well as a team, with Weidhaas being the driver of the clinical and cancer aspects of studies and Slack the driver of the next novel directions from the scientific microRNA perspective. After about 6 months, they received funding for their first joint project to investigate how *let-7* and *KRAS* communication, or miscommunication, may lead to lung cancer. With the help of a graduate student researcher, Lena Chin, Slack and Weidhaas began by examining lung cancer tissue samples that Weidhaas had dug up in the freezer of one of Yale's basement-level tissue banks with the help of a research-minded pathologist. They soon found what they were looking for, a mutation in approximately 20% of their lung cancer patient samples that prevented appropriate communication between *let-7* and *KRAS*, likely leading to the patients' cancer (see Fig. 1). What they didn't expect to find, however, was that this mutation was inherited, which meant it was present in all cells, and was relatively common, presenting

---

[1] *KRAS* stands for Kirsten rat sarcoma viral oncogene homolog.

- *let-7* targets the *KRAS* 3' UTR
- 10 predicted *let-7* complementary sites

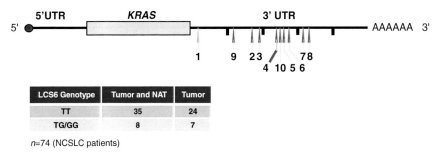

LCS6 Genotype	Tumor and NAT	Tumor
TT	35	24
TG/GG	8	7

n=74 (NCSLC patients)

G-allele present in ~ 20% of lung cancer patients (*KRAS* ORF WT)

Fig. 1 Diagram of the discovery of the *KRAS*-variant. Sequencing of the *KRAS* 3'UTR led to the identification of a binding site mutation in let-7-conserved sequence 6, which was found in 20% of lung cancer patients

in 5–7% of the population. At this time, scientists and clinicians were focused on mutations only found in cancers, or tumor-acquired mutations, primarily because so few inherited cancer-causing mutations had ever been discovered, and those that had been were exceedingly rare.

Weidhaas and Chin next looked at the patient charts associated with the lung cancer samples, and, according to a *Discover* magazine article about their work, "What Weidhaas found was startling—and chilling. The 20 percent of lung cancer patients who carried the *KRAS*-variant developed multiple different cancers, not just lung cancer." As Weidhaas explained, "We'd go through their charts and see the same things over and over. They'd beat lung cancer, but then they'd get head and neck cancer, or breast cancer, or colon cancer or pancreatic cancer. I remember thinking, 'Holy cow—this is real.'"[2]

From Academia to Market

One night while falling asleep, Weidhaas told her husband, AJ, about the exciting finding and the discovery of the *KRAS*-variant as a predictor of lung cancer. Weidhaas' husband, also a private equity attorney, kept her up late into the night, asking questions and thinking through the potential business angles of such a discovery. Over the next couple weeks, he began to investigate the process of licensing the intellectual property from Yale to build a stand-alone business, and formed MiraDx, with Weidhaas and Slack as co-founders. Through one of AJ's business

---

[2] Linda Marsa, "True Believer," Discover, December 2014, p. 41.

contacts, Weidhaas was introduced to John Oteri,[3] the former CEO of a genetic diagnostics company. Oteri was very excited about the potential opportunity and said he wanted to be involved. He quickly recruited two colleagues who had experience in the diagnostics space to begin scoping out the business model and finding funders. While Weidhaas had truly never thought about starting a business before, she felt strongly that their findings needed to get to patients, so agreed to see where things could go with the team Oteri suggested.

The Market for Genetic Testing

In 2009, the market for molecular diagnostics was booming, with 35% growth over the previous year, annual revenues of $5.5 billion, and an annual test volume of 400 million.[4] Molecular diagnostics gained momentum in the early 2000s after the completion of the Human Genome Project, the international effort to map all the genes in the entire human genome. According to an article in *Managed Care Magazine*, "In 2008, [molecular diagnostic] testing volume broke down into the following categories: infectious disease, 55 percent; blood screening, 23 percent; genetic testing, 13 percent; and cancer, the most expensive and fastest growing area, 7 percent."[5] At this time, there were a handful of genetic testing companies on the market using genetic information as tools for risk assessment, with 23andMe, Navigenics, and Myriad Genetics among the best known. 23andMe and Navigenics had both adopted a direct-to-consumer model to sell a test whereby consumers could have their DNA analyzed for more than 90 traits and conditions, ranging from Parkinson's disease and macular degeneration to baldness and obesity, after providing a saliva sample. Though both companies were relatively new to the scene, they had already received significant traction in the marketplace and media hype, with *Time* magazine bestowing its Best Invention of 2008 award on 23andMe's $399 "retail DNA test."[6]

Alongside the newcomers in the personal genomics space, Myriad Genetics, founded in 1991, represented one of the most well-established genomics companies and the 800-pound gorilla in the marketplace. By 2008, Myriad had achieved annual revenues of over $200 million for its molecular diagnostics business alone, which included genetic tests for hereditary melanoma, colon cancer, breast cancer, and ovarian cancer. Myriad employed a large salesforce to sell its tests through physicians, and relied on insurance company reimbursement to help patients cover the steep price point, ranging upward of $3500. In 1996, Myriad introduced the first

---

[3] Most names contained here have been fictionalized in the interest of privacy.

[4] Emad Rizk, MD, "Molecular Diagnostic Testing Presents $5 Billion Conundrum," April 2009, http://www.managedcaremag.com/archives/0904/0904.moleculartesting.html (June 17, 2015).

[5] Emad Rizk, MD, "Molecular Diagnostic Testing Presents $5 Billion Conundrum," April 2009, http://www.managedcaremag.com/archives/0904/0904.moleculartesting.html (June 17, 2015).

[6] Anita Hamilton, "Best Inventions of 2008," TIME, October 29, 2008, http://content.time.com/time/specials/packages/article/0,28804,1852747_1854493_1854113,00.html (June 17, 2015).

molecular diagnostic test for hereditary breast and ovarian cancer, known as BRACAnalysis, based on recently discovered inherited gene mutations in the *BRCA1* and *BRCA2*[7] genes. As it is normally expressed, the *BRCA* gene plays a key role in repairing a cell's damaged DNA and/or destroying cells in which the DNA cannot be fixed. However, a mutation in the *BRCA* gene impairs the gene's ability to repair the damage, leading to increased risk of cancer due to the loss of proper DNA repair. Though *BRCA* mutations are quite rare, found in only 0.25% of the population, they are important indicators of increased cancer risk, particularly for those individuals with strong family histories of cancer.

Testing the Waters

By late 2008, based on additional data generated by Weidhaas, the small MiraDx team, which at this point included Weidhaas and Slack in founder/advisory roles and Oteri and his team as the business group, agreed that MiraDx's best go-to-market strategy was genetic diagnostics in women's health, as they had found that women who carried the *KRAS*-variant were at a significantly increased risk of ovarian cancer [1]. With Myriad's $2 billion market capitalization as proof that there was a business to be had in genetic testing for women's cancer risk, Oteri arranged meetings with several venture capitalists (VCs) throughout the fall of 2008 to raise a Series A round of funding. In early 2009, Weidhaas presented the latest *KRAS*-variant findings at the annual meeting of the Society of Gynecologic Oncology in Austin, showing that the *KRAS*-variant was a strong predictor of ovarian cancer risk, and explained family cancer in over 50% of BRCA-negative patients. This presentation resulted in a term sheet from an Austin-based VC firm that had attended her talk. Weidhaas recalled her first encounter with the firm: "The term sheet was very aggressive, and I got the sense they were real sharks. I just did not get a good feeling from them, and I told AJ that my gut was telling me this was a bad idea."

Though the opportunity to obtain financing was attractive, Weidhaas was concerned that the Austin firm was not interested in developing the *KRAS*-variant to its full potential to help as many people as possible. As a cancer physician, her top priority was to ensure that providing an individual with knowledge that they carried this genetic mutation could help them make the best decisions for their health. As a result, Weidhaas, with Slack's agreement, decided to turn down the term sheet, hopeful that the company would find additional investors whose philosophy was more in line with her own. Weidhaas recalled after her decision, "I had shared the term sheet with my uncle (the former CEO of Merck). After I informed him that I was not going to move forward with the deal, he said, 'Oh, thank God you didn't sign that! I will help you, please never agree to terms like that.'"

---

[7] *BRCA* stands for "breast cancer susceptibility."

Though Weidhaas was confident in the decision, Oteri was understandably very disappointed to let the deal go, as he had delivered what he promised, a VC term sheet to fund the company. At the same time, he was based in Texas, while Weidhaas and Slack were located in New Haven, which ultimately led to their decision to part ways. True to his promise, Vagelos contributed seed money to help fund MiraDx's launch, Weidhaas put in her own capital, and they were soon joined by other friends and family who were excited about the potential opportunity to build a great company based on this novel gene mutation. Over the course of 2009, Weidhaas was able to raise a significant amount of additional seed capital to fund MiraDx, though she now needed to find a new solid business team to help build the company from the ground up.

Building a Team

In the summer of 2009, Weidhaas reached out to Stacy Palmer, a former venture capitalist who also lived in Westport and whom Weidhaas knew through overlapping social circles. Palmer was an electrical engineer by training who had achieved personal financial wealth after a 15-year-long career as a technology investor. A few years prior, Palmer had left venture capital to explore other interests, and had recently been let go from the foundation she had been working for in the role of CFO. Palmer was excited at the prospect of taking a lead role in MiraDx, and Weidhaas was anxious to place someone with business experience at the helm, particularly now that they had raised a significant sum of money that needed to be put to work.

Palmer assumed the role of COO, and among her first efforts were securing office and lab space and assembling a small lab team in New Haven. While Palmer had tremendous passion for MiraDx's mission, and Weidhaas loved having a woman involved in leading the company, it soon became clear that the new COO was in over her head, with no prior experience and little understanding of the diagnostic space or a reasonable plan for going to market. More importantly, potential investors were skeptical of Palmer and came to Weidhaas directly to tell her she needed someone with diagnostic experience or she would never be able to raise additional funds.

Weidhaas' husband helped source another outside advisor, Romy Nagel, who had recently retired after a lengthy career as an executive in the biotech and diagnostics space. Nagel recommended the former head of sales, Brad Davies, from his previous company as a strong leader who could step in as president to help Palmer steer the ship. Weidhaas had some reservations about Davies after their first two meetings, recalling, "Again my gut was just telling me that this was not the right fit, but we were anxious and I was the scientist, not the business person, so I again deferred." Davies joined MiraDx in early 2010 with the goal of helping the company bring its *KRAS*-variant ovarian cancer test to market.

PreOvar

Among Davies' first orders of business was to hire a small salesforce, and develop a solid plan by which he and his two sales representatives could most effectively penetrate the market. Davies believed that MiraDx could sell its "PreOvar" test, named for its ability to predict risk for ovarian cancer before it happened, in the same way Myriad Genetics had gained such a broad footprint. While Myriad sold its BRACAnalysis test for upward of $3000–$4000, it relied on insurance to reimburse approximately 50% of the cost. Weidhaas wanted to keep the cost of the test low, but Davies pointed out that they had a fiduciary responsibility to return capital to her investors, combined with the need to employ an increasingly large salesforce to market the test, all of which would contribute to the expense of the test itself. Initially the team, under Davies' guidance, directly submitted claims to insurers, but after 6 months, during which time 90% of the claims were rejected, it became clear that this strategy was not going to work to support the company. In his defense, Davies had come from a large and powerful diagnostics company where this strategy had worked time and time again, but it appeared an easy reimbursement path was not possible for a startup company with no insurer relationships.

The first target for selling the test would be genetic counselors who were trained to advise individuals about the consequences and nature of genetic disorders for which they had been tested. In addition, MiraDx would reach out to obstetrician-gynecologists (OBGYNs), physicians who specialized in women's health. With the help of Davies' two sales reps, he was able to compile a list of the genetic counselors who represented high-volume purchasers of Myriad's *BRCA* test. Davies sent out a mass mailing to these counselors to market the pending launch of the PreOvar test, with the goal of reaching the women with whom the counselors were already working (primarily women with strong family histories of breast and ovarian cancer) to offer PreOvar in addition to BRACAnalysis. While Davies' outreach met the goal of informing genetic counselors about MiraDx's test, it also raised a red flag with the Food and Drug Administration (FDA), the federal body responsible for regulating all medical and drug-related products and devices. Fortunately, after calling a meeting with MiraDx, the FDA realized that the startup was a very small and benign player in the genetics LDT market, and subsequently informed MiraDx that it should proceed responsibly with its testing, but did not need to follow up. However, this misstep by Davies convinced Weidhaas that someone with startup experience would likely be a better fit to lead the charge at MiraDx.

The Search for a New CEO

In July 2010, with less than one million dollars in the bank, and a burn rate of $250,000 a month, Weidhaas began the search for a new CEO to run the company. Among the candidates she interviewed was Mark Stadheim, a chemical engineer by training with a 25-year career in molecular diagnostics and life science research tools. After serving in various senior management roles in midsize biotech companies, Stadheim most recently held the position of CEO of a molecular diagnostics startup focused on tumor-based screening. Stadheim had been let go from his previous company shortly after raising Series B venture capital funding, an event which Weidhaas admitted "should have been a red flag, or at least something to investigate a little more thoroughly. But he seemed intelligent and was a nice person at heart who worked hard."

Stadheim was hired as MiraDx's CEO in November 2010, with the promise to make significant cuts to the operating budget, largely through layoffs, once he got a better understanding of the company dynamics. Unlike Davies and Palmer, who regularly shared their opinion that Weidhaas should be less involved with company operations, Stadheim welcomed and asked for more of her input, as he recognized that her deep knowledge and understanding of the patient population was critical to success.

At the time of Stadheim's hiring, MiraDx was selling approximately 25–30 tests per month, largely to OBGYNs, but with little to no reimbursement. Among Stadheim's stated goals from the beginning was to initiate conversations with Myriad, believing there were opportunities to partner with the testing company and to leverage its salesforce to sell the PreOvar test. Weidhaas remembered feeling skittish about this approach at the time, particularly given Myriad's monopoly status in the market. However, she had hired Stadheim to set the strategic direction as CEO, so in early 2011, Weidhaas and Stadheim had their first meeting with the president and CSO of Myriad in MiraDx's New Haven office. Over the course of the discussion, Stadheim freely shared the details about the partners with whom the company was working, several academic groups with large clinical data sets which they would use as validation, as well as the various avenues of research Weidhaas was pursuing. Although Weidhaas felt uncomfortable with the level of disclosure, she could not have anticipated the firestorm involving Myriad and these projects that would follow.

The Politics of Women's Cancer

In 2009, Weidhaas approached a group of investigators known as the Ovarian Cancer Association Consortium (OCAC) to discuss collaborating, after learning that they had started studying the *KRAS*-variant after seeing her abstract at a cancer conference. This group pooled large numbers of ovarian cancer samples together for study, applying a research platform developed in 2002 called genome-wide association studies (GWAS) to try to identify inherited genetic markers that predicted ovarian cancer risk. Weidhaas supplied the group with information on how to test for the

KRAS-variant, in addition to all that she had learned about this gene mutation, in the spirit of academic collaboration. In return, OCAC agreed she would be the first author on the study, and sent her information on the cohorts of patients they would include in the analysis. It was immediately obvious to Weidhaas that the data they planned to use was clinically inappropriate: "There were entire studies where they used men as their controls, and almost 20 percent of the samples classified as 'ovarian cancer' were not clinically documented as cancer. While their approach sounded good in concept, it soon became clear that the poor quality of samples trumped the quantity. And this was just the tip of the iceberg." Weidhaas pointed out these concerns to the leaders of the consortium, but was quickly shut down with the claim that none of these details would matter given the large number of samples being evaluated.

After receiving results on the full data set, she analyzed the data with a statistician with whom she worked closely at Yale. They found that the results of the analysis validated the positive correlation between the *KRAS*-variant and ovarian cancer, not just for women with a family history of cancer but for all women. However, the impact was being diluted by inclusion of some of OCAC's poorly constructed sample sets. Weidhaas asked about the appropriateness of including these data sets in the final analysis, but in response was attacked by the leader of the group. Weidhaas recalled, "I suddenly realized that if my data was confirmed to show that a single, functional biomarker could predict ovarian cancer, and that their approach had completely missed it, it would invalidate their genome-wide approach. They just wouldn't or couldn't have it, and they actually ended up kicking me off the paper and adding even more flawed data sets." Although Weidhaas knew that the OCAC group was putting together their results into a negative paper, she had meanwhile completed a second analysis showing that women with the *KRAS*-variant with ovarian cancer were resistant to platinum agents, and significantly more likely to die of their ovarian cancer, which cemented the importance of this variant in ovarian cancer. This work was selected as the first plenary session at an upcoming conference, the Society of Gynecologic Oncology (SGO). However, the conflict with OCAC came to a head in March 2011, days before the conference, when Weidhaas learned that her talk had been pulled, apparently for a technical reason. Only at the meeting did she find out that her talk had been replaced by one of the leaders of OCAC who would be presenting the consortium's paper regarding the *KRAS*-variant, which put Weidhaas' work in an extremely negative light.

Shortly after the SGO conference, the discussant of the OCAC paper, a previous collaborator of Weidhaas', became a vice president at Myriad Genetics, and Myriad subsequently distributed the OCAC paper to its 300-person salesforce as a means to invalidate the *KRAS*-variant findings among a broad-based clinical audience. Though Weidhaas had at one point anticipated her SGO talk would be a pivotal turning point to get this information to women, she now questioned whether the company would be able to survive this devastating turn of events.

Marching On

Though MiraDx had received two VC term sheets in early 2011 through connections Stadheim had helped generate, all leads went cold after the SGO conference's negative presentation. MiraDx's test volume quickly tapered off to nothing, and Stadheim had yet to conduct layoffs to reduce MiraDx's burn rate. At Weidhaas' insistence, he finally let Palmer, Davies, and one of the sales reps go in April 2011, leaving only one sales rep and the two-person laboratory team remaining. With cash in the bank at almost zero, Weidhaas returned to her initial investors to raise a bridge round of financing based on MiraDx's new data regarding the use of the *KRAS*-variant to predict chemotherapy response. Together with capital provided by Weidhaas and her husband, she was able to secure enough additional capital to keep the company afloat.

By the summer of 2011, the future of MiraDx seemed bleak, with a few exceptions. In March, Weidhaas and a large group of collaborators published a paper in the esteemed journal *Lancet Oncology* describing the role of the *KRAS*-variant as a biomarker for the development of triple-negative breast cancer[8] in premenopausal women [2]. The findings were important, as they provided further validation of the *KRAS*-variant's significant role as a functional biomarker for predicting cancer risk, especially in women. Additionally, later that year a large independent validation study was published showing the *KRAS*-variant was found in approximately 50% of women with multiple primary breast and ovarian cancers who were *BRCA*-negative, tying her findings together [3]. Weidhaas' study on how the *KRAS*-variant could be used to predict chemotherapy resistance was also published, further proving the ability of this new class of mutations to be used to direct cancer treatment [4].

The Power of Personalized Medicine

Over the previous decade, genetic information increasingly had been utilized as a way to gauge an individual's response to treatment, leading to the growth of an entirely new field known as personalized medicine. Rather than give an entire population of individuals the same drugs to treat their disease and hope for the best, research in the field of molecular diagnostics was helping to provide physicians with the data they needed to individually tailor treatment to their patients, based on each person's unique genetic makeup. Weidhaas' finding indicating that cancer patients with the *KRAS*-variant responded poorly to cisplatin was somewhat paradigm shifting, as previously only tumor-acquired mutations, as opposed to inherited mutations like the *KRAS*-variant, had been used to direct cancer therapies.

---

[8] There are several types of breast cancer, classified as being either receptive or non-receptive to estrogen and/or progesterone. Triple-negative breast cancer is so called because it tests negative for three factors: estrogen receptors, progesterone receptors, and human epidermal growth factor (HER2) receptors. Women with triple-negative breast cancer therefore do not respond to standard hormone therapies such as tamoxifen or aromatase inhibitors due to the nature of their cancer.

With this new data in hand, Stadheim and Weidhaas began reaching out to various groups in the pharmaceutical space to gauge their interest in using the *KRAS*-variant to streamline the lengthy and costly drug development process. Weidhaas envisioned utilizing the *KRAS*-variant in a clinical trial, for example, to segment out those 6–10% of patients who tested positive for the variant since they would likely have a differential response to the drug under study. Pharmaceutical companies could thus use this biomarker as one tool to more quickly evaluate a drug's efficacy for a specific population, potentially resulting in cost savings of up to hundreds of millions of dollars over the life of a trial. Rather than shelving an expensive and potentially useful drug for eternity because a large subset of individuals did not respond well during clinical trials, the pharmaceutical company may find that segmenting out the *KRAS*-variant individuals changed the outcome enough to bring the drug to market (i.e., as one that worked well either *for* patients with the *KRAS*-variant or for those without it). Despite the compelling data, Weidhaas achieved little traction with this approach. After extensive discussions and limited progress with multiple pharmaceutical companies, she wondered if resistance stemmed from their reluctance to engage any tool that would threaten to indicate that the market was smaller than previously believed. Regardless of the reason for resistance, Weidhaas soon accepted that pharma partnerships would not be a viable funding or development path for the company or the *KRAS*-variant.

A New Direction

By early 2012, it had become clear to Weidhaas that Stadheim was not going to be able to find avenues to keep MiraDx funded, and thus could not continue on as MiraDx's CEO. In addition, Weidhaas had to lay off "one of the best employees we ever had," Brenda Pritchard, the remaining sales rep who had remained creative and flexible throughout the turbulence of the preceding months. After paying off the debt Stadheim had accrued and reducing the monthly burn rate to $20,000 (the cost to run the lab), Weidhaas found herself once again facing the question of how to get this important information about the *KRAS*-variant and mutations like it to patients and doctors. She felt like in the previous two-and-a-half years since launching MiraDx, she had been defeated at every turn by market forces that often felt out of her control. It was at this time Weidhaas received news that she had been accepted into the Stanford Graduate School of Business' Sloan program, a 1-year full-time masters of science program in business, designed for experienced professionals who wanted a deeper understanding of business fundamentals. Weidhaas did not consider herself an "experienced" business person; however, given the numerous market challenges MiraDx had faced in the previous few years, she hoped that the Sloan program could provide her with the tools she needed to help MiraDx achieve its true potential. Although it was an incredible leap of faith, she took a leave from her position at Yale, and she and AJ moved their family to Stanford, CA, where she started the program in July of 2012.

New Opportunities, New Challenges

In June 2013, Weidhaas completed her coursework at Stanford, after having spent the previous year studying accounting, finance, and strategic marketing, among other topics. She also learned about the complexities of the US medical system through several classes which explored the then relatively new Affordable Care Act. While at Stanford, she consulted with numerous faculty members and fellow students, many of whom had experience in the health-care or finance space, to gain their insights on her company's most viable direction. Overwhelmingly, she received feedback that she should focus exclusively on the personalized medicine side of the business, based on the belief that there were too many challenges to building a business around cancer prevention given how the US health-care system was currently structured. She was told more times than she could count, "No one pays for prevention." Though Weidhaas' heart was dedicated to women's health and cancer prevention, she also had to face the reality that she must build a business that could both return capital to its investors and become self-sustaining if she were ever going to do the work to which she was truly committed.

As she began planning for the year ahead, she knew that she wanted to get back to her translational research while trying to relaunch MiraDx after its yearlong hiatus. However, there were several events that would happen in the months to come that would significantly impact the market dynamics for the struggling company.

The Supreme Court Ruling

In June 2013, the Supreme issued a landmark ruling in the case of the *Association for Molecular Pathology* vs. *Myriad Genetics* that would forever impact the future of molecular diagnostics and genetic research. Myriad acquired patents on the *BRCA*1 and *BRCA*2 genes in the mid-1990s, allowing it an effective monopoly on genetic testing for those genes over the subsequent 20 years. The Supreme Court's 2013 ruling held that because genes were products of nature, they were not patentable, thus invalidating Myriad's intellectual property for the *BRCA* genes. The shock waves of this decision resounded throughout the scientific and business community, with many hailing it as a turning point and others viewing it as an impediment to the commercialization of genetic discoveries. In an ABC News report, Professor Lori Andrews of the Illinois Institute of Technology Chicago-Kent College of Law said, "Today's decision allows any doctor or scientist to use the breast cancer gene for diagnosis or treatment. This means all genetic tests will become affordable and more researchers will be able to look for cures."[9] On the flip side, companies in the diagnostic testing space argued that the economic incentives

---

[9] Ariane de Vogue, "Supreme Court Strikes down *BRCA* Patent," June 13, 2013, http://abcnews. go.com/Politics/supreme-court-strikes-*BRCA*-gene-patent/story?id=19392299 (June 19, 2015).

to commercialize tests would disappear without patent protection, thereby stymying consumers' ability to access this important information.

While MiraDx held method patents that protected the *process* of identifying the *KRAS*-variant, as opposed to patents on the genetic mutation itself, the recent ruling did not bode well. It was felt that this was just the first of several such rulings from the court in this realm, leaving intellectual property and the value of patents in an incredibly tenuous state. What made this especially risky for MiraDx was that the *KRAS*-variant was a single marker, and thus very easy to test by others. In the fall of 2013, Weidhaas went out to the market to engage several companies in partnership deals, all of whom cited interest, but at an absurdly low price or to revisit discussions in 12–24 months when the intellectual property landscape became clearer.

The FDA Fully Steps In

Over the previous few years, the FDA had begun to place more scrutiny on diagnostic tests, largely in response to the proliferation of genetic tests being offered direct to consumers. In 2011, roughly 25 direct-to-consumer (DTC) genetic testing companies were sent warning letters from the FDA. The letters explained the agency's desire to meet with each company "to discuss whether the service [they] are promoting requires review by FDA and what information [they] would need to submit in order for [their] product to be legally marketed."[10]

After the FDA's initial review of these 25 companies, the agency's scrutiny of laboratory-developed tests (LDTs) only increased, resulting in a dramatic dictate to one of the best-known players in the market at that time. In the fall of 2013, the FDA instructed 23andMe to cease the sale of its personal genetic test until further notice. At issue was 23andMe's delayed response to the FDA's requests for documentation, as well as the administration's concerns that sensitive genetic information was being delivered to consumers without the engagement of a medical professional. In its letter to the company, the FDA stated that its regulators "still do not have any assurance that the firm has analytically or clinically validated the [personal genome service] for its intended uses."[11] While MiraDx continued to engage a physician in the communication of all test results, the FDA's announcement completely eliminated the direct-to-consumer option as a commercialization strategy, and also presented an additional risk that the FDA would only continue to increase its scrutiny of diagnostics. If MiraDx wanted to reach a broad audience, was its only option to engage a large and costly salesforce to reach out to physicians and genetic counselors, similar to the Myriad model?

---

[10] "Consumer Testing and Future of DTC Testing," Kalorama Information, April 2012, p. 44.

[11] James O'Toole and Aaron Smith, "FDA Orders Genetic Testing Firm 23andme to Halt Sales," http://money.cnn.com/2013/11/25/technology/fda-23andme/ (June 19, 2015).

Too Much Money

In addition to the regulatory and intellectual property challenges the company now faced, MiraDx faced market challenges stemming largely from its predecessors in the genomics space. Genomic Health was founded in 2000 with the goal of using the genetic information found in a cancer patient's tumors to personalize cancer treatment. The company's first test to market, Oncotype DX, provided a breast cancer assay which helped predict the likelihood of breast cancer recurrence as well as chemotherapy benefit for early-stage breast cancer patients. In 2010, the company introduced its colon cancer assay and, in 2013, a prostate cancer assay which helped guide cancer treatment. Though the company achieved much acclaim, its underwhelming year-over-year performance soured investors who had put millions of dollars into the company over the years.

Similarly, Foundation Medicine, founded in 2009, was a genomic testing company that promised to utilize the genetic information found in cancer patients' tumor samples to personalize treatment. By early 2013, the company had already raised $100 million in capital but had delivered little return to its investors and struggled to achieve profitability. The result for MiraDx was limited access to capital, since the financing community had largely pulled back from the space, having grown weary of investing in companies that required such intense time and capital to achieve revenue milestones.

Charting a Path Forward

As 2013 came to a close, Weidhaas weighed her options. She knew there were numerous research studies she wanted to conduct to further validate the *KRAS*-variant's role in women's health, as well as its role as a companion diagnostic. She also wanted to ensure that women would have access to their personal *KRAS*-variant results if they chose. As well, she and Slack had sequenced the microRNA regions of the genome, identifying numerous additional mutations, like the *KRAS*-variant. She was anxious to apply this knowledge to other pain points in oncology. Although capital sources from the investment community were not widely available, the research community had begun to embrace the significance of the *KRAS*-variant. This enabled her to tap into a variety of funding sources through such organizations as the National Cancer Institute and the National Institutes of Health, opening the door to several potential research paths and additional career options.

MiraKind

Among the studies in Weidhaas' pipeline was the Army of Women (AoW) study, conducted in collaboration with Dr. Susan Love Research Foundation's Army of Women program which enabled breast cancer survivors to enroll in active research. In early 2014, Weidhaas formed MiraKind, a nonprofit with the goal of "uniting patients with groundbreaking research to transform women's health." Given the myriad of challenges she had faced in bringing the *KRAS*-variant test to market through MiraDx, MiraKind would allow her to effectively provide women interested in participating in her research with access to the *KRAS*-variant test, which to her was of ultimate importance as it gave them critical genetic information which could inform their cancer diagnosis and treatment. The study was supported through an NIH grant that Weidhaas held, while the testing was performed at the MiraDx laboratories to allow reporting to patients. A webinar of the study results was organized through MiraKind.

Back to Academia

Although MiraKind served as a patient education and outreach platform, as a nonprofit, it was not equipped to advance the research that came out of studies like the Army of Women. Weidhaas had learned an incredible amount over the past 5 years, but she truly missed the collaborative spirit of academia and the opportunity to care for patients. As well, she wanted to conduct further research to apply the additional genetic mutations she and Slack had discovered to answer other cancer treatment challenges. She thus felt very fortunate to find an opportunity to return to academics as head of translational research in the Department of Radiation Oncology at UCLA. Everything that was described to her about the position felt like the right fit—they were enthusiastic to bring important findings to patients, and with appropriate management of conflict of interest, they were very supportive of company founders, viewing her startup and business school training as positives. She therefore proposed to the hiring committee that she would like to apply the new class of genetic markers she and Slack had discovered to radiation oncology, a field with amazing technologic advances, but in need of treatment personalization based on patients' personal genetics. Her proposal to develop a radiogenomics program was met with great enthusiasm. After many productive and open discussions with her new chair and the dean of the medical school about her goals, she accepted the position at UCLA.

As a vice-chair in radiation oncology, Weidhaas has learned to walk the tight rope of being a company co-founder with an academic appointment at UCLA. She holds an advisor role at MiraDx, which allows her to participate in high-level strategy setting for the company and promote its mission of improving care for cancer patients while also caring for patients and pursuing her research interests at UCLA. MiraDx has obtained significant SBIR funding to perform genetic testing for several clinical trials led by other principal investigators at UCLA, which allows Weidhaas and her peers to collaborate with the company she founded. Reflecting on her journey, Weidhaas is happy to be back in academics, but also appreciates all she learned through her unconventional detour into entrepreneurship. "I have landed exactly where I want to be, although it was certainly a long and arduous route to get here."

Summary Bullet Points

- There are many unknown obstacles and market forces that can be roadblocks when trying to move research findings to market through the startup path.
- Everyone will have their own path to entrepreneurship.
- Be aware that your goals may be quite different than the goals of funders or other medical companies. Success requires finding alignment between these various stakeholders.
- Advancing translational work through academics and access to like-minded companies has many potential benefits to advancing patient care.

For Discussion with a Mentor or Colleague

- If you are interested in founding a company, why and what role do you envision yourself playing?
- What does success look like for you?
- What trade-offs might you have to make as an entrepreneur?
- Do you have business experience or close contacts with business experience to advise you?
- Are there other avenues to advance your findings that you would be comfortable with?
- Are you at an institution where they are open to academic founders and can help manage conflicts of interest?

References

1. Ratner E, Lu L, Boeke M, et al. A KRAS-variant in ovarian cancer acts as a genetic marker of cancer risk. Cancer Res. 2010;70(16):6509–15.
2. Paranjape T, Heneghan H, Lindner R, et al. A 3′-untranslated region KRAS variant and triple-negative breast cancer: a case-control and genetic analysis. Lancet Oncol. 2011;12(4):377–86.
3. Pilarski R, Patel DA, Weitzel J, et al. The KRAS-variant is associated with risk of developing double primary breast and ovarian cancer. PLoS One. 2012;7(5):e37891.
4. Ratner E, Keane F, Lindner R, et al. A KRAS-variant is a biomarker of poor outcome, platinum chemotherapy resistance and a potential target for therapy in ovarian cancer. Oncogene. 2012;31(42):4559-66. https://doi.org/10.1038/onc.2011.539. Epub 2011 Dec 5.

An Approach to the Management of Selected Personnel and Ethical Problems in Academic Radiation Oncology

Edward C. Halperin and Jennifer Riekert

What makes an organization complex? A complex organization has multiple stakeholders such as customers or patients, providers of services, suppliers, regulators, and owners; multiple organizational structures such as divisions, teams, or joint ventures; multiple people who are involved in completing a task; and multiple steps that must be completed in order to get a job done. By all of these criteria, an academic radiation oncology department is a complex organization.

An academic radiation oncology department's stakeholders include patients and their family members, referring physicians, the medical school, the affiliated hospital(s), the cancer center, the suppliers of radiation oncology equipment, and physicians, physicists, dosimetrists, nurses, radiation therapists, business managers, patient transporters, receptionists, cancer biologists, and administrative assistants. The department often has disease-based or location-based divisions and treatment teams. The administration of external beam radiation therapy or brachytherapy is a multistep process involving many people. Regulators and accreditors oversee the operation of the department.

It is no surprise that in a department of radiation oncology, the daily interactions of a large number of people performing consequential tasks in the treatment of cancer patients lead to multiple personnel and ethical problems that require solutions. In this chapter we will describe five of these problems. For each problem we will offer our thoughts on a managerial approach.

E. C. Halperin (✉)
New York Medical College, and Provost for Biomedical Affairs, Touro College and University System, Valhalla, NY, USA
e-mail: Edward_Halperin@nymc.edu

J. Riekert
New York Medical College, Valhalla, NY, USA
e-mail: Jennifer_Riekert@nymc.edu

© Springer Nature Switzerland AG 2021
R. A. Chandra et al. (eds.), *Career Development in Academic Radiation Oncology*, https://doi.org/10.1007/978-3-030-71855-8_26

The Case of the Distressed Staff Member

The Case

For many years Anitha has been a highly productive cancer biologist in the department of radiation oncology, with an enviable list of publications and track record of external grant funding. One day, however, Charles, the department vice-chair, hears that Anitha is considering a job at another university and makes an appointment with her to discuss the rumor.

"I have heard rumors that you are considering leaving us for a new position," Charles begins the conversation. "Is there something you'd like to discuss?"

Anitha looks across the desk at Charles and bursts into tears.

"Oh my," the flustered Charles responds. "This is obviously not a good time to talk. I will come back another time." He beats a hasty retreat.

That evening Charles tells his wife what happened at work. When he gets to the part of the story where Anitha burst into tears, his wife interjects, "Well I certainly hope you didn't do something insensitive and patronizing like say I'll come back when you have composed yourself."

"But that's exactly what I did," Charles says.

"Well then you were wrong," his wife tells him.

Concerned about the way he handled his meeting with Anitha, Charles returns to work the next day and goes to visit the most senior of the clinical department chairs, Robert, the chair of the department of obstetrics-gynecology. Robert listens silently as Charles describes the situation. When Charles has finished telling the story, he asks Robert what might be a better approach than the one he took.

"Charles," Robert intones in a sonorous Southern accent, "what do you see on my credenza behind me?"

"A large box of tissues," Charles replies.

"That's right. Now what I would do in the situation you described is reach back, take that box of tissues and set it in front of the faculty member, then fold your hands, and sit silently. When your employee is done crying, you resume the conversation."

After thanking Robert, Charles walked back to his office and looked at his long-time office assistant. "Ruth," Charles says, "please order a half a dozen boxes of tissues."

What Are the Lessons of the Case Regarding Academic Management?

When faced with a tearful subordinate, you cannot, at first, be sure of the etiology of the tears. Is the individual crying because they are facing a distressing personal problem, because they trust you, or because they are trying to engender a sense of sympathy? When you're an academic manager, however, you need to manage. You might consider the following guidelines:

1. Be aware of what the trigger was for the tears. What part of the conversation launched the tearful reaction?
2. Don't overreact to the tears. Allow a nonjudgmental recovery period and resume the meeting.
3. Don't try to play the role of psychiatrist. Be prepared to manage, in a thoughtful and kind way. Keep your focus on work-related concerns. Do not offer to make everything all right. Leave the psychological/psychiatric counseling to professionals.
4. This is not the time to tell the crying individual about some problem in the past that made you tearful. It's not about you. It's about them and their impact on the organization.
5. End the meeting with a clear conclusion. "This is what is expected to happen next."
6. Afterwards, question yourself. Are you, as a manager, really paying attention to your subordinates and their needs? Could you have anticipated the situation and addressed it earlier? [1, 2]

The Case of the Unfaithful Spouse

The Case

For many years Dolores has been a highly productive medical physicist in the department of radiation oncology. She is married to Ralph, a successful plastic surgeon. Dolores becomes pregnant. Unfortunately, as the pregnancy progresses, Dolores becomes increasingly ill. She is afflicted with serious medical problems which necessitate her being confined to the hospital for the last three months of her pregnancy Charles, her department vice-chair, makes it a point to stop and see her in the hospital regularly, bring audiobooks, and try and keep her spirits up. Dolores survives the pregnancy and gives birth to a healthy baby.

About a year later, Dolores is back at work in the radiation oncology department and asks for a meeting with Charles.

"I have learned that while I was hospitalized during my pregnancy, my husband was having an affair," Dolores tells Charles. "What would you advise I do?"

Charles demurs and asks Dolores to give him some time to think the matter over. He makes another appointment to go see Robert.

"Perhaps you have faced problems like this before in your long career as a department chair?" Charles asks Robert. "What do you advise I do?"

Robert fixes Charles with a long look. "Charlie, do you have a marriage counseling certificate on your wall?"

"Of course not," Charles replies.

"Then that's your answer," Robert replies. "You have no expertise in marriage counseling. You tell your physicist that you'll find out who is the best qualified person to help her, that you'll give her whatever time off she needs to work through this issue, but don't you dare start giving out marital advice. If she listens to you and something goes wrong based your uninformed advice, then it's going to be your fault."

What Are the Lessons of the Case Regarding Academic Management?

One can envision a long list of reasons why a faculty or staff member's work performance is impaired because of troubles outside of the office: an unfaithful spouse, divorce, a medical illness in the family, drug addiction in a family member, or legal difficulties. When problems at home interact with work in the radiation oncology department, then it's time for thoughtful and compassionate management of the situation.

The radiation oncology department is in the business of the diagnosis and treatment of cancer patients. The personal problems of physicians and staff must never be permitted to compromise the quality of patient care. To that end, it is worth keeping several principles in mind:

1. As a manager you need to be empathetic and compassionate while maintaining the highest possible clinical standards and keeping the department focused on its primary mission.
2. Invest the time and effort to make it clear to your subordinates that you are open and available to hear about their problems at home, but don't pry. Your job is to manage, not to act as the departmental psychiatrist.
3. Spend more time listening than suggesting.
4. Know what you can and cannot offer. Familiarize yourself with institutional policies on leaves of absence or changes in work scheduling so that you don't offer an employee accommodations which you are not authorized to offer.
5. Remember that your actions as a manager will be observed. Be consistent in handling situations so that you are not viewed as showing favoritism toward one subordinate and their problems compared to another's [3].

The Case of "The Doctor Who Gives Me the Creeps"

The Case

Chiu-an, the clinical service line director of the department of radiation oncology, is sitting at his desk when his senior medical physicist, Jennifer, comes in to see him. Over the year Chiu-an has come to rely on Jennifer to help in day-to-day departmental clinical management. Jennifer wants to talk about the new assistant professor, George, who they hired a year ago. George's job assignment is to cover the breast cancer and gynecological cancer clinical services.

Slowly and methodically Jennifer tells Chiu-an that she has been investigating several allegations regarding George. One of the dosimetrists and one of the radiation therapists says George "gives them the creeps" because they have witnessed him making sexually suggestive and inappropriate comments to female patients during breast or pelvic examinations. George has also made what are perceived as sexually provocative comments to the female dosimetrists and radiation therapists. Jennifer has interviewed all potential eyewitnesses to these allegations, including the involved patients, and finds that all of the stories are consistent. Jennifer has documented everything she's done regarding the investigation.

Chiu-an thinks things over, consults with university counsel, and brings George in for a talk. Confronted with the allegations, George admits that this is the type of language he does use with his patients and co-workers. He thinks "some humor in the clinic helps put the patients and co-workers at ease."

After George leaves, Chiu-an starts thinking. "George came to us from a prestigious academic department. His letters of reference said nothing about this type of behavior," Chiu-an muses. He picks up the phone and calls the chair of the department who wrote George the recommendation. He promptly confirms that the other department had the same kinds of problems with George and told him to resign and try to restart his career elsewhere. He didn't mention this pattern of behavior in his letter of reference to Chiu-an on advice of his own university counsel.

What Are the Lessons of the Case Regarding Academic Management?

Patients may become dissatisfied with their physician for alleged failure to fulfill expectations for diagnosis and treatment, failure to promptly diagnose, rudeness, producing excessive pain, practicing outside their area of expertise, or inappropriate behavior regarding billing [4]. Sexual misconduct is among the most serious reasons for patient dissatisfaction. Physician sexual misconduct is a behavior that exploits the physician-patient relationship in a sexual way. There are two types of physician sexual misconduct. Sexual impropriety includes behavior, gestures, or expressions that are seductive, sexually suggestive, disrespectful of patient privacy, or sexually demeaning to a patient. Sexual violation includes physical sexual contact between a physician and a patient [5, 6].

The best way for a radiation oncology leader to deal with physician sexual misconduct by a subordinate is to be well-prepared via leadership training. It is essential to be familiar with the relevant institutional policies and reporting requirements of the state medical board. At least one trusted member of the department faculty should undergo yearly training in how to conduct the initial assessment of an allegation of sexual misconduct within the department. Prompt involvement of experienced legal counsel is also essential.

This case also raises the issue of the interpretation of letters of reference. Out of fear of litigation, some letter writers produce useless documents. Others convey their negative messages using code language. Two examples of code language negative letters of reference are:

Example 1
Dear Anand,

In response to your request for a letter of reference for Dr. John Doe, he served as a member of the faculty here from July 1, 2016, to June 30, 2017.

Sincerely yours,

Or

Example 2
Dear Anand,

On the advice of hospital counsel, I am unable to provide any information in response to your request for a letter of reference for Dr. John Doe.

Sincerely yours,

Often nothing can take the place of a telephone or a face-to-face conversation when an honest reference is desired.

The Case of the Moving Price

The Case

Sophia, the associate professor of radiation oncology who has been selected to lead the equipment selection committee of the department of radiation oncology, is chatting with the sales representatives of a major linear accelerator manufacturer. The hospital system is going to buy a new linear accelerator and own the machine. The hospital system CEO is relying on Sophia to recommend a vendor.

The sales representatives explain that either they can price the equipment for the hospital system at $4.2 million and make a $200,000 donation to Sophia's discretionary research account "to support her academic needs in the department" or they can price it at $4 million with no donation to the research account.

Puzzled, Sophia calls a senior faculty member at another major medical center. "It happens all the time," she is told. "What do you care? It's not your money; it's the hospital's money."

Sophia makes an appointment to speak to his hospital's CEO. "I think I have been offered a bribe," she begins, "and I want to talk to you about it."

What Are the Lessons of the Case Regarding Academic Management?

The linear accelerator manufacturer is proposing a transfer of $200,000 of the hospital's money to the department budget under the ruse of the pricing of the equipment. This sort of behavior helps drive up the costs of health care. No amount of rationalization about "helping research" justifies immoral conduct. Whether in the guise of "supporting research," payments for attending "equipment users' meetings" at luxury resorts, or "consultant's fees," real or apparent conflicts of interests must be acknowledged, disclosed, and honestly addressed.

The Case of the Unexpected Arrest

The Case

Diane Garcia is an assistant professor in the department of radiation oncology. She is covering one of the satellite clinics for the department and is at her desk working on a report after the staff has left for the day. She has been waiting for a call regarding a patient's laboratory results, so when the phone rings, she is quick to answer.

"Hello, Dr. Garcia, radiation oncology, may I help you?" she says–expecting to hear about the laboratory results she has been awaiting.

"This is Keiko Masumoto and I am a reporter with the *Spring Valley Post*. Do you have a Dr. Bazyler on your staff?"

Diane confirms that Dr. Bazyler is on staff at the satellite clinic but not available at the moment.

"Are you aware that Dr. Bazyler was arrested two days ago and is out on bond? I have been unable to reach him directly," the reporter tells Diane. "Can you give me a statement?"

Startled, Diane tells the reporter she has no knowledge of the situation and asks what the charges behind his arrest were.

"Domestic violence," the reporter says. "Dr. Bazyler assaulted a minor living in his home." Ms. Masumoto's tone of voice becomes a bit more arched. "Are you telling me, Dr. Garcia, that as a physician in your department you don't even know that a colleague on your own medical staff has been arrested?"

"We will have to look into this and get back to you," Diane responds. "Can you please give me your contact information?"

Taken off guard and flustered by the unexpected call, Diane decides she should arrange a conference call with the heads of the medical center's legal and the public relations departments.

What Are the Lessons of the Case Regarding Academic Management?

As a manager, when an employee runs into legal issues, you must consider the rights and needs of the employee as well as the reputation and operation of the organization. It is not your job to judge if they are innocent or guilty. You will need to give them the appropriate resources and services while also ensuring your organization's policies are followed and the crisis is effectively managed.

Given the trusted and high-profile persona of physicians and professors, any criminal accusations leveled against them are likely to result in media attention. While the best advice is to avoid situations that will result in negative consequences, crises do happen and you have to be prepared to manage them.

Depending on the size of your organization and your specific responsibilities, your role in crisis communications may vary. Having a plan and assembling a crisis management team will ensure you are prepared to address issues as they arise. The legal department will gather facts and make sure policies and laws are followed. The public relations team will vet all media requests to confirm the legitimacy of media inquiries. Diane, for example, has no way of knowing if the voice on the phone claiming to be a reporter, Keiko Masumoto, actually is a reporter or is someone posing as a reporter. A public relations professional can make that determination. The public relations team can also create a response strategy, draft and issue statements, and monitor news coverage. The human resources department will ensure the rights of the employee are upheld.

Be prepared to deal with different channels of mass media, including: broadcast (television and radio), print, and digital. When contacted for an interview that will appear in print or digital media, it is acceptable to ask for questions in advance of the interview so you can prepare your responses. For broadcast interviews, speak in a strong clear voice. Don't be surprised if a lot of your interview "ends up on the cutting room floor." The final segment, which will actually be broadcast, is likely to only feature a short clip of your overall interview, so be sure to keep responses brief and to the point. Be prepared to summarize your key point in less than 60 seconds.

In a crisis situation, you may walk out of your office and, on the way to your car in the parking lot, be confronted by a reporter with a microphone backed up by a cameraperson asking rapid-fire questions. Rather than blurting "no comment" and racing away with the cameraperson in pursuit, state the known facts at the time of the inquiry, acknowledge the seriousness of the situation, and, if you do not know the answer to a question, say, "I don't know and I'll get back to you when I do know."

Similarly, whether confronted with an unexpected telephone call from the media or asked a potentially difficult question during a planned interview, it is advisable to respond "I do not know that answer at this time. I will have to get back to you." Be aware that reporters may rephrase a question or continue to ask the same question repeatedly to try get the interviewee to stray from their prepared statement and provide a detailed response [7, 8].

Table 1 Crisis communications using the RESPOND technique

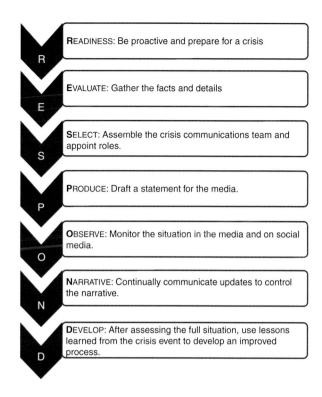

R — READINESS: Be proactive and prepare for a crisis

E — EVALUATE: Gather the facts and details

S — SELECT: Assemble the crisis communications team and appoint roles.

P — PRODUCE: Draft a statement for the media.

O — OBSERVE: Monitor the situation in the media and on social media.

N — NARRATIVE: Continually communicate updates to control the narrative.

D — DEVELOP: After assessing the full situation, use lessons learned from the crisis event to develop an improved process.

When faced with a crisis communication situation, follow seven steps, which can be remembered with the acrostic RESPOND (Table 1).

Readiness: The first step in crisis communication is ensuring the organization is prepared and equipped with a crisis communications plan to prepare for a crisis before it occurs. To develop an effective plan, identify the key members of leadership who will be involved in managing the crisis and meet with them to brainstorm potential crisis situations and map out ways to respond before a crisis hits. When a crisis first presents itself, it can be a stressful time for management, and having a plan laid out in advance will serve as a roadmap to navigate the situation.

Evaluate: Once faced with a potential crisis, gather all the facts and information regarding the situation. Before rushing to respond, take the time to learn as much as possible, assess the situation, and determine if it is a crisis that could affect the reputation and/or operation of your organization. Sometimes, when it comes to dealing with the media, one must make a judgment that it is more important to get it right than get it fast.

Select: The crisis communication team members are the ones that make decisions and manage the crisis. After a situation has been deemed a crisis, the team needs to be assembled to carry out their different roles. The crisis communication team will vary given the size of the organization but ideally will include either the department chair or, depending upon the severity of the situation, the dean, hospital

CEO, or vice president, a designated spokesperson, as well as the heads of public relations, legal counsel, security, and facilities.

Produce: In a crisis situation, it is vital to communicate information in a timely and accurate manner. Since there are often few details at the early stages of a crisis, a brief holding statement is frequently used until you can "get it right." This statement should include only the known facts, provide necessary details, be compassionate, and take responsibility for the situation. The statement should not offer opinions, personal statements, or unnecessary details. A sample holding statement for the above case is:

Spring Valley Academic Medical Center learned on December 16, 2019, that a member of the medical staff in the department of radiation oncology, Dr. Bazyler, was arrested in Suffolk County, Montana, on December 14, 2019. We take this allegation seriously, and, in accordance with our policies, we have placed him on administrative leave pending an institutional investigation. The Medical Center will, of course, fully cooperate with law enforcement authorities.

Observe: After the initial media statement has been issued, the situation will need to be monitored in the print and electronic media as well as on social media. Alerts can be set up to send notifications whenever your organization is mentioned in the media and on social media. Stakeholders will often reach out to an organization directly on social media for information on a crisis. The leadership of the radiation oncology department must be certain that stakeholders higher up in the organization structure (such as the dean or university president) are never blindsided by media inquiries. Be sure to keep such people informed.

Narrative: As more information becomes available and the crisis evolves, these details need to be continually communicated via the designated spokesperson to the media and stakeholders. In an attempt to control the narrative, the communications should be customized for the various channels including print media, press conferences, social media, and emails to stakeholders.

Develop: Once the dust settles, the crisis team should once again convene to discuss lessons learned, what worked, what could have been handled better, and ask if the crisis could have been avoided. The crisis communications plan as well as any relevant policies and processes should then be updated as needed.

Summary Bullet Points

- The missions of a radiation oncology department are to deliver the highest-quality care to its patients, generate new knowledge, and teach its trainees. When problems at home appear in the workplace, a supervisor must manage them professionally and compassionately while staying focused on the mission. The supervisor must, however, be a manager and not attempt to be a psychiatrist, marriage counselor, or personal advisor.
- Physician misconduct must be dealt with immediately, firmly, and in accordance with institutional policies with the assistance of legal advice.

- No matter how it is dressed up by radiation oncology equipment manufacturers, a bribe is a bribe.
- Crisis communication situations will arise, so be ready to respond.

For Discussion with a Mentor or Colleague

- Training to be a radiation oncologist is distinct from training to manage a radiation oncology department. How did you learn to do the latter?
- What managerial moral dilemmas have you faced in your career and how did you deal with them? With the benefit of the passage of time, do you think you could have handled them differently?

References

1. Gallo A. What to do when an employee cries at work. Harvard Bus Rev. 2013; https://hbr.org/2013/06/what-to-do-when-an-employee-cries-at-work accessed on April 2, 2021.
2. Kislik L. How to manage an employee who cries easily. Harvard Bus Rev. 2018; https://hbr.org/2018/03/how-to-manage-an-employee-who-cries-easily accessed on April 2, 2021.
3. O'Hara C. How to manage an employee who's having a personal crisis. Harvard Bus Rev. 2018; https://hbr.org/2018/07/how-to-manage-an-employee-whos-having-a-personal-crisis accessed on April 2, 2021.
4. Halperin EC. Grievances against physicians: 11 years' experience of a medical society grievance committee. West J Med. 2000;173:235–8.
5. Federation of State Medical Boards. Addressing sexual boundaries: guidelines for state medical boards. Dallas: Federation of State Medical Boards of the United States, 2006.
6. Stacy SC. The misuse of power: professional sexual misconduct: Professional Renewal Center; 2003; https://www.fclb.org/Portals/7/Home/MisuseofPower.pdf accessed on April 2, 2021.
7. Anges M. When designing controls around your crisis communications, don't do this. [Blog Post]. Retrieved from /melissaagnes.com/when-designing-controls-around-your-crisis-communications-dont-do-this/. 2019.
8. Seeger MW. Best practices in crisis communication: an expert panel process. J Appl Commun Res. 2006;34(3):232–44. https://doi.org/10.1080/00909880600769944.

Approaching Strategic Planning

Brian D. Kavanagh

The best-laid schemes of mice and men
  Go oft awry
  --Robert Burns, "To a Mouse, on Turning Her Up in Her Nest With the Plough, November, 1785," translated from the original Scots language

Culture eats strategy for breakfast
  Peter Drucker

Everybody has a plan until they get punched in the mouth
  Mike Tyson

Introduction

Strategic planning is often applied in an effort to improve the chance of achieving individual and institutional professional goals. However, the literature on the topic is prodigious. It can be daunting to try to process the myriad scientific and lay publications on this process. To narrow the focus for the purpose of providing a digestible volume of insights within a single book chapter, examples of challenges in radiation oncology to which principles of strategic planning have been systematically applied will be presented. Next, a selected sample of high-profile thought leaders whose work on business strategy has been applied to medicine will be identified, and key tenets of their philosophies will be acknowledged. Finally, strategic planning on an individual level will be explored.

B. D. Kavanagh (✉)
Department of Radiation Oncology, University of Colorado, Aurora, CO, USA
e-mail: BRIAN.KAVANAGH@CUANSCHUTZ.EDU

© Springer Nature Switzerland AG 2021   373
R. A. Chandra et al. (eds.), *Career Development in Academic Radiation Oncology*, https://doi.org/10.1007/978-3-030-71855-8_27

Strategic Planning in Radiation Oncology: Macro to Micro Examples

The American Society for Radiation Oncology (ASTRO) most recently updated its strategic plan in 2017, and the summary can be found on the society's website [1]. There had been a prior strategic plan initially approved 5 years previously and updated once in the interim, but it was felt that the continued rapid evolution in the field and in the larger landscape of oncology in general prompted a need to restate and modernize the central purpose of the organization and lay out a roadmap in the broadest sense of how to achieve intermediate- and longer-term objectives. Whereas the ASTRO is an organization with over 10,000 members, the strategic plan revision process took over a year to complete. The final product was informed by many stakeholders from multiple forms of interaction, including but not limited to the following: a general membership survey probing what members found most helpful from the organization; statements from various committees expressing perspectives on directional priorities; and a 2-day in-person retreat and numerous conference calls with the organization's board members facilitated by an outside professional business strategy consultant to crystallize statements of the society's core values and major areas of focus to achieve success according the overall vision.

Individual departments of radiation oncology periodically review their operations and opportunities to align efforts for maximum group achievement. The Princess Margaret Hospital team published the methods and results of a strategic planning initiative conducted in 2015 "to ensure that program priorities reflect the current health care environment, enable nimble responses to the increasing burden of cancer, and guide program operations until 2020" [2]. Their methods involved surveying staff regarding implementation of the prior strategic plan, interviewing key external stakeholders, and convening a number of focus groups plus two larger (30–50 persons) retreats. The final work product was a document that articulated the department's vision statement, mission statement, strategic priorities, and core values. The authors described an implementation process that called for regularly scheduled progress assessments with metrics intended to gauge the success of the initiative.

That final point is worth emphasis. There is not universal consensus that strategic planning is likely to yield the desired organizational outcomes as stated, at least not without proper cultural change. In a commentary published in 2019, William Mallon tackles the question of whether strategic planning is helpful in an academic medical setting [3]. Mallon points out that strategic plans can be criticized at times for being fatuous recitations of universal platitudes, in effect simple affirmations of high ideals. He notes that academic medical institutions have enjoyed the privilege of growth and prosperity in the last 50 or more years without necessarily having to map out detailed strategies, though in recent decades a variety of external forces have certainly added economic and other pressures that do demand more decisions about where limited resources should be directed. Nevertheless, to the well-known observation from Peter Drucker quoted at the beginning of this chapter, namely, the suggestion that the working environment of an organization often overrides whatever specific plans leadership might propose, Mallon responds by turning that notion around: perhaps the true value of a strategic plan is actually the possibility that repeated emphasis of core values and aspirational goals might in fact help shape the culture rather than the other way around, nudging everyone along toward better places.

Popular Business Strategies Applied in the Healthcare Arena

Jim Collins has authored several best-selling books analyzing why some companies survive and thrive but others fade away. Perhaps the most famous is *Good to Great*, published in 2001, which has sold millions of hardcover copies [4]. The challenge of moving up from competence to excellence at an individual or organizational level has been the theme of many educational sessions at American Society for Radiation Oncology (ASTRO) and American Society of Clinical Oncology (ASCO) educational presentations, many of which have invoked the catchphrase *Good to Great* [e.g., 5, 6]. One key message of *Good to Great* is that perhaps counterintuitively, highly successful leaders do not always start with a strategic roadmap and then add in people to take along for the ride. In fact, it is argued that just the opposite approach might be important: first get the right people on the proverbial bus, and then decide to go somewhere great together as a team.

Other thought leaders have looked at strategies for addressing the overarching problems in healthcare rather than individual institutional operational issues. In 2012 Michael Porter delivered a keynote address at the ASTRO Annual Meeting entitled "Value-based Healthcare Delivery." Dr. Porter is a professor at the Harvard Business School whose extensive work in the area of competition and strategy has addressed corporate and national perspectives. In the realm of healthcare, Dr. Porter has long advocated for a value-based system, and his 2009 essay on this topic in the *New England Journal of Medicine* has been cited over 800 times [7]. Teckie and Steinberg incorporated Porter's work in drafting a proposed framework for assessing value in radiation oncology [8].

Although many other experts in the application of strategic planning to healthcare-related issues have contributed greatly to current doctrines in this area, one final example of an individual with lasting influence is Clayton Christensen, who is credited as the first to call attention to the challenges of what is known as "disruptive innovation" [9]. The concept of disruptive innovation refers to a revolutionary advance in technology that is less costly or more efficient in such a way that an entire market is overturned: businesses formerly leading a sector are suddenly struggling to keep up unless they modify their approach to include the savings advantages to average consumers afforded by the new technology. Accordingly, strategic plans can be thwarted by the surprise introduction of a competitor's novel software and hardware that render older processes obsolete.

Hwang and Christensen considered the issue of disruptive innovation in healthcare in an article published in 2008 that has now been cited over 500 times [10]. A major difference the authors noted between typical businesses and healthcare is the fact that disruptive innovation as defined by Christensen requires that a market of incentivized consumers, i.e., patients, can shop for products and services that best meet their need, a situation unlike the current US healthcare system. Regardless, throughout all areas of medicine, there is a frequent tendency to identify and label new developments as disruptive innovation. Yu and Bortfeld enjoyed a spirited debate on which if any advances in radiation oncology could be classified as disruptive innovation per the Christensen definition as well as the likely source of any future disruptive innovations in the field, each offering thoughtful opinions [11].

Career Planning Strategies on an Individual Level

The preceding sections touch mostly on strategic planning for institutions and large sectors in medicine. However, individual physicians must still try to chart a course for their own personal career evolution. And so, the question remains: how might an early career academic radiation oncologist plan strategically for satisfaction in their chosen professional domain?

Lowenstein and colleagues surveyed over 1400 medical school faculty members using a 75-question instrument intended to understand what factors are associated with professional dissatisfaction [12]. Among the 532 respondents, over 40% indicated that they were seriously considering leaving academic medicine within the next several years. The predictors of this viewpoint included difficulties balancing work and family life, inability to comment on institutional leaders, absence of faculty development programs, lack of recognition of clinical work and teaching in promotion evaluations, and failure of chairs to evaluate academic progress regularly.

In a study focused specifically on career development challenges for women in academic medicine, Chang and colleagues analyzed Association of American Medical Colleges (AAMC) data to assess the effect of career development programs (CDPs) on the chance of retaining women faculty in their current institution [13]. The three specific CDPs included were the ones sponsored by the AAMC and Drexel University School of Medicine. Key observations were that CDP participants were less likely to leave academic medicine than peers who had not participated in a CDP, and the impact was especially strong for women at an earlier career stage at the time of participation.

Ayyala and colleagues conducted semi-structured interviews with School of Medicine participants (protégés) and sponsors (department chairs) in an executive leadership program in in an effort to characterize the nature of effective "sponsorship," defined here as "active support by someone…who has significant influence on decision-making processes or structures and who is advocating for, protecting, and fighting for the career advancement of an individual" [14]. The interviews illuminated numerous themes such as the acknowledged difference between sponsorship and mentorship (though occasionally the same person can serve in both roles); the recognition that effective sponsors are established and well-networked "talent scouts"; and that trust, respect, and weighing risks are key to successful relationships between sponsors and their protégés. Of note the interviewees believed that women are less likely to seek sponsorship than their male peers.

Conclusions

The process of strategic planning at a department or large organizational level is often conducted with the input of many stakeholders to seek consensus and a sense of community. It is possible that the team-building, culture-reinforcing aspects of the exercise of strategic planning are even more important than the specific goals and objectives articulated in the final plan. Thought leaders from the world of corporate business have offered insights of possible value in the world of healthcare, but the fundamental structural differences between healthcare and free markets are substantial. Disruptive innovations can sometimes reshape the quickly landscape in either sector. Strategic planning for career stability and success in an academic medical setting on an individual level should incorporate looking for environments conducive to personal satisfaction and a sense of being appreciated. Structured career development programs can be valuable, and both mentors and sponsors are likely needed to maximize career advancement.

For Discussion with a Mentor or Colleague

- How should I make decisions when trying to achieve a good work-life balance?
- Are there opportunities to participate in a structured career development program? Would that be beneficial in my specific case?
- Who might serve as a helpful sponsor to improve the chances of upward career trajectory via strategic networking?
- In my current institution, am I performing with a balance of clinical and academic work that will be favorable for promotion to the next rank?
- *For those who have not done so already*, should I write down a 3–5-year individual strategic plan?

References

1. https://www.astro.org/About-ASTRO/Strategic_Plan. Accessed 14 July 2020.
2. Hamilton JL, Foxcroft S, Moyo E, et al. Strategic planning in an academic radiation medicine program. Curr Oncol. 2017;24(6):e518.

3. Mallon WT. Does strategic planning matter? Acad Med. 2019;94(10):1408–11.
4. Collins J. Good to great. New York: HarperCollins Publishers; 2001.
5. Going from good to great: improving doctor-patient communication in radiation oncology, ASTRO annual meeting 2016, Boston, Massachusetts, 27 Sept 2016.
6. Moving from good to great—training oncology clinicians in palliative care skills. American Society of Clinical Oncology Annual Meeting, Chicago, IL, 2018.
7. Porter ME. A strategy for health care reform—toward a value-based system. N Engl J Med. 2009;361(2):109–12.
8. Teckie S, McCloskey SA, Steinberg ML. Value: a framework for radiation oncology. J Clin Oncol. 2014;32(26):2864.
9. Christensen CM. The innovator's dilemma: when new technologies cause great firms to fail. Boston: Harvard Business School Press; 1997.
10. Hwang J, Christensen CM. Disruptive innovation in health care delivery: a framework for business-model innovation. Health Aff. 2008;27(5):1329–35.
11. Yu CX, Bortfeld T, Cai J. In the future, disruptive innovation in radiation oncology technology will be initiated mostly by entrepreneurs. Med Phys. 2019;46(5):1949–52.
12. Lowenstein SR, Fernandez G, Crane LA. Medical school faculty discontent: prevalence and predictors of intent to leave academic careers. BMC Med Educ. 2007;7(1):1–8.
13. Chang S, Morahan PS, Magrane D, et al. Retaining faculty in academic medicine: the impact of career development programs for women. J Women's Health. 2016;25(7):687–96.
14. Ayyala MS, Skarupski K, Bodurtha JN, González-Fernández M, Ishii LE, Fivush B, Levine RB. Mentorship is not enough: exploring sponsorship and its role in career advancement in academic medicine. Acad Med. 2019;94(1):94–100.

Part V
Contextual Issues and Special Topics

Handling Burnout

Bhishamjit S. Chera, Stanley L. Liauw, Kate Hardy, Charles R. Thomas Jr., and Daniel T. Chang

Introduction

Burnout has become a ubiquitous term used frequently as a descriptor of medical professionals' frustration with their work, and is often misconstrued as depression. However, burnout is experienced by all individuals of any field of work – it is a natural occurrence. Burnout is included in the 10th and 11th revision of the International Classification of Diseases as an occupational phenomenon, but is not classified as a medical condition. The World Health Organization is currently developing evidence-based guidelines on mental well-being in the workplace. Burnout appears to disproportionately affect physicians; many burnout experts state that it is an epidemic which represents a public health crisis with negative impact on individual physicians, patients, and healthcare organizations and systems [1]. It may have characteristics of a contagion, as clinicians who are burned out increase the risk that others around them feel the same [2, 3]. In this chapter we will discuss the causes, prevalence, consequences, and management of burnout.

B. S. Chera
Department of Radiation Oncology, University of North Carolina, Chapel Hill, NC, USA

S. L. Liauw
Department of Radiation and Cellular Oncology, University of Chicago, Chicago, IL, USA

K. Hardy
Department of Psychiatry and Behavioral Sciences, Stanford University, Stanford, CA, USA

C. R. Thomas Jr.
Department of Radiation Medicine, Knight Cancer Institute, Oregon Health & Science University, Portland, OR, USA

D. T. Chang (✉)
Department of Radiation Oncology, Stanford Cancer Institute, Stanford, CA, USA
e-mail: dtchang@stanford.edu

© Springer Nature Switzerland AG 2021   381
R. A. Chandra et al. (eds.), *Career Development in Academic Radiation Oncology*, https://doi.org/10.1007/978-3-030-71855-8_28

What Is Burnout?

Burnout is a syndrome conceptualized as resulting from occupational stress that has not been successfully managed. It is a reaction to chronic job-related stress characterized by physical, emotional, and mental exhaustion. Burnout has been described as occurring in stages, beginning early on with high levels of job satisfaction and energy but, through lack of proper coping mechanisms, can progress to frustration, stress, anxiety, and dissatisfaction that impacts individuals professionally and personally [4]. It was first conceptualized in 1974 by Freudenberger [5] and subsequently developed by Maslach and colleagues [6], whose work has established the most accepted definition of burnout, which include three dimensions: emotional exhaustion, depersonalization, and a decreased sense of personal accomplishment (Fig. 1):

- Emotional exhaustion: the individual experiences physical and emotional exhaustion, sleeps poorly, and is prone to headaches and colds. The person becomes over-involved emotionally, and feels overwhelmed by the demands of other people. The individual feels he or she can no longer "give" to others.
- Depersonalization: the individual becomes cynical toward co-workers, clients, and themselves, which sets the stage for a detached and dehumanized response whereby the person wishes other people were out of his or her life.
- Reduced personal accomplishment: the individual feels a low self-esteem and has a lack of self-worth. At this stage, an individual is at risk of leaving his or her job.

The most widely accepted standard for burnout assessment is the Maslach Burnout Inventory (MBI), which also includes a Human Services Survey (HSS) applicable to healthcare professionals. The MBI-HSS is comprised of 22 items each scored from 0 to 6 based on self-reported frequency of the feeling addressed by each item. There are three domains of the survey which correspond to the three phases of burnout: (1) emotional exhaustion domain (9 items, total score range of 0–54), (2) depersonalization domain (5 items, total score rage of 0–30), and (3) personal

Fig. 1 Venn diagram of the three dimensions of the burnout syndrome: emotional exhaustion, depersonalization, and reduced personal accomplishment

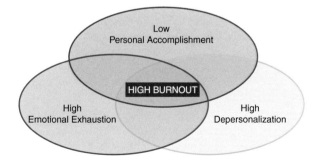

accomplishment domain (8 items, total score range of 0–48). The quantitative total (i.e., composite score) for all three domains should be reported; however, the data can be classified into tertiles where emotional exhaustion scores ≥27, depersonalization scores ≥10, and personal accomplishment scores of ≤33 are considered as high levels of burnout. In most of the published literature overall, burnout has commonly been defined as a high level of either emotional exhaustion or depersonalization.

Physician Burnout

Over the past three decades, burnout in medicine has become an avid area of research. The prevalence of burnout among physicians in training and practicing physicians has been reported to be as high as 50–70%, but there is substantial variability in prevalence estimates of burnout, burnout definitions, assessment methods, and study quality [7]. Burnout rates are markedly higher among physicians as compared to other professions, even after adjusting for confounding factors (e.g., work hours). Physicians may be predisposed to developing burnout due to inherent personality traits of compulsiveness, guilt, and self-denial, and a medical culture that emphasizes perfectionism, denial of personal vulnerability, and delayed gratification [8]. Across specialties, the rates of burnout vary (e.g., lower in occupational medicine and higher in emergency medicine). Some have reported higher rates of burnout in private practice physicians as compared to academic physicians. In addition, female physicians have been consistently shown to have higher rates of burnout compared to men, with women more likely to experience emotional exhaustion [9], which may be due to a number of reasons including primary parenting responsibilities [10] and gender bias and discrimination in the workplace [11]. While women may be more challenged with balancing the demands of work and family, recent work suggests that the primary culprit is rather the culture of overwork, which may disproportionately impact women [12].

An exhaustive summary of all the literature would be beyond the scope of this chapter. A recently published study in *The New England Journal of Medicine* is worth mentioning. Hu and colleagues conducted a cross-sectional national survey of general surgery residents, assessing mistreatment, burnout (modified Maslach Burnout Inventory), and suicidal thoughts [13]. The survey was administered immediately after the 2018 American Board of Surgery in-training examination. Among the 7409 residents that took the surgical in-training examination, the response rate was 99%. Regarding mistreatment, 32% reported discrimination based on their self-identified gender, 17% reported racial discrimination, 30% reported verbal and/or physical abuse, and 10% reported sexual harassment. Rates of mistreatment were higher among women (65% reporting gender discrimination and 20% sexual harassment). Patients and patients' families were the most frequent sources of gender discrimination and racial discrimination, whereas attending surgeons were the most frequent sources of sexual harassment and abuse. Weekly burnout symptoms were reported by 39% of residents, and those who reported exposure to discrimination, abuse, or harassment were more likely to have symptoms of burnout (odds ratio, 2.94; 95% confidence interval [CI], 2.58–3.36) and suicidal thoughts (odds ratio, 3.07; 95% CI, 2.25–4.19). Women were more likely than men to report burnout symptoms. Interestingly, this difference did not persist after adjustment for bias and discrimination. These data suggest that gender bias (by patients, patients' family members, and superiors in the workplace) occurs frequently, especially in women.

Burnout in Radiation Oncology

There have been several burnout studies in the United States (USA) conducted in radiation oncology residents, program directors, and chairs. All of these studies conducted cross-sectional surveys using the MBI-HSS. Ramey et al. conducted a survey of 232 of 733 radiation oncology residents (31% response rate) in the USA in 2017 [14]. Approximately one third of residents reported a high level of burnout which is consistent with previous oncology literature but lower levels than residents of other medical specialties. Aggarwal et al. conducted a survey of 47 of 88 program directors (53% response rate) in 2015 [15]. Only 6% reported high burnout rate (83% reported moderate burnout rates). The most commonly cited stressors were satisfying Accreditation Council for Graduate Medical Education/Residency Review Committee requirements (47%), administrative duties (30%), and resident morale (28%). Having more years on faculty prior to becoming program director correlated with less emotional exhaustion and depersonalization. Dedicated time for program director duties correlated with less emotional exhaustion. Kusano et al. surveyed 66 of 87 radiation oncology chairpersons (76% response rate) in 2013 [16]. Twenty-five percent of respondents met the MBI-HSS criteria for low burnout, 75% for moderate burnout, and none for high burnout. These results compare favorably to reported burnout by chairpersons in other specialties; anesthesia chairpersons, for example, reported a 28% rate of high burnout in a survey of 102 faculty reported in 2011 (response rate 87%) [17]. Reported major stressors were budget deficits and human resource issues. Approximately a quarter reported that it was at least moderately likely that they would step down in the next 1–2 years, and these individuals reported significantly higher emotional exhaustion. Burnout has also been assessed among radiation oncologists outside of the USA, primarily focused on radiation oncology residents [14]. From these data we can conclude that during the professional lifetime of a radiation oncologist, burnout is at its highest during residency training; however, in contrast to other medical specialties, particularly medical oncology and surgical oncology, overall burnout is less prominent in radiation oncology.

Understanding the Causes, Consequences, and Solutions for Physician Burnout

In 2019, a consensus study report was released by the National Academy of Sciences to address professional well-being and burnout (Fig. 2) [18]. Physicians work in complicated healthcare systems where multifactorial work and personal factors contribute toward professional well-being or burnout and their respective consequences. Collective, coordinated actions across all levels of the healthcare system

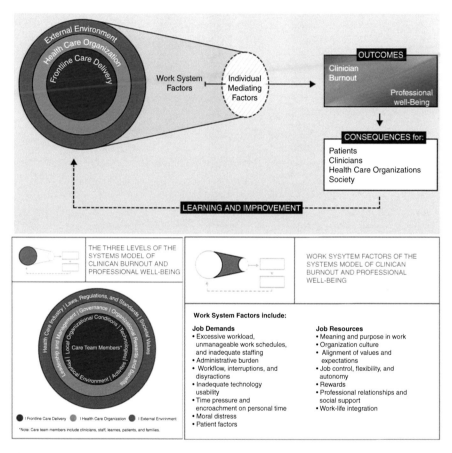

Fig. 2 A systems model for clinical burnout and professional well-being. Multilayer system issues both inside and outside the healthcare system produce work system factors which are mediated by individual factors of the physician which either result in burnout of physician well-being and thus the respective consequences to the patients, physicians, healthcare organizations, and society. (Adapted National Academy of Sciences: Taking Action Against Clinician Burnout: A Systems Approach to Professional Well-Being; Figures S-1, S-2, S-3 [18])

are necessary to prevent, reduce, and ideally eliminate clinician burnout. Using established methods and principles in human-centered design, human factors and systems engineering, organizational design, and change management, the committee identified six areas of opportunity for healthcare system stakeholders to pursue: (1) create positive work environments; (2) create positive learning environments; (3) reduce administrative burden; (4) enable technology solutions; (5) provide support to clinicians and learners; and (6) invest in research on clinician professional well-being.

Causative and Contributing Factors of Burnout (Fig. 2)

The major drivers of physician burnout can be found in the healthcare organizations and systems in which physicians work (Fig. 2 and Table 1): heavy workloads, inefficiencies in processes and workflows, clerical and administrative burdens, human resource investigations, the need to negotiate with healthcare payers, and a feeling of lack of control in an uncertain and ever-changing healthcare environment and changing reimbursement models [1]. As such, patients, their family members, colleagues, and healthcare administration may play causative and/or contributing roles [13].

The implementation of electronic medical records (EMRs) may also contribute to increased physician burnout. In the EMR era, tasks that were previously spread across the healthcare team (medical assistant, nurse, etc.) have now been added to the physician workload such as order entry and documentation. The accessibility of the EMR may have a negative impact on work-life balance. In a recent study, 79% of community oncologists reported accessing the EMR outside of clinical work hours [19]. A related issue is that suboptimal design of workflows, workspaces, and environmental factors contributes to burnout. Healthcare systems' physical structures (e.g., inpatient wards, outpatient clinics) are never large enough to accommodate all required physical space for patient care. Patient spaces are prioritized resulting in overcrowded physician workspaces that have poor ergonomical design, resulting in excessive cognitive and physical burden.

The increasing regulatory and documentation requirements and financial/reimbursement landscape for physicians also significantly contribute to burnout. These requirements come from many authorities: federal government, state government, healthcare organizations, professional organizations, and board-certifying organizations, which have resulted in an ever-rising number of online courses, surveys, and data entry for physicians. Newer alternative payment models are centered around reimbursing for quality and paying a lump bundle for an episode of care. Quality is measured by physicians reporting certain metrics (increased clerical burden), and healthcare systems' solution to bundle payments is to use economies of scale (i.e., do more with less; see more patients). Physician salary models also affect

Table 1 Contributing factors to physician burnout and organizational- and individual-level solutions

Driver	Organizational-level solutions	Individual-level solutions
Workload excess	Fair productivity targets Duty hour limits Appropriate distribution of job roles	Part-time status Informed specialty choices Informed practice choices Stress management training
Inefficiencies in workflows	Nonphysician staff (e.g., scribes) to off-load clerical burdens Care redesign Human factor engineering	Prioritize tasks and delegate work
EMR burden	Optimize electronic health records	Maximize knowledge and training with EMR functionality Avoid using EMR afterhours
Regulatory requirements	Accurate interpretation of regulatory requirements	
Patient and patient family member mistreatment	Provide ways to report patient/patient family member mistreatment	
Superiors and colleague mistreatment	Fair and just human resource program	Recognition of mistreatment of others and obligation to protect
Work-life balance	Respect for home responsibilities in setting schedules for work and meetings Include all required work tasks within expected work hours Support flexible work schedules, including part-time employment	Reflection on life priorities and values Attention to self-care
Loss of control and autonomy	Engaging physicians at all levels of leadership Prioritizing physician buy-in with all decision-making	Stress management Coaching: resiliency training, positive coping strategies, mindfulness
Loss of meaning from work	Promote shared core values Protect physician time with patients Promote physician communities Offer professional development Opportunities Leadership training and awareness around physician burnout	Coaching: resiliency training, positive coping strategies, mindfulness Engagement in physician small-group activities around shared work experiences

Adapted from Table 2 of West et al. [1]

burnout, with physicians on performance-/incentive-based programs reporting higher burnout than their counterparts who are salaried [1]. Younger physicians [20] and physicians with partners/spouses that are in a nonphysician medical field may also be at increased risk of burnout, perhaps due to not having a partner with a similar work experience with whom to share common challenges [1].

Table 2 Examples of coaching dialogue with a burned-out physician

Burned-out physician's issues	Coach's input	Burned-out physicians' responses	Results
Fatigue, low sense of accomplishment: "The demands on my time are too much; I'm exhausted and not accomplishing anything"	"Can you think of anything that you have accomplished recently that was meaningful" "What's a new viewpoint?"	"I guess I helped my patients; that's true. And, I felt good to find out my manuscript was accepted for publication" "Maybe that I don't need to be so hard on myself?"	Focus shifts from overwhelmed to appreciation of accomplishments Sense of engagement with his work is fostered Realistic emphasis on the positive decreases stress and contributes to life balance
Self-doubt: "I don't have NIH funding. I don't have what it takes. I'm not smart enough"	"I'm hearing a 'not-good enough' message. How are you experiencing this right now?" "What academic work are you most proud of?"	"I'm worried that I won't be promoted on tenure track" "I have published several seminal research papers in high-impact journals, and my chair is happy with my work"	1. Focusing experience in the present leads to awareness of the source of the belief 2. Orienting toward the reality, the coach helps institute a more affirming internal message
Cynicism, decreased sense of purpose: "I'm like a hamster on a wheel. Why go on?"	"What gives your work value and meaning?" "What energizes you?"	"My relationships with patients have always been what is meaningful for me" "Playing piano brought me peace and energy, but I just don't have any time"	1. Existing sources of professional meaning are highlighted 2. Physician finds a source of calm and revitalization. The coach encourages playing 15 min a day, helping the physician glimpse control he can exert over his time, as well as his ability to effect change

Adapted from Table 1 of Gazelle et al. [8]

Consequences of Burnout (Fig. 2)

Physician burnout is associated with negative consequences on patient care, physician workforce and healthcare system cost, and physician's personal health and safety. A meta-analysis by Panagioti et al. showed that physician burnout was associated with an increased risk of patient safety incidents, poorer quality of care due to low professionalism, and reduced patient satisfaction [21]. Using mathematical modeling, Han et al. estimated the attributable cost of physician burnout in the USA at approximately $4.6 billion (range $2.6 billion–$6.3 billion) [22]. Burnout may negatively impact physical and mental health, job performance, and job turnover. Premature turnover is an important issue, given that the estimated cost of replacing one physician ranges from hundreds of thousands to over a million depending upon specialty, practice location, and other factors [1].

Physical signs of burnout include exhaustion, headaches, fatigue, gastrointestinal problems, and insomnia [1, 23]. The emotional response to burnout includes job distancing, depression, paranoia, a negative self-image, a sense of powerlessness, and detachment from work [1, 23]. Behavioral responses to burnout include alcohol and drug abuse; physical withdrawal from co-workers; increased absenteeism; altered work patterns, such as arriving for work late and leaving early or arriving early and leaving late; employee turnover; accidents; and suicide [1, 23].

Managing Burnout

Lee and Mylod have conceptualized a *seesaw* framework of burnout as a balance between rewards and stress, and the causes and contributors are from both the organization and the physician (Fig. 2) [3]. Variation in these organizational and individual rewards and stresses determines the burnout experience for the physician. Some rewards and stresses are inherent to being a physician, such as patient care, and thus cannot be easily eliminated or even mitigated. Such factors could potentially be managed by what Lee and Mylod consider a first area of opportunity: to increase the impact of inherent rewards. For example, professional/peer coaching may help physicians rediscover the rewards of patient care (see below section on Coaching). Another intervention may be for physicians to form peer groups where they can discuss their work-related experiences and stresses and form social bonds through shared activities. A small randomized trial showed that physicians who participated in small groups had a ~16% reduction in depersonalization symptoms [24].

Other stresses and rewards may be external, such as workflow inefficiencies, metric-based performance evaluations, or EMR documentation requirements. Lee and Mylod state that there is little to no association between added rewards and stresses: for example, added income does not mitigate the challenges with using the EMR [3]. They suggest that the second major area of opportunity is for organizations to seriously address the added stressors they place on physicians.

The third major opportunity to improve the burnout experience is to teach and develop resiliency in physicians. Resilience (i.e., the capacity to recover quickly from difficulties; toughness; elasticity) is the moderating influence that nudges the fulcrum of the *seesaw* framework of burnout to a point where more stress is bearable (Fig. 2).

There have been many studies of organizational and individual interventions to ameliorate burnout in physicians, which suggest that both individual-focused and structural or organizational strategies can result in clinically meaningful reductions in burnout among physicians. A meta-analysis of 15 randomized trials and 37 cohort studies of 2914 physicians which evaluated interventions to reduce burnout observed that overall burnout decreased from 54% to 44% [25]. The most commonly studied interventions have been mindfulness-based training (i.e., resilience), stress management, small-group discussions (to promote community, connectedness), and duty hour restriction polices. Table 1 lists the common causes/factors contributing to burnout and suggested organizational and individual countermeasures.

Coaching [8]

Professional coaching is a strategy that has long been utilized in the business world to provide a results-oriented and stigma-free method to address burnout. The primary result of coaching is to help the burned-out individual develop self-awareness and resiliency. Most individuals already have the strength and skills to handle personal and professional challenges; however, self-defeating thoughts and beliefs and negative perspectives prevent them from responding in a healthy way. Coaching utilizes techniques to increase one's sense of accomplishment, purpose, and engagement. Elements of positive psychology, mindfulness, and self-determination theory and cognitive-behavioral therapy can help the individual examine how thoughts and actions impact emotional state. The coaching method relies on an iterative process of open-ended questions that enable the burned-out individual self-examine fixed and unhelpful thoughts and behaviors. The person being coached learns to question these unhelpful automatic thoughts and beliefs, and identify cognitive distortions (unhelpful thinking patterns) that contribute to emotional distress, thus consciously shifting his or her perspective, revealing new options for action, and ultimately increasing choice and control. Coaches also help the burned-out individual clarify values and align them with professional and personal goals. Table 2 contains a hypothetical case study of a burned-out physician being coached. The coaching strategy has been adopted by many healthcare systems and medical schools. Some physicians in training and in practice receive specialized training in how to be a "peer coach." There is evidence that coaching by physicians to address burnout in colleagues and trainees may be effective [26, 27] potentially drawing on the importance of shared experience to also support the individual to make changes to reduce burnout. However, it is important to note that on occasion, individuals who experience extreme or continued burnout may also experience thoughts of self-harm and suicidal ideation. We strongly encourage physicians that experience these thoughts to reach out for professional help or contact the local emergency room for assistance to ensure safety and access to appropriate treatment.

Work-Life Balance

Giving your body what it needs is the foundation of burnout prevention. You can help reduce the energy depletion associated with burnout and facilitate restoration by prioritizing three universal core needs: sleeping, eating, and moving. Most adults need 7–9 hours of sleep, and studies have shown that insufficient sleep predicts for burnout [28]. A healthy diet and taking the time to eat are important to daily well-being and performance at work. The portmanteau "hangry" (blended words of hungry and angry) is a common reality for physicians who are often too busy with clinical, academic, and personal duties to pause and nourish. An often-referenced study of judicial decisions by Israeli judges illustrates how the effects of breaks for nourishment during the workday may affect performance [29] (Fig. 4). In this observational study, the judicial rulings for parole for Israeli judges were recorded in relation to the two daily food breaks, which resulted in segmenting the deliberations of the day into three distinct "decision sessions." The percentage of favorable rulings dropped gradually from ~65% to nearly 0 within each decision session and returned abruptly to ~65% after a break (Fig. 3). The health benefits of regular physical exercise are well described. In addition to the cardiovascular and metabolic benefits, there are tangible psychological benefits that positively influence common burnout symptoms: depression, stress, anxiety, etc. Any amount of exercise is good,

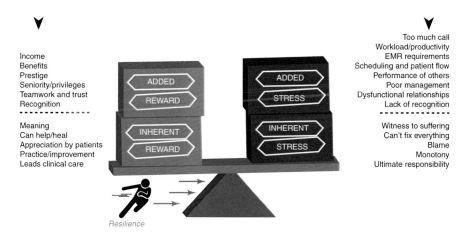

Fig. 3 Framework for deconstructing burnout (with permission from Mylod et al.). This framework distinguishes rewards and stresses inherent to the role of caring for patients (*bottom boxes*) from those that are added (*upper boxes*). Resilience is a moderating influence that nudges the fulcrum to a point where more stress is bearable. EMR indicates electronic medical record. (This figure was created by Dr. Mylod while working at Press Ganey and has been published with permission. Copyright: Press Ganey [3])

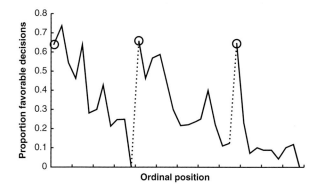

Fig. 4 Israeli judicial ruling study (with permission from Danziger et al.). Proportion of rulings in favor of the prisoners by ordinal position. Circled points indicate the first decision in each of the three decision sessions; tick marks on x-axis denote every third case; dotted line denotes food break. Because unequal session lengths resulted in a low number of cases for some of the later ordinal positions, the graph is based on the first 95% of the data from each session [29]

and a regular regimen is even better. The current Centers for Disease Control and Prevention (www.cdc.gov) recommendation for adults is at least 150 min of moderate-intensity aerobic physical activity (i.e., walking) or 75 min of vigorous-intensity physical activity, or an equivalent combination each week.

Organizational Interventions

Experts in burnout and national physician societies agree that organizations need to seriously take action to address physician burnout in their institutions [1, 3, 30, 31]. Organizations are well versed in tracking performance measures via dashboards, and some have suggested that burnout assessment should be tracked as a quality measure and leadership performance metric [1, 32]. Organizations should foster a culture that values physicians and protects against having physicians feel like "relative value unit machines" [3]. Ultimately, organization leaders should understand that physician burnout has a direct negative impact on the healthcare system performance (increased medical errors, decreased patient satisfaction, increased costs with recruitment to replace physician turnover – see consequences of burnout section). Studies have shown that healthcare organizations that empower physicians with increased control of workplace issues lead to improved physician job satisfaction [1]. The ever-increasing subtext in healthcare is to "do more with less"; namely, see more patients with inefficient workflows to maintain revenue. Some organizations have successfully reduced burnout in the "do more with less" healthcare environment by improving physician work processes, mostly through increased support for clinical work, often referred to as care redesign [33]. National and international efforts are also needed to address the regulatory burden on physicians.

One final point regarding managing burnout is that waiting until an individual is burned out may be too late, and more resources and effort should be directed at identifying the early stages of burnout in order to prevent it, an idea advocated by Back and colleagues [34]. The early stages of burnout actually look quite different from the classic symptoms described in the Maslach Inventory and are marked by high levels of job satisfaction as accomplishments leading to recognition, rewards, added responsibilities, and promotions. However, as the individual begins to face challenges and, more importantly, frustration and failure, stress begins to build. How the individual responds to this stress plays a critical role in determining the progression toward classic burnout. He or she may start to neglect personal care, sacrifice personal time with family, sleep fewer hours, and devote less time toward hobbies and interests, all of which may lead to increasing levels of isolation and resentment toward others, thus beginning the path toward full-blown burnout without intervention. Therefore, deployment of the above techniques such as resilience training, coaching, and managing work-life balance may be most effective in the immediate early stages of one's career, long before classic burnout symptoms emerge.

Post COVID-19 Era

At the time of this writing, the ongoing COVID-19 pandemic has presented unique and extraordinary challenges that will likely exacerbate and accelerate burnout. With the transition to the remote workplace, there is a potential loss of social connection and bonding with co-workers, colleagues, and friends. Working from home carries the threat of loss of personal time as the physical barrier of work is removed and constant access to emails, phone, text, and other communications prevents workers from completely disconnecting from their jobs. Virtual medicine brings many advantages and conveniences for both patients and physicians, but it may also impede the development of the doctor-patient relationship, which, according to a recent survey by the Physicians Foundation, was rated as the greatest source of job satisfaction in 79% of physicians [35]. The cancellation or conversion of major scientific meetings and conferences to the virtual format has led to a significant reduction in travel, social bonding with colleagues and friends, and opportunities for presenting knowledge and receiving professional acknowledgment and recognition. Institutions and departments have made the transition to virtual meetings, which may erode camaraderie among co-workers, friends, mentors and mentees, and many others who make up a regular and crucial part of the daily social network, leading to feelings of isolation. Closures of schools have added additional burden for parents to arrange childcare or address educational needs while still balancing work responsibilities. As discussed earlier, working women in particular may be higher risk of burnout given that they more often bear primary parenting roles. The inability to plan for the future has led to the phenomenon of living in an "infinite present" and fear of the unknown as people mourn the loss or cancellation of important milestones and personal events such as weddings, graduations, birthday celebrations, and family vacations. Finally, regular stress relief through travel, socializing with friends and family, recreational activities, and entertainment has suddenly become unavailable, while concerns of health and financial uncertainty for self and loved ones continue to persist.

For these reasons, the need to address and prevent burnout is even greater. However, traditional efforts such as those outlined above may be even more challenging or even impossible under social distancing restrictions during a pandemic. It will be imperative for burnout experts to understand the effects of the COVID-19 on burnout and develop new tools for how to overcome these new challenges. Simple measures to restore meaningful communication and connection to prevent the feeling of social isolation may be a first step that can be immediately implemented. Longer-term steps could range from slight workflow adjustments all the way to complete redesigns of the workplace that must also carefully balance patient safety and quality.

Conclusions

Burnout is a natural syndrome experienced by all workers. Most radiation oncologists are likely to experience low to moderate burnout during their professional careers, with the highest levels of burnout experienced during residency training. However, compared to other medical specialties, the prevalence and severity of burnout in radiation oncology is less. The radiation oncologist has a responsibility to mitigate burnout through individual interventions, mentoring colleagues and trainees, and participating in organizations as physician leaders.

Summary Bullet Points

- Burnout is experienced by all individuals of any field of work – but it does appear to disproportionately affect physicians.
- The prevalence of burnout varies among physician specialties (~20–70%), and is ~30% in radiation oncology.
- The causative and contributing factors for burnout are multifactorial and range from systems and organizational issues to patients themselves.
- Physician burnout has significant consequences to the healthcare system (including cost, quality of care, patient safety) and to the well-being of the physician workforce.
- The individual physician and healthcare/national/professional organizations all have roles to play in managing burnout.

For Discussion with a Mentor or Colleague

- Name some factors which can cause a higher rate of physician burnout.
- What three phases of burnout are assessed in the Maslach Burnout Inventory?
- Identify what current work factors currently contribute to your risk of burnout.
- Identify one potential intervention to implement on a personal level to reduce your risk of burnout.
- Identify one potential intervention to implement on an organizational level to reduce your risk of burnout.
- What factors might contribute toward lower burnout rates among physicians in radiation oncology compared to medical or surgical oncology?

References

1. West CP, Dyrbye LN, Shanafelt TD. Physician burnout: contributors, consequences and solutions. J Intern Med. 2018;283(6):516–29. Epub 2018/03/06. https://doi.org/10.1111/joim.12752.
2. Bakker AB, Schaufeli WB, Sixma HJ, Bosveld W. Burnout contagion among general practitioners. J Soc Clin Psychol. 2001;20(1):82–98. https://doi.org/10.1521/jscp.20.1.82.22251.
3. Lee TH, Mylod DE. Deconstructing burnout to define a positive path forward. JAMA Intern Med. 2019;179(3):429–30. Epub 2019/02/05. https://doi.org/10.1001/jamainternmed.2018.8247.
4. Kraft U. Burned out. Scientific American Mind. 2006:5.
5. Freudenberger HJ. Staff burn-out. J Soc Issues. 1974;30(1):159–65. https://doi.org/10.1111/j.1540-4560.1974.tb00706.x.
6. Maslach C, Jackson SE. The measurement of experienced burnout. J Organ Behav. 1981;2(2):99–113. https://doi.org/10.1002/job.4030020205.
7. Rotenstein LS, Torre M, Ramos MA, Rosales RC, Guille C, Sen S, Mata DA. Prevalence of burnout among physicians: a systematic review. JAMA. 2018;320(11):1131–50. Epub 2018/10/17. https://doi.org/10.1001/jama.2018.12777.
8. Gazelle G, Liebschutz JM, Riess H. Physician burnout: coaching a way out. J Gen Intern Med. 2015;30(4):508–13. Epub 2014/12/21. https://doi.org/10.1007/s11606-014-3144-y.
9. Spataro BM, Tilstra SA, Rubio DM, McNeil MA. The toxicity of self-blame: sex differences in burnout and coping in internal medicine trainees. J Womens Health (Larchmt). 2016;25(11):1147–52. Epub 2016/10/13. https://doi.org/10.1089/jwh.2015.5604.
10. Cinamon RG, Rich Y. Gender differences in the importance of work and family roles: implications for work–family conflict. Sex Roles. 2002;47(11):531–41. https://doi.org/10.1023/A:1022021804846.
11. Bruce AN, Battista A, Plankey MW, Johnson LB, Marshall MB. Perceptions of gender-based discrimination during surgical training and practice. Med Educ Online. 2015;20:25923. Epub 2015/02/06. https://doi.org/10.3402/meo.v20.25923.
12. Ely R, Padavic I. What's really holding women back? Harvard Bus Rev. 2020.
13. Hu YY, Ellis RJ, Hewitt DB, Yang AD, Cheung EO, Moskowitz JT, Potts JR 3rd, Buyske J, Hoyt DB, Nasca TJ, Bilimoria KY. Discrimination, abuse, harassment, and burnout in surgical residency training. N Engl J Med. 2019;381(18):1741–52. Epub 2019/10/29. https://doi.org/10.1056/NEJMsa1903759.
14. Ramey SJ, Ahmed AA, Takita C, Wilson LD, Thomas CR Jr, Yechieli R. Burnout evaluation of radiation residents Nationwide: results of a survey of United States residents. Int J Radiat Oncol Biol Phys. 2017;99(3):530–8. Epub 2017/12/28. https://doi.org/10.1016/j.ijrobp.2017.06.014.
15. Aggarwal S, Kusano AS, Carter JN, Gable L, Thomas CR Jr, Chang DT. Stress and burnout among residency program directors in United States radiation oncology programs. Int J Radiat Oncol Biol Phys. 2015;93(4):746–53. Epub 2015/11/05. https://doi.org/10.1016/j.ijrobp.2015.08.019.
16. Kusano AS, Thomas CR Jr, Bonner JA, DeWeese TL, Formenti SC, Hahn SM, Lawrence TS, Mittal BB. Burnout in United States academic chairs of radiation oncology programs. Int J Radiat Oncol Biol Phys. 2014;88(2):363–8. Epub 2013/11/06. https://doi.org/10.1016/j.ijrobp.2013.09.027.
17. De Oliveira GS Jr, Ahmad S, Stock MC, Harter RL, Almeida MD, Fitzgerald PC, McCarthy RJ. High incidence of burnout in academic chairpersons of anesthesiology: should we be taking better care of our leaders? Anesthesiology. 2011;114(1):181–93. Epub 2010/12/24. https://doi.org/10.1097/ALN.0b013e318201cf6c.

18. Medicine NAo. National Academies of sciences E, medicine. Taking action against clinician burnout: a systems approach to professional Well-being. Washington, DC: The National Academies Press; 2019. 334 p.

19. Gajra A, Bapat B, Jeune-Smith Y, Nabhan C, Klink AJ, Liassou D, Mehta S, Feinberg B. Frequency and causes of burnout in US Community oncologists in the era of electronic health records. JCO Oncol Pract. 2020;16(4):e357–e65. Epub 2020/04/11. https://doi.org/10.1200/JOP.19.00542.

20. Marchand A, Blanc ME, Beauregard N. Do age and gender contribute to workers' burnout symptoms? Occup Med (Lond). 2018;68(6):405–11. Epub 2018/06/19. https://doi.org/10.1093/occmed/kqy088.

21. Panagioti M, Geraghty K, Johnson J, Zhou A, Panagopoulou E, Chew-Graham C, Peters D, Hodkinson A, Riley R, Esmail A. Association between physician burnout and patient safety, professionalism, and patient satisfaction: a systematic review and meta-analysis. JAMA Intern Med. 2018;178(10):1317–30. Epub 2018/09/08. https://doi.org/10.1001/jamainternmed.2018.3713.

22. Han S, Shanafelt TD, Sinsky CA, Awad KM, Dyrbye LN, Fiscus LC, Trockel M, Goh J. Estimating the attributable cost of physician burnout in the United States. Ann Intern Med. 2019;170(11):784–90. Epub 2019/05/28. https://doi.org/10.7326/M18-1422.

23. Ahn SM, Chan JY, Zhang Z, Wang H, Khan Z, Bishop JA, Westra W, Koch WM, Califano JA. Saliva and plasma quantitative polymerase chain reaction-based detection and surveillance of human papillomavirus-related head and neck cancer. JAMA Otolaryngol Head Neck Surg. 2014;140(9):846–54. Epub 2014/08/01. https://doi.org/10.1001/jamaoto.2014.1338.

24. West CP, Dyrbye LN, Rabatin JT, Call TG, Davidson JH, Multari A, Romanski SA, Hellyer JM, Sloan JA, Shanafelt TD. Intervention to promote physician Well-being, job satisfaction, and professionalism: a randomized clinical trial. JAMA Intern Med. 2014;174(4):527–33. Epub 2014/02/12. https://doi.org/10.1001/jamainternmed.2013.14387.

25. West CP, Dyrbye LN, Erwin PJ, Shanafelt TD. Interventions to prevent and reduce physician burnout: a systematic review and meta-analysis. Lancet. 2016;388(10057):2272–81. Epub 2016/10/04. https://doi.org/10.1016/S0140-6736(16)31279-X.

26. Palamara K, Kauffman C, Chang Y, Barreto EA, Yu L, Bazari H, Donelan K. Professional development coaching for residents: results of a 3-year positive psychology coaching intervention. J Gen Intern Med. 2018;33(11):1842–4. Epub 2018/07/25. https://doi.org/10.1007/s11606-018-4589-1.

27. Palamara K, Kauffman C, Stone VE, Bazari H, Donelan K. Promoting success: a professional development coaching program for interns in medicine. J Grad Med Educ. 2015;7(4):630–7. Epub 2015/12/23. https://doi.org/10.4300/JGME-D-14-00791.1.

28. Soderstrom M, Jeding K, Ekstedt M, Perski A, Akerstedt T. Insufficient sleep predicts clinical burnout. J Occup Health Psychol. 2012;17(2):175–83. Epub 2012/03/28. https://doi.org/10.1037/a0027518.

29. Danziger S, Levav J, Avnaim-Pesso L. Extraneous factors in judicial decisions. Proc Natl Acad Sci U S A. 2011;108(17):6889–92. Epub 2011/04/13. https://doi.org/10.1073/pnas.1018033108.

30. Association AM. Physician burnout [cited 15 Apr 2020]. Available from: https://www.ama-assn.org/topics/physician-burnout.

31. Hlubocky FJ, Taylor LP, Marron JM, Spence RA, McGinnis MM, Brown RF, McFarland DC, Tetzlaff ED, Gallagher CM, Rosenberg AR, Popp B, Dragnev K, Bosserman LD, Dudzinski DM, Smith S, Chatwal M, Patel MI, Markham MJ, Levit K, Bruera E, Epstein RM, Brown M, Back AL, Shanafelt TD, Kamal AH. A call to action: ethics committee roundtable recommendations for addressing burnout and moral distress in oncology. JCO Oncol Pract. 2020;16(4):191–9. Epub 2020/04/01. https://doi.org/10.1200/JOP.19.00806.

32. Wallace JE, Lemaire JB, Ghali WA. Physician wellness: a missing quality indicator. Lancet. 2009;374(9702):1714–21. Epub 2009/11/17. https://doi.org/10.1016/S0140-6736(09)61424-0.

33. Wright AA, Katz IT. Beyond burnout - redesigning care to restore meaning and sanity for physicians. N Engl J Med. 2018;378(4):309–11. Epub 2018/01/25. https://doi.org/10.1056/NEJMp1716845.
34. Back AL, Steinhauser KE, Kamal AH, Jackson VA. Why burnout is so hard to fix. J Oncol Pract/Am Soc Clin Oncol. 2017;13(6):348–51. Epub 2017/05/12. https://doi.org/10.1200/JOP.2017.021964.
35. Foundation TP. 2018 Survey of America's physicians practice patterns & perspectives 2018 [cited 18 May 2020]:74 p. Available from: https://physiciansfoundation.org/wp-content/uploads/2018/09/physicians-survey-results-final-2018.pdf.

Preparing for Retirement and Career Transitions

Leonard L. Gunderson

I will chronologically discuss the various "career transitions" that occurred in my life, and the influence that earlier paths had on my final career choice as a surgically oriented, clinical, and academic radiation oncologist [1–4]. Following that, I will share some personal reflections on "preparing for retirement" combined with insights from other physician authors [5–7].

Career Transitions

When a career in medicine is initially anticipated, what is envisioned is often not what transpires. Having been raised on a farm and ranch in northern Montana, veterinary medicine seemed my most likely medical career. As I progressed through high school, however, my paternal grandmother and high school English teacher and coach (football, basketball) encouraged me to consider medical school, and I was impressed by the dedication of the general practitioner who served our rural Montana community for many years.

Medical School Versus MS-PhD Anatomy

During my senior year at Montana State University (MSU; 1963–1964), I applied to medical school, but was not accepted. My premed counselor at MSU encouraged me to consider an MS-PhD program in anatomy, and I was accepted as a graduate student at the Univ. of N Dakota 2-year med school (UND, Grand Forks).

L. L. Gunderson (✉)
Department of Radiation Oncology, Mayo Clinic Arizona/Rochester, Scottsdale, AZ, USA

© Springer Nature Switzerland AG 2021
R. A. Chandra et al. (eds.), *Career Development in Academic Radiation Oncology*, https://doi.org/10.1007/978-3-030-71855-8_29

While in my Master's in Science program in Anatomy (MS Anatomy, 1964–1966), I had a wonderful mentor, Dr. Frank Lowe, who definitely influenced my career. He taught me a scientific method of inquiry and critical evaluation of the literature. There is little doubt that once I decided to become involved with academic radiation oncology, my time with Dr. Lowe influenced both my clinical research efforts and scholarly activities and production.

During year 2 in the Master's program, I realized that I still preferred to be an MD rather than an Anatomy professor. I applied to the UND medical school as a second year student in the spring of 1966, having completed all of the first year med school class materials in my 2-year MS program. I was quickly accepted but was soon informed that they had to withdraw my medical school acceptance at the request of the Anatomy Chair. The Dean informed me that five other US medical schools were willing to accept individuals as second year students, and I was subsequently interviewed by and accepted at the University of Kentucky (UKY) in Lexington.

Medical School/Surgery Internship/Residency Surgery Versus Radiation Oncology

The transition from MS Anatomy student at UND to second year med student at UKY went well. I knew for certain that I had made the correct choice with the transition to the year 3 and 4 clinical rotations. While I enjoyed each rotation, my favorite was the general surgery rotation and a dog surgery elective (UKY had a very strong surgery program and a dynamic chair, Dr. Ward Griffen).

During clinical year 4, I applied for straight surgery internships in Chicago, Oregon, California, and Utah. I ranked the University of Utah (Salt Lake City, SLC) as my #1 choice in the matching program and was one of the six individuals accepted into that program. My goal was to complete a 4-year residency in general surgery and have a subsequent general surgery practice that included gastrointestinal (GI) cases. The straight surgery internship (June 1969–1970) included 6–9 months on general surgery rotations, rotations in urology and orthopedic surgery, and an elective month in anesthesiology.

Another straight surgery intern, Dr. Richard Brown, spent his elective month with Dr. Henry Plenk, Chair of Radiation Oncology at LDS Hospital/Intermountain Health Care (IHC) in SLC. Dr. Brown was surprised to find that he wanted to become a radiation oncologist instead of a surgeon, and suggested that I should also spend a month with Dr. Plenk. Since I had already done my months elective in anesthesiology, a 1-month elective with Dr. Plenk was not an option. I was able to spend the occasional half-day seeing patients with him and also became intrigued with the field of radiation oncology. After in-depth discussions with my wife regarding a medical career in radiation oncology versus various surgical subspecialties, I met with the head of the Department of Surgery internship and residency program and was released from the commitment to the surgery residency program.

I became a first year resident in Dr. Plenk's 4-year radiation oncology training program at LDS Hospital/IHC in June 1970 along with Dr. Brown. The LDS Hospital/IHC RadOnc residency program was awarded an NIH training grant that allowed residents the opportunity to spend a portion of their training outside the parent institution. My year of elective time included 6 months at the University of Utah (radiation oncology, 3 months, with Dr. Robert Stewart, Chair and Dr. James Eltringham; medical oncology, 3 months) and 3 months at MD Anderson Cancer Center (MDACC) for additional exposure to patients with head and neck cancer (with Drs. Robert Lindberg and Gilbert Fletcher) and gynecologic cancer (with Dr. Luis Delclos).

The remaining 3 months of elective time was spent at the University of Minnesota reviewing the re-operative data on patients with prior surgery for various abdominal/pelvic cancers. I had become aware of this data during a third or fourth year surgery rotation in medical school at UKY. The UKY chair of surgery, Dr. Ward Griffen, had been on the surgery staff at the Univ. MN during the re-operative era, and occasionally discussed the data from a surgical perspective. Dr. Griffen facilitated my time at Univ. MN by interacting with Dr. Henry Sosin who was still on staff in the Univ. MN Department of Surgery. When I communicated with Dr. Sosin about reviewing the data, he preferred that it be done by one of the Univ. MN surgery residents. When they had no interest, Dr. Sosin approved my project and essentially said "well, I'm not sure there's much there, but if you want to come, you can do so."

Dr. Owen Wangensteen, a prior chair of surgery at Univ. MN, had developed the re-operative procedures for patients with prior surgery for gastrointestinal (GI) or gynecologic (Gyn) cancers. He felt that for patients who were at high risk for tumor relapse, a reoperation should be performed 3–6 months after the first surgery to find early evidence of cancer relapse that could be surgically removed. This would potentially change patients from a non-curative to a curative state. However, if a GI or Gyn cancer is so locally advanced that the initial surgery does not prevent relapse, a second surgery is unlikely to do a better job.

The 3-month period at the Univ. MN comprised an extensive review of the available records, extraction of pertinent findings onto written flow sheets, and duplicating copies of both the original and re-operative records (both operative and pathology reports). Dr. Sosin also gave me permission to communicate with physicians of those patients to get additional information on patterns of relapse and other information including patient status (alive with disease, DOD, etc.). I analyzed the data when we returned to Utah. Following the analysis, I decided to work with an artist to put the patterns of relapse in diagrammatic fashion and illustrate/indicate potential radiation fields.

Review and analysis of the Univ. MN re-operative data yielded intriguing information on patterns of relapse for colorectal and gastric cancers and how to design radiation fields to encompass those potential areas of relapse. This early scholarly activity as a resident led to important findings and helped get radiation oncology more involved in the treatment of patients with GI cancers. It was also the basis for future recruitment to Massachusetts General Hospital/Harvard as a subspecialized radiation oncologist for patients with GI Cancer.

RadOnc Private Practice: Northwest US Versus LDS Hospital/IHC

When residency was coming to a close, had there been a good private practice opportunity in the Northwest, I likely would have proceeded in that direction. I wasn't actually thinking of an academic career at that time. I accepted an offer from Dr. Henry Plenk to be on staff at LDS Hospital/IHC where I spent 2 years on staff with Drs. Henry Plenk and Richard Brown (1974–1976) functioning as a general radiation oncologist. I evaluated and treated patients with every type of malignancy and served as the GI cancer expert for our group of three physicians.

RadOnc MGH/Harvard

While on staff at LDS Hospital/IHC, I was invited by Dr. Herman Suit to give a lecture at Massachusetts General Hospital/Harvard as part of their residency-training course in radiation oncology. Two weeks before I came he said, "Oh, by the way, I want you to look at a staff position to be the MGH GI cancer radiation oncologist."

Dr. Suit's unexpected proposal did not result in "and the rest is history" immediately because my wife and I weren't planning to move. We had just built a new home in Salt Lake. I was planning to try out for the Mormon Tabernacle Choir (now known as "The Tabernacle Choir at Temple Square"), a continuation of my musical interests. But Herman was a very tenacious and creative recruiter; we received packets of material from him every few days. After much consideration including everything from flow chart analysis of pros and cons to the use of fasting and prayer to receive spiritual input, we ended up deciding that a move east could be a good opportunity. Although the position at MGH/Harvard was of clinical and academic interest, the initial financial offer was not competitive, which was resolved satisfactorily with Dr. Suit.

The time spent on staff at MGH/Harvard (Mar 1976–Nov 1980) was extremely valuable from both a professional and personal perspective. I functioned as the MGH/Harvard GI radiation oncologist and developed close working relationships with both surgeons and medical oncologists who had subspecialty interest in patients with GI cancer. Although we saw patients in separate clinics, we communicated closely in developing multidisciplinary approaches to the care of our common patients. I also saw select soft tissue sarcoma patients with Dr. Suit that initiated my subsequent interest in evaluating and treating patients with sarcoma.

My professional schedule at MGH, per discussion with Dr. Suit at the time of recruitment, was to be an 80/20 split of clinical practice (4 days/week) and clinical research (1 day/week) [2, 3]. However, my actual schedule ended up being clinical practice 5 day/week and clinical research from 9 pm to 12 pm or 2 am, since I felt the need to make sure my new MGH colleagues knew that I was a compassionate, available clinician. This unwise schedule ultimately resulted in a bleeding ulcer and a permanent need for good sleep habits to avoid recurring symptoms. I felt the need to renegotiate my professional work schedule of 80/20 with a return of the 20% clinical research time. Dr. Suit's response was "Len, I never took away your research day, you just didn't use it!" Subsequently, I spent 1 day/week in my home office doing clinical research while fresh and alert, and found I could see the same number of new and follow-up patients in 4 day/week by being more efficient [2–4].

I learned early in my time at MGH, that when one transfers from one institution to another, it takes time to develop working relations with new physicians, and one needs to be careful not to push preferred treatment approaches/concepts/biases onto referral colleagues too quickly. I came to MGH with a personal preference/bias toward treating high-risk rectal cancer patients with postoperative irradiation or chemoradiation (as I had done at LDS Hospital/IHC in SLC), since the extent of disease was not known preoperatively. That bias was challenged by one of the referring MGH surgeons (Dr. Steven Hedberg) who preferred preoperative adjuvant treatment. Dr. Hedberg ended up being the largest referral source of rectal cancer patients during my MGH/Harvard tenure. Had I been unwilling to deliver full-dose preoperative adjuvant treatment to his patients, I would possibly have lost a valuable referral source, and/or patients may not have been referred for adjuvant treatment pre- or postoperatively.

The use of intraoperative irradiation (IORT) with electrons as a component of treatment for patients with locally advanced abdominal or pelvic cancers was instituted at MGH in May 1978 (second IORT program in the USA, preceded only by Howard University). Involved radiation oncologists (Drs. Suit, Bill Shipley, and me) worked closely with our colleagues in surgery and anesthesiology, since transfer from the surgical ORs to the radiation oncology department was necessitated. Initial patients were those with either select GI cancers (locally unresectable rectal; locally unresectable pancreas) or retroperitoneal sarcoma.

IORT combined my surgical and radiation oncology interests. I always felt very comfortable in the operating room because of my straight surgery internship. IORT is also a fantastic way to develop working relationships with surgeons. You demonstrate your willingness to interact with them on their turf and make team decisions based on surgical/pathological findings.

In addition to my clinical responsibilities, I had the opportunity to serve as director of the resident training program in RadOnc from 1977 to 1980. During that time, cross rotation of residents from the two Harvard training programs in radiation oncology (MGH, Joint Center for Radiation Oncology) was established in conjunction with Dr. Samuel Hellman, Chair of RadOnc at the Harvard Joint Center.

RadOnc Mayo Clinic Rochester

I did not go to MGH planning to stay long term, as we were a "Western family." We went to MGH/Boston with the idea of staying there for five-plus years. My parents' and my grandparents' major medical institution was Mayo Clinic in Rochester MN.

In early 1980, Drs. Charles Moertel (Chair of Oncology) and John Earle (Chair, Radiation Oncology) inquired about my interest in joining Mayo Clinic Rochester as a GI Radiation Oncology replacement for Dr. Donald Childs who was planning to retire later that year. Dr. Moertel and I had made contact early in my career because I was invited, as a young Jr. staff, to be one of several speakers on GI cancer panels at regional or national meetings along with Dr. Moertel. While I had interest in the Mayo Rochester position, I needed assurance that Mayo was willing to commit to IORT as a component of treatment for appropriate patients and that I could have the 80/20 clinical practice/clinical research schedule that worked well at MGH. Drs. Earle and Moertel were totally supportive of an IORT program, along with the Chair of Surgery, Dr. Donald McIlrath. After agreement was reached on all critical issues, we moved our family to Rochester MN in August 1980, and I continued to see and treat patients at MGH until late November.

A major difference at Mayo Clinic Rochester was that Dr. Moertel had already instituted multidisciplinary clinics long before my arrival. I essentially saw all of my new and follow-up GI cancer patients 3 half-days a week in multidisciplinary clinics side by side with the medical oncologists, and separate surgeons would join us as indicated. Each new GI cancer patient had the benefit of being part of an individual patient's tumor conference. For patients with extremity soft tissue sarcoma, I went to the orthopedic floor and saw them together with the orthopedic surgeons.

Patients who were candidates for IORT were seen jointly with the involved surgeon in the department of radiation oncology before starting pre-op RT or chemo-RT. We saw each IORT patient with the surgeon again, just before the subsequent surgical resection and IOERT but after the restaging workup was completed.

In addition to clinical responsibilities with GI and sarcoma patients at Mayo Clinic Rochester from 1980 to 2001, I held a variety of administrative positions in the Division of Radiation Oncology and Department of Oncology (Divisions of RadOnc, MedOnc, and Oncology Research). In RadOnc, I was chair of the education committee from 1981 to 1986 (responsibility for the residency training program) and chair of clinical practice from 1986 to 1989. I became vice-chair of radiation oncology in 1986 (with Dr. John Earle, Chair) and transitioned to Chair of RadOnc in 1989 (1989–1996). I served as vice-chair of the Department of Oncology from 1994 to 1996, and became chair of oncology in 1996 (1996–2001). I was the only radiation oncologist to serve as chair of the Department of Oncology at Mayo Clinic Rochester.

I was recruited to Mayo Rochester at the level of Assistant Professor of Oncology and Consultant in Radiation Oncology and was advanced to Associate Professor in 1981. In 1985, I was advanced to the level of Professor of Oncology.

In the spring of 1988, the life of our oldest daughter Valerie (HS senior, age 17) was taken by a former boyfriend. We wanted to leave Rochester before he was eligible for parole. Accordingly, in 2000 we began to evaluate professional options at both Mayo Clinic Arizona and IHC/Salt Lake City. We again relied on spiritual input after carefully considering both personal and professional aspects of both opportunities and chose Mayo Clinic Arizona.

RadOnc/Mayo Clinic AZ

I was willing to consider a move to Mayo Clinic AZ as a member of the RadOnc staff with Dr. Michele Halyard serving as chair. However, Dr. Halyard preferred that she step aside as chair to allow me to be recruited to and function in that position. She had been functioning as Chair of RadOnc and a member of the Mayo Clinic Arizona Board of Governors at the assistant professor level and needed the opportunity to become academically productive.

I shifted from Mayo Clinic Rochester to Mayo Clinic Arizona in 2001 (Sept 2001–May 2009) where I served as chair of radiation oncology and as deputy director for Clinical Affairs at Mayo Clinic Cancer Center-Arizona. In the latter capacity, I had the opportunity to organize disease-site working groups for all major cancer disease sites. At the time of my arrival, there were no functioning disease-site groups, including breast cancer, even though breast cancer multidisciplinary clinics had been occurring for several years.

From a clinical perspective, I continued to evaluate and treat patients with GI cancer, soft tissue sarcoma, and recurrent gynecologic cancer in conjunction with surgery and MedOnc colleagues. I also helped initiate an IOERT program with surgery colleagues and RadOnc physicians and physicists using the new technology of a mobile electron accelerator.

Preparing for Retirement

When asked by Dr. Thomas to write this chapter, I told him that if he was willing to accept "personal reflections" on the topic, I could accomplish the task. In the past 6 months, I also found some short articles in MDLinx on the topic of physician retirement by Drs. Murphy, Meszaros, and Saleh that add some nice insights on the topic [5–7].

Retirement Insights from MDLinx Authors

Dr. Murphy noted that "The one thing doctors must do before retirement" is to find a new job; find something as satisfying to do in your retirement years as in the decades of employment [5]. Options could include volunteering, counseling, teaching, or even a reduced work schedule in the current job. A theme he expanded on was "Don't take it as a loss." He also stated the obvious need to make a sound financial plan before retirement and figure out an exit strategy.

Dr. Meszaros reported results of a MDLinx survey on physician retirement plans [6]. Many who participated in the survey were not ready to retire, for varied and interesting reasons. Of those planning retirement, reasons quoted included government bureaucracy, medical-legal entrapment, the drudgery of paperwork, reaching financial security, and burnout. Many wanted to *retire to have time for the finer things in life*, such as family, hobbies, travel, and leisure. When asked what *age they intend to retire*, only 14% said before 60, 49% noted between ages 65 and 70, 19% said after age 70, and 7% said never.

Dr. Saleh discussed briefly "7 great gigs for retired (or semiretired) docs" [7]. These included locum tenens, consulting, telemedicine, teaching, healthcare administration, writer and editor, and international volunteerism. Dr. Saleh also noted the AMA recommendation of "a gradual transition to retirement with a tapering of professional responsibilities" and pursuit of meaningful activities that will offer a sense of purpose during retirement.

Personal Reflections on Retirement and Transitions to Retirement

From a personal perspective, my retirement strategy, just as my career transitions, has been a phased affair. This was affected by personal journeys along the way and accomplished in conjunction with my wife Katheryn.

If "work-life balance" exists in your life before retirement, as it did in mine, the transition into life after retirement is much easier [2–4]. My wife and I found it both helpful and necessary to create goals (prioritize them in each of our areas of interest – family, profession, home, spiritual, hobbies/interests, personal health, other) and then calendar our lives in order to achieve a healthy "work-life balance." This was especially important while raising our six children. We valued family time centered on family meals, kid's activities (school, extracurricular), vacations, and church. We enjoyed having fun together (boating, tennis), but also benefitted from working together (gardening, raking fall leaves). Date nights were important, for my wife and me, to nurture and maintain our relationship in preparation for "life after children."

Personal lessons in calendaring/prioritizing and achieving balance in my life have been gained over the years in both personal and professional settings. While serving as a lay church leader, I received valuable calendaring advice from another ecclesiastic leader (also a physician) on how to balance my time and responsibilities [3, 4]. The calendaring schedule and learning to say no selectively within each aspect of my life helped me maintain work-life balance (note: it's not OK to say no only to your family/partner). The combination of an 80/20 professional schedule and use of 2 nights per week for scholarly activity allowed me to meet many goals for academic productivity during my professional career.

Clinical Retirement/Professional Transitions: Mayo Clinic Rochester Versus Arizona

I had a wonderful working relationship with my radiation oncology colleagues as well as the surgeons (thoracic, oncology, colorectal, general, and orthopedic), medical oncologists (gastrointestinal and sarcoma), and gynecologic oncologists at Mayo Clinic Rochester. Barring the tragedy of our daughter's death, we likely would have chosen to remain in Rochester MN at least until retirement.

At the time of my recruitment to Mayo Clinic Arizona, I intended to function as an active clinician and chair of the department of radiation oncology until age 70. However, in the spring of 2003, I was admitted to the hospital for a subarachnoid hemorrhage with CT findings of associated hydrocephalus. The neurosurgeon consultants felt I would likely need two surgical procedures (decompressive shunt, surgical ligature of suspected burst aneurysm based on the volume of intracranial blood on CT). Subsequent imaging studies did not reveal an aneurysm, and I responded to intensive intravenous fluids plus medications intended to prevent vasospasm and associated death (no surgeries needed). While I recovered completely from a clinical perspective and continued to function as Chair of RadOnc at the time of discharge, I had to take 4 h of neurocognitive tests before I was allowed to see patients and participate in IORT cases with surgery colleagues.

A number of professional transitions were initiated as a result of my subarachnoid hemorrhage. The Mayo Clinic Arizona CEO, Dr. Victor Trastek, and I agreed that I would continue to serve as Chair of RadOnc with the provision that we would have annual reviews to determine whether I should continue to function in that role. Soon after my return to clinical practice and administrative responsibilities, I asked Dr. Steven Schild, one of the five other RadOnc MD staff, to become vice-chair of the RadOnc department. From that point forward, Dr. Schild and I functioned as a RadOnc Executive Committee in making critical RadOnc decisions. At that time, we requested permission from institutional committees and the Mayo AZ CEO to recruit a new RadOnc physician that would have similar clinical interests to me regarding patients with GI cancer and soft tissue sarcoma (Dr. Matthew Callister, who did his residency at MDACC, was recruited to that position).

I decided to step aside as Chair of RadOnc in Dec 2007 in consultation with Dr. Trastek, and Dr. Schild was asked to serve as the new chair. Dr. Schild asked me to remain on the RadOnc Exec Committee until I chose to retire from clinical practice in May 2009 (age 65½). Dr. Jonathan Ashman (RadOnc residency at Memorial Sloan Kettering) was recruited to fill my position, and for purpose of clinical transition and training in IORT with electrons, we overlapped for ~3 months.

Retirement Transitions: Writer and Editor and ASTRO
President-Chair Track

While I retired from clinical practice in 2009, my transition to full retirement was eased by involvement with one of Dr. Saleh's "7 gigs," that of "writer and editor." Dr. Joel Tepper and I had served as Sr. editors for the first two editions of *Clinical Radiation Oncology* prior to 2009 and two subsequent editions after that date (CRO3 in 2012, CRO4 in 2016). CRO4 had a new feature of periodic clinical/content updates of disease-site chapters in the online version of the textbook. Although I was heavily involved in the clinical/content updates for CRO4 in conjunction with disease-site associate editors and chapter senior authors, I promised my wife, Katheryn, that I would not edit further editions of *Clinical Radiation Oncology*. When the decision was made to proceed with CRO5, Joel and I selected two new Sr. editors (Drs. Robert Foote and Jeff Michalski) to assist Joel in the editing process, and at Joel's request, I was involved with the three of them in the planning process for CRO5. Another writer/editor effort after clinical retirement was publication of a second edition of a textbook on *Intraoperative Irradiation: Techniques and Results* in 2011 in conjunction with co-editors Drs. Christopher Willett, Felipe Calvo, and Louis Harrison and many chapter authors. I also had major involvement with the lower GI cancer chapters (anus, colon/rectum) for the seventh and eighth editions of the *AJCC Cancer Staging Manual* (Ed'n 7 published in 2010 and Ed'n 8 in 2017).

An additional transition to full retirement was ASTRO leadership involvement (along the lines of the AMA recommendation of "a gradual transition to retirement with a tapering of professional responsibilities"). I served an initial term on the ASTRO Board of Directors (BOD) as secretary-treasurer from 2003 to 2008. In early 2009, I received a call from Dr. Louis Harrison, chair of the ASTRO nominating committee, to ask if I would be a candidate for ASTRO 2009 president-elect (4-year term as president-elect, president, chair, past-chair). I said "Lou, I am retiring in May." Lou's response was along the lines of "Len, that means you can do a better job." I agreed to be a candidate, was elected, and served in the ASTRO president/chair leadership track from 2009 to 2013, a very rewarding 4 years, both personally and professionally. The most personally rewarding aspect of the 4-year term was to serve as chair of the 2011 Annual Meeting and Program Committee and give the ASTRO 2011 Presidential Address "Work-Life Balance and Effective Communication." I continued to receive comments about that presentation for over 8 years, which never occurred with any of my GI cancer or IORT talks at local, regional, national, or international meetings.

Financial Planning/Family/Service to Others/Physical Activity

Financial planning is an essential part of getting ready for and surviving life both before and after retirement. Early in our marriage, we created our first will with legal assistance and subsequently established a living trust that is periodically updated with our personal trust/estate attorney. We also have both a financial planner available through Mayo Clinic (a rare but appreciated employee benefit) and a separate personal financial planner. We meet periodically with both financial planners on about a yearly basis since retirement in 2009 to get advice on both investment options and strategies and when to file necessary documents from an IRS perspective (i.e., on which retirement annuities does one need to start withdrawals at age 70½?).

For those who are married or have a partner, one of the things that occur after retirement is getting used to being around each other on a more continuous basis. When I was still seeing patients and was gone from home 4–5 days/week, I considered the home my wife's domain and rarely expressed opinions about home-oriented things, except when asked for input. Accordingly, 1 day during the first year of spending more time at home, my wife asked *"Why do you have an opinion about this?"* with some degree of exasperation! Both of us remember the occasion, but not the issue. ☺ That example notwithstanding, I have always felt strongly about my roles and responsibilities as husband and father and the need to achieve work-life balance in my life in order to function well in those roles [2–4].

After retirement, there is certainly more time available *"for the finer things in life*, such as family, hobbies, travel and leisure" as noted in the MDLinx 2019 survey. We have certainly enjoyed traveling with our extended family and spending more time with our 17 grandkids (and their parents).

Retirement also brings the option of spending a block of time committed to serving others.

In 2016–2017 my wife and I served as senior missionaries for our church for 12 months in the mission office of the California Fresno Mission. We assisted the Mission President and wife in caring for the needs of 130–175 young missionaries (most ages 18–22).

Physical activity to help maintain body function and weight is an important part of life before and after retirement. The difference after retirement is the ability to choose the time of day for walks or other physical activities, dependent on weather and other issues or commitments.

Summary Comments

- While many situations in life benefit from careful planning and preparation, others require flexibility in response to life's events and unforeseen circumstances, and the willingness to seek spiritual input, as indicated.
- My career as a surgically oriented, clinical, and academic radiation oncologist was far different from initial expectations (large animal veterinarian or general practitioner) and was influenced by a number of events and mentors along the way (Dr. Frank Low, Anatomy Professor, UND Medical School; Dr. Ward Griffen, Chair of Surgery, UKY Medical School; RadOnc: Drs. Henry Plenk and Charles Votava, LDS Hospital/IHC; Drs. Robert Stewart and James Eltringham,

Univ UT; Drs. Gilbert Fletcher, Robert Lindberg and Luis Delclos, MDACC; Drs. Herman Suit, CC Wang and Sam Hellman, MGH and Harvard).
- Retirement including retirement transitions was definitely altered by life's events (daughter's death, subarachnoid hemorrhage, ASTRO BOD president-chair track, writer and editor responsibilities).

For Discussion with a Mentor or Colleague

- How did you decide it was time to start planning your retirement?
- What would you have done differently in your personal life and medical career to prepare for retirement?

Bibliography

1. Allison R, Gressen E, Gunderson LL. ASTRO History Committee interview. 2018.
2. Johnson D. Becoming more productive. Education session on work-life balance. ASCO; 2011.
3. Gunderson LL. Work-life balance and effective communication. Presidential Address, ASTRO; 2011.
4. Gunderson LL. Work-life balance. Chairman's Update. ASTRO News. 2012, pp. 7–8.
5. Murphy J. The one thing doctors must do before retirement. MDLinx. 2019.
6. Meszaros L. MDLinx survey results: 2019 retirement plans. MDLinx. 2019.
7. Saleh N. 7 great gigs for retired docs. MDLinx. 2020.

Personal Finance and Work–Life Balance

Monica E. Shukla and Carmen R. Bergom

Personal Finance

In this section, we will provide a list of resources to help you become financially literate and/or learn more about advanced financial planning topics. We then will discuss key issues for physicians, including paying off student loans, managing earnings, retirement planning, asset protection, estate planning, and giving.

Get Educated

> We should remember that good fortune often happens when opportunity meets with preparation. — *Thomas A. Edison*

The term personal finance is enough to give most medical school graduates a pit in their stomach. Why? Because we know so little about it. It is important to fight your instinct to bury your head in the sand. Start reading and/or listening to whatever you can starting *now*, even if it is in very short periods of available time. We are fortunate in that so many resources exist today; you can select what you need in terms of format and the desired level of detail.

Some recommended books on the general topic of personal finance are:

- *The Richest Man in Babylon* by George Clason
- *The Millionaire Next Door* by Thomas Stanley

M. E. Shukla (✉)
Department of Radiation Oncology, Medical College of Wisconsin, Milwaukee, WI, USA
e-mail: mshukla@mcw.edu

C. R. Bergom
Department of Radiation Oncology, Washington University of Medicine in St. Louis,
St. Louis, MO, USA

© Springer Nature Switzerland AG 2021
R. A. Chandra et al. (eds.), *Career Development in Academic Radiation Oncology*, https://doi.org/10.1007/978-3-030-71855-8_30

- *The Bogleheads' Guide to Investing* by Larimore, Lindauer, and LeBoeuf
- *Think and Grow Rich* by Napoleon Hill – many see this more as a self-development book
- *The White Coat Investor, A Doctor's Guide to Personal Finance and Investing* by James M. Dahle, MD – physician-specific, but also relevant to other high-income professionals

It may be difficult to consider how to make time to read books on finance. Luckily, many of the above are available in audiobook format which you can listen to during your work commute or other downtimes. Alternatively, you can try out financial podcasts.

Here are a several frequently recommended podcasts on personal finance and retirement planning:

- *Money for the Rest of Us*
- *The Dave Ramsey Show*
- *Radical Personal Finance*
- *Afford Anything*
- *Mad Fientist*
- *ChooseFI Podcast*

Here are a few financial podcasts that are physician-specific:

- *The White Coat Investor*
- *Financial Residency*
- *Doctor Money Matters*

There are hundreds of personal finance websites. Here are a few well-curated websites that are ideal for the those with a beginner to intermediate level of personal finance knowledge:

- https://www.investopedia.com
- https://www.thesimpledollar.com
- https://www.nerdwallet.com
- https://www.khanacademy.org/economics-finance-domain/core-finance   –   The content here is not solely on personal finance, but available free and in a video format

There are also several excellent physician-focused websites:

- https://www.whitecoatinvestor.com
- https://www.physicianonfire.com
- https://passiveincomemd.com

Paying Off Your Student Loans

According to the 2019 AAMC report, 73% of students graduated with a student loan debt, with a median amount owed of $200,000. There are many ways to attack student loans, you just need a plan.

If you are still in medical school and have some time left until graduation, the key for you is to not take out more money than you absolutely need to. Graduate student loans generally carry a higher interest rate. For 2019–2020, the interest rate on Direct Federal Loans for graduate or professional students was 6.08% (versus 4.53% for federal undergraduate loans). Also, graduate loans are not subsidized, and thus they start accruing interest even while you are a full-time student. Here are some tips to help you incur the least amount of graduate student loan debt:

1. Choose to live as inexpensively as possible with regard to housing, food, entertainment, and travel.

   • This does not mean to pick an unsafe place to live, but you should not choose to live in the most upscale place to impress your friends.
   • Host potlucks with friends instead of eating out at expensive restaurants.
   • Forgo trips to expensive, faraway resorts in favor of driving to nearby attractions such as beaches or National Parks.
   • Keep discretionary expenditure to a minimum.

2. If possible, borrow money from family members instead of banks (e.g., interest-free loans).
3. Apply for any grants, scholarships, tuition support, research fellowships, etc., that you can.

For radiation oncology residents, the main thing to avoid is forbearing or deferring payments on student loans at all, or at least, for any extended period of time. In the end, the capitalized interest will make the debt burden much higher. Currently, if you have Direct Federal Loans you can enter into one of four federal income-driven repayment (IDR) programs: Income-Based Repayment (IBR), Income-Contingent Repayment (ICR), Pay As You Earn (PAYE), or Revised Pay As You Earn (REPAYE). All of these programs have benefits and drawbacks, but payments are a percentage of your discretionary income and further adjusted for family size. Under any of the four plans, with regular payments, any balance remaining after 20–25 years (depending on the plan) will be forgiven.

Another option is the Public Service Loan Forgiveness Program, which forgives the Direct Loan balance after 120 qualifying payments *IF* you are working for a federal, state, local, or tribal government or a not-for-profit organization. Qualifying payments are generally those that are made on one of the above-mentioned income-driven repayment plans. While there has been recent discussion about ending this program, at the time this chapter was written, this program was still active. For residents with interest in this program, you should join an IDR program and start making payments as soon as possible. For those with private loans, they should be refinanced to the lowest possible interest rate that provides a realistic payment schedule. Some companies will offer a great rate with a payback over 5 years, but that may not be feasible for many, especially early on.

For those entering an academic radiation oncology practice, most organizations have not-for-profit 501(c)(3) status. If you are interested in Federal Public Student

Loan Forgiveness (PSLF) and have made payments for several years on an income-driven plan as a resident, keep making payments and in many cases, there will be a portion of your student loans that can be forgiven after 120 payments. It would be very difficult for you participate in the PSLF Program if you were not making regular qualifying payments during residency. If you deferred or forbore payments for part or all of your time in residency and only went into repayment as an attending, 120 qualifying payments on your new and improved full-time attending salary (full-time employment is a requirement) would in most cases have the remaining balance paid off before 120 payments. If you do not qualify for PSLF or it doesn't make sense for you, then as above, loans should be refinanced to the lowest possible interest rate available (watching the fees) in order to pay down debt quickly. Many discuss the idea of making minimum payments on student loans and using the extra cash on hand to invest (e.g., if you're loans are at 4% and you could be making 6–8% on the market with a semi-aggressive to aggressive portfolio). This might be the right move for some, but many will instead choose to simplify their lives and pay down their student debt quickly.

Earnings

> It is good to have money and the things that money can buy, but it's good too, to check up once in a while and make sure you haven't lost the things money can't buy. – *George Horace Lorimer*

How much you earn is important. It is in your best interest to not settle for less than what you should be making based upon your level of training and experience (see below resources). However, salary is only one part of the very complex decision of selecting a position. If you are considering a position with an exceptionally high salary, the salary may be high to compensate for some undesirable features of the job, or there could be something regarding your job expectations that you are missing. If you are considering an academic position, there may be less variability between contracts and fewer points that can be changed despite negotiations. Academic contracts are fairly standard and surprisingly short. Many of the fine details are in the institution's clinical practice policies and medical staff bylaws, which the contract often refers you to. If you are in heavily involved in research, there may be much more to negotiate in terms of laboratory space, personnel support, start-up funding, and research time. This is covered in other sections.

Aside from salary, here is non-comprehensive list of other important things to consider when selecting a position, from a financial perspective only. Consider reviewing your contract with a lawyer specializing in medical contracts before signing.

- Salary (% base vs. incentive; what is the incentive component based upon; are there clinical/research productivity benchmarks?)
- Contract length, termination language

- Health insurance (medical, dental, vision, plan options)
- Other insurance benefits (medical malpractice (occurrence vs. claims-made – thus potential need for "tail insurance" on exit), group life insurance, group disability)
- Other general benefits (healthcare spending account (HSA), healthcare flexible spending account (FSA), dependent care FSA, among others)
- Retirement accounts (403b, 457b, employer matching, and vesting schedule).
- Provision of time and funds for continuing medical education (CME), coverage of society membership fees
- Opportunities for advancement, average time to promotion (e.g., Instructor to Assistant Professor, etc.)
- Stability of the practice (insurance pool, market share, threats from other hospital systems or practice, etc.)
- Financial health of the practice
- Location and length of daily commute
- Call expectations and any additional compensation
- Restrictive covenants (noncompete clauses)

Physician Compensation Resources

- AAMC Faculty Salary Report: Compensation data from faculty at 151 U.S. medical schools broken out by specialty, degree, rank, and region. The full report is available for purchase on the AAMC website for $1150. Faculty/staff at member institutions may purchase for $43 (https://store.aamc.org/aamc-faculty-salary-report-fy19-online.html). It may also be available from your institutional library.
- Medical Group Management Association (MGMA) data
- Talk to your colleagues at other institutions
- CareerNavigator (Doximity)
- Medscape Survey

Saving, Spending, and Emergency Funds

Do not save what is left after spending, but spend what is left after saving. – *Warren Buffett*

Budgeting

We cover spending and saving under the same heading as they are two sides to one coin. The first step to optimizing your savings is to create a budget. This can be tedious and is put off by many. It may help to think about a budget as actually allowing you to do the things you love the most. A budget will set the groundwork for future financial growth. Only money saved can be invested, and thus have the opportunity to grow. Here is a general process to create and adhere to a budget:

1. Assess your spending:

    (a) Try to be as granular as possible and figure out where every dollar is coming in and going out. Do this for 1–3 months, as there may be some variance in month-to-month expenses. Several programs and apps can make this easier: Mint, YouNeedABudget (YNAB), Mvelopes, Personal Capital, Quicken, etc.

2. Analyze where your money is going by grouping expenses into different categories. The above apps may do this automatically. Also categorize by fixed, variable, and discretionary expenditures.
3. Readjust where you spend your money. Cut certain categories that appear to be in excess and allocate more to others if needed.

    (a) Several popular budgeting methods exist, such as the envelope method, the zero-sum budget, the 50/30/20 budget, etc. Select the one that makes sense for you. Several personal finance resources advocate at least a 20% savings rate (or more if possible). Your savings rate is calculated from your disposable personal income (after-tax income).

4. Stick to the budget and reevaluate spending on a regular basis to make sure the budget is working for you. This should be done more frequently at first; later it can be spaced out as your budget is optimized. This is very important and will pay off in the long run!

Saving

The most important action to ensure proper savings is to automate your contributions to your various accounts (including retirement accounts, 529 plans, personal investment accounts, savings account, among others). The only thing that should trump meeting the 20% target savings rate is paying off high-interest debt. Another equally important item for maintaining a healthy saving-to-spending ratio is to change your mindset about money. You may (or soon will) have a lot of high-income friends. Avoid the temptation to keep up with them and buy expensive cars and take up expensive hobbies. The goal is to live like a resident as long as you can in the beginning. Hopefully, it will not be long until you can max out all your contributions, cover all your expenses, and still have money left over. Importantly, while adhering to your budget, buy things and partake in hobbies you like, instead of what others around you like or what is trendy. It is okay if those things are expensive, as long as the expenditure is intentional, and you have accounted for it in your budget.

Emergency Fund

Everyone needs an emergency fund. No one knows what the future holds and you should have a relatively liquid fund available to help you weather these unanticipated storms, particularly early on in your career. So how much do you need? The typical answer is 3–6 months' worth of expenses. That means that the emergency fund that was adequate for you as a resident may not be enough to cover your new and improved attending lifestyle. How much you need to set aside requires having a pulse on your month-to-month expenses (see Budgeting). This sum of money should be *available quickly without incurring major penalties for withdrawing* that money, which can occur with methods such as selling an heirloom, selling part of your portfolio at a loss, withdrawing from retirement accounts, spending money on a high-interest credit card, etc. Many individuals keep this sum of money in a high-interest earning savings account. This is also a good place to set aside money being saved for a down payment on a house or other large purchase you are anticipating in the near future.

As of the writing of this chapter, we are going through the COVID-19 pandemic. Especially for us as radiation oncologists in an academic practice (employed by a medical school or hospital system), we think our salaries are guaranteed, right? We signed a contract after all. The COVID-19 pandemic has taught us otherwise. Patient volumes were down dramatically in the clinics and operating rooms due to postponing elective procedures and non-essential treatments. No money coming in means that eventually no money can go out. Several major institutions have recently announced salary reductions and employee furloughs, with many soon to follow suit. Most physicians with a pay cut will still be doing okay, but individual circumstances vary. Even as an attending radiation oncologist, if you are the sole earner, have a large family, dependent elderly parents, are paying for childcare and/or have other financial responsibilities, things could be tight financially for quite a while. This highlights the importance of living within your means, budgeting, and keeping an adequate emergency fund.

Retirement Planning

In investing or retirement planning, time is your greatest asset. – *Unknown*

This is a vast topic. We will cover the basics, but will refer you to other sources for more detail. Our advice should not replace your personal research into these topics, being in contact with your benefits manager, and/or the advice of a financial professional.

403(b)

In academic radiation oncology, your prospective or current employer is most likely a 501(c)(3) organization or a not-for-profit organization. If so, they are likely offering a 403(b) retirement account in your benefits package. A 403(b) is a type of tax-advantaged account that allows you to contribute pre-tax dollars up to a set limit. The contribution limit for 2020 was $19,500. If your employer's plan allows, contribution limits can be higher for those over 50 years old (called "catch-up" contributions) and for those individuals with over 15 years of service to the same employer. That money can then grow tax-deferred over time. When you withdraw funds from this account in retirement (called a distribution), the money is taxed at the rate of your annual gross income at that time. In addition to the benefit of your earned dollars growing tax-deferred over time, in most cases, your tax rate in retirement will be lower than your current tax rate. You can start taking distributions at age 59.5. Any withdrawals prior to that are assessed a 10% tax penalty, unless you have a prespecified exception (e.g., disability, qualifying economic hardship, severance from employment, etc.).

Some employers offer a match on retirement contributions, which you should certainly take advantage of. Anything that you contribute to your 403(b) is yours. Employer contributions generally have a vesting period before you are entitled to the matching funds (i.e., you can take them with you if you move jobs). If you are not fully vested and you change jobs, you may need to give all or part of those employer-contributed funds back. The vesting schedule is employer-specific. The total contribution limit from both employers and employees in 2020 is $57,000. In comparison to a 401(k), options for types of investments within a 403(b)s are more limited in terms of asset classes, and the options available may have higher expense ratios which can erode at the tax-deferred benefit.

Individual Retirement Accounts (IRAs)

An IRA or an individual retirement account is an account that you would open through a brokerage firm (TD Ameritrade, Fidelity, Charles Schwab, etc.). The maximum yearly contribution limit in 2020 is $6000 (or $7000 per year if you are 50 years or older). The main upside of an IRA is that you have much more flexibility with regard to investment options (stocks, bonds, annuities, exchange-traded funds (ETFs), index funds, target-date funds, etc.), and you can find those options at a much lower cost whereas you would be limited to what your employer is offering in your 403(b).

There are many types of IRAs, but two that are frequently used are the traditional IRA and the Roth IRA. Both are tax-advantaged. With a Roth IRA, contributions are made with post-tax dollars and distributions in retirement (after age 59.5 years) come out tax-free. With a traditional IRA, contributions are made with pre-tax dollars. Distributions in retirement are taxed at the rate of your annual gross income at that time. Neither have age limits on contributions, but the Roth IRA has an income limit of $139,000 for individuals and $206,000 for a couple. Another difference is that a traditional IRA requires minimum distributions starting at age 72, while a Roth IRA has no stipulations of when or how much money you need to withdraw. Before retirement, you can take money out of a Roth IRA without penalty up to the amount you contributed (not earnings). If you withdraw earnings prior to age 59.5, a 10% tax penalty is assessed on the earnings only (remember contributions were made with post-tax dollars), and that sum is counted as normal income and taxed at your adjusted gross income rate. There are exceptions to this rule, however (e.g., acquired disability, first-time home buyer, etc.). With a traditional IRA, if you withdraw *any* funds prior to retirement, you will be assessed a 10% penalty (again there are exceptions), and you will owe taxes on the entire sum, as the contributions were made with pre-tax dollars.

A Roth IRA is a particularly attractive option for those earlier in their medical career (e.g., in medical school, residency, and as an early attending), as these individuals are generally below the upper income limit allowed to make contributions. You will likely become ineligible for Roth contributions the year or year after you start your first attending job. For those above income limits, there is a way to *legally* contribute post-tax dollars to a non-deductible IRA and then convert that money to a Roth IRA, called a "back-door Roth." This option has been available since 2010 due to a revision in the tax code that did not set income caps for those wanting to make a conversion from a traditional IRA to a Roth IRA. Although this option is available now, it may not be in the future. You will need to run the numbers yourself or with the help of a financial professional to see if this option makes sense for you. You'll also need to appropriately follow the pro-rata rule if you have other IRAs and finally, submit the proper paperwork with your tax returns on a yearly basis.

457(b)

A 457(b) is another tax-deferred retirement account offered to government and not-for-profit employees. The 2020 contribution cap is $19,500. Unlike a 403(b), this cap is for both employer and employee contributions. Above limit contributions can be made if you are over 50 years old. Additionally, if you are within 3 years of normal retirement age, you can double your yearly contribution. A major upside to the 457(b) is that you can start withdrawing funds from the account prior to retirement without penalty, as long as you no longer work for the employer that provided the plan. This is nice feature if one retires early either by choice or due to an unforeseen circumstance. For the minority of our readership, if offered a 457(b), it will be a governmental type, which is not subject to the creditors of your organization. If you have funds in a non-governmental 457(b), the funds in this account can be lost if your organization files for bankruptcy. You can clarify this with your organization's benefits office. 457(b) accounts, like 403(b)s, and in contrast to IRAs or 401(k)s, can have limited investment options.

Health Savings Accounts (HSA) and Healthcare Flexible Spending Accounts (FSA)

Employers may offer a healthcare flexible spending account (FSA) or a healthcare savings account (HSA). In these accounts, employees can set aside pre-tax dollars to be used for eligible medical, dental, and vision expenses not covered insurance (e.g. co-pays, co-insurance, eligible medical supplies). If you elect to use an HSA, it is generally contingent upon you also carrying a high deductible health insurance plan. With an FSA, funds not spent by the year end are lost (some may allow grace period to spend down funds or small roll-over limit). With an HSA, money left over at years end can be rolled over to the following year. For the year 2020, the maximum contribution limit to an HSA for personal coverage is $3550 and goes up to $7100 for family coverage. For FSAs, the 2020 limit is $2750. Money kept in an HSA can grow over time, and its earnings are not taxed. Money in an HSA can usually be invested (this is a major benefit). Investment choices vary by HSA administrator (generally mutual funds, although some now offer exchange-traded funds (ETFs), individual stocks, and bonds through a self-directed brokerage platform). As long as the funds are pulled out and used for healthcare-related expenses, they are not taxed. If money is withdrawn and used for non-healthcare-related expenses, it will be taxed at the normal rate and essentially functions as another tax-deferred investment. You are only allowed to contribute to an HSA until age 65, at which time you would be Medicare-eligible. Another perk is that HSAs are portable, meaning you can take them with you if you change jobs.

Due to scope and space limits, we are unable to cover several other important topics including, but not limited to, taxable investment accounts, investment strategy within retirement and taxable accounts, tax efficiency, 529 accounts for higher education, and/or passive income pursuits, including real estate. Please see resources listed under the heading "Get Educated" to read more about some of these topics.

Asset Protection

Disability Insurance

Disability policies protect you from lost wages if you become disabled and can no longer work in the capacity you are trained for. This is far more likely to occur than death. This is why disability insurance policies are expensive, and term life insurance policies are much more affordable. Disability policies carry the most value in your earlier years of practice, when a career-limiting injury or illness would devastate your lifetime earning potential. The best policies are the ones that cover your "own occupation" and are "specialty-specific," meaning that if you could not work as a radiation oncologist, you would be compensated as such. It is also important to understand whether your policy covers mental illness- and/or substance abuse–related disability. No one plans on having these challenges, but when choosing a policy it seems logical to cover all the ways in which you may be rendered unable to work in your current capacity. The younger and healthier you are, the lower your premium will be. Therefore, you should consider obtaining a small policy in residency (with a premium you can afford) to lock in a good rate and upgrade this over time. The bottom line is that you should purchase a plan with an inclusive definition of disability from a reputable company from an independent insurance agent.

Many use a percentage of their current income as a guide to how much disability insurance they need to carry, but most of us can live comfortably on much less than our salaries. The level of benefit you need depends upon your expenses, how much you need to save regularly to fund your retirement (most policies do not pay out after retirement age), and other income streams you may have that could support you in the event of disability. Hopefully, the more stable the financial ground you find yourself on as time goes on, the more you should consider whether it is worth continuing to pay your monthly premiums. Many will consider allowing policies to lapse when they are in their late 50s or early 60s, when they are approaching financial independence.

Your employer may provide a group disability benefit as well. You will need to look at your individual needs, what your employer is providing, and how much would need to be made up with an individual policy. The upside of your individual policy is that it will stay with you. Your employer's policy will terminate if you leave that job. If the group policy premium is being paid for by your department, of course, accept this benefit during open enrollment. If a group benefit is offered, but you would need to pay the premium, you will need to understand the level of benefit and the language on the policy to see if it makes sense for you.

Malpractice Insurance

In academic radiation oncology, the institution that you will be working for will almost certainly provide malpractice insurance. Medical malpractice insurance covers any claims brought against you for negligence in medical care that led to harm or injury of a patient. Malpractice insurance would cover any damages if awarded, but it also covers fees associated with any litigation/arbitration. The biggest factors that will influence the cost of your malpractice insurance are the state that you work in, specifically tort reform, the legal culture in your state, and of course your specialty.

There are two major types of medical malpractice insurance policies: a claims-made policy or an occurrence-based policy. The latter covers any incident that occurred while the policy was active, no matter when the claim was put forth (this can be many years after the policy has lapsed), while the former would only cover an incident that occurred while the policy was active, with the claim also being made during that time. With a claims-made policy you will need to obtain "tail" coverage once you leave that position to cover any potential claims that would be brought forth after that policy has lapsed. Tail insurance can be expensive, in the range of 1.5–2.5× the annual premium. There are also other liabilities of being in medical practice aside from patient care. Many recent claims brought forth deal with cyber-liability and HIPAA. You can purchase riders on your policy to cover these special circumstances.

There are generally two coverage limits associated with a malpractice policy. The first number is the award limit per claim made and the latter value is a limit for all claims on the policy (a common combination is $1 million/$3 million). Limits are usually determined by your specialty, scope of practice, and geography.

Umbrella Insurance

This is an insurance policy that covers claims and litigation fees that would arise from a claim that exceeds the value of what another policy that you own would cover (i.e., auto insurance or homeowner's insurance). While some people opt out of this coverage, umbrella insurance is an inexpensive additional policy that can help alleviate worry about financial catastrophe from a claim made against you. For example, what would happen if a delivery person slips and gets injured on your not-so-clean driveway in the winter months, and a 1-million-dollar award is granted to the person filing a claim against you? If your homeowner's insurance caps at $300k, then you would have to come up with the remaining $700k from your savings, retirement, etc. Umbrella insurance would cover the extra $700k in this situation. How much umbrella insurance to get depends upon how much exposure you have to a possible lawsuit and how many assets you have that are exposed beyond what each of your existing policies would cover (homeowners, auto, boat, etc.). Examples of items that would increase your risk of exposure are household employees, children (especially other people's children coming over to your house to use your trampoline or pool), a dog (or a pet tiger, which people apparently have). One thing to note about an umbrella policy is that is usually requires you to max out your liability coverage on your other policies (home, auto, etc.). There are some concerns that a large umbrella policy may invite a lawsuit from someone seeking a large payout. That may be true, but on the flip side, the more coverage you have, the more "on the hook" the insurance company is to make that payout if a judgement is made in the claimant's favor. The insurance company's corporate lawyers will be hard at work defending both themselves and you to prevent/limit any potential payout. Bottom line: insure properly depending upon the value of your assets at risk and your level of exposure.

Many will consider obtaining an LLC for protection of assets instead of, or in addition to, an umbrella policy. The nuances of this are beyond the scope of this chapter. See web resources below for further information:

1. https://www.investopedia.com/articles/personal-finance/040115/how-umbrella-insurance-works.asp
2. https://www.themoneycommando.com/umbrella-policy-vs-llc-asset-protection-part-1/

Will/Estate Planning and Life Insurance

Death is complicated and difficult for those you are leaving behind. Making arrangements in advance will make the transition less painful, less chaotic, and your heirs will be able to better enjoy the assets you intended them to have. In general, is not hard to pass assets to a spouse, and these assets are not typically subject to estate taxes. It becomes complicated when transferring assets to your children, other family members, or friends.

Last Will and Testament

Anyone over the age of 18 can create a will or trust, but it is not critical until one has a positive net worth, gets married, or has dependents. A last will and testament is a legal document that states how you would like your property to be distributed upon your death. An executor of your estate is also named whose responsibility it is to distribute your assets per your wishes. If you have children, the named guardian would be responsible for raising them. Wills are relatively inexpensive to draft and are considered public documents. They require probate (the court-supervised legal procedure by which assets are passed from deceased to the beneficiary). With a clear and up-to-date will, probate can be a mere formality. If you die "intestate," that is, without a will, your estate will also go through probate, but items in your estate will be distributed according to your state's inheritance law. It can be a long and difficult process to identify all the assets of the deceased and to find an appropriate place for all assets to go. Probate is a matter of public record so if you are averse to a stranger pouring over your records at the local courthouse once you are deceased, you may consider a revocable living trust.

Revocable Living Trust

The topic of trusts can get complicated, but to keep the topic simple, an alternative to a will is a revocable living trust. It takes a bit more effort and cost to set up on the front end, but the major advantage is that your assets pass directly to your named beneficiaries outside the courts, without any lawyers or fees. It is called a living trust as it is created while you are alive and is enduring after you pass on. All the assets that you wish to bequeath go into the trust. You, as the trustor, maintain ownership/control while you are alive. Similar to an executor in a will, you will name a trustee that is responsible for the distribution of the assets to your beneficiaries as described in the trust. The reason why this works outside of the courts is that your agreement is with the trust. If you pass, the trust is still living and can operate per your prior documentation. You as the trustor can changes its terms at any time (beneficiaries, structure) or revoke it altogether.

If you've hired a lawyer to assist in establishing your trust or drafting your will, have your Healthcare Power of Attorney paperwork drafted at the same time. This is not a financial item, but as a healthcare provider you know important this is.

Life Insurance

The basics of life insurance are fairly simple. Most opt for a term life insurance policy with a reputable company when they are relatively young, in good health, and have dependents or a partner or family that they provide for. Most commonly, a term policy with a level premium is purchased. Fewer opt for an annual renewable policy where the premium starts out less expensive than a level premium term policy, but the cost increases over time. This option works best for those planning to cancel their policies early after achieving financially independence. Your employer will often provide a group life insurance, though the benefit is usually not large enough to cover your needs if you are the sole earner in your family. You will need to consider taking out a policy large enough to cover the expenses for those that you are leaving behind. For example, a 40-year-old female physician with a stay-at-home husband and two young children may want to leave behind enough money to allow her husband and their children to maintain a similar standard of living for the next 20 years and also leave enough to pay for higher education for both children. You may need to budget for more or less depending on whether your spouse can return to work.

Many will consider stacking plans as the need for the life insurance benefit, in most cases, will decrease over time as you build your nest egg and most dependents become independent. For example, one might consider having two $1 million policies, one for a 20-year term and the other for a 10-year term; in all, $2 million worth of coverage for the first 10 years which would drop to $1 million for the second 10 years.

Many financial professionals that you will encounter (and they will often seek you out) will try to sell you various forms of life insurance than can be used as an investment vehicle. There are plenty of articles written on this topic, but to summarize, reviews are mixed on whether or not this is a wise thing to pursue.

Giving

No one has ever become poor by giving. Anne Frank

Although most of this chapter focuses on strategies to protect and grow your own wealth, you are probably better off than most. It is important to consider charitable giving for several reasons:

1. Giving to others improves your own sense of well-being.
2. Giving supports causes/values that are important to you.

3. If giving locally, it transforms your community into a better place for you to live in.
4. It teaches your children and those around you to be charitable as well.

How much to give and where to give is not always straightforward. You will have to decide, with other members of your household, what causes are the most important to you. Once you identify what causes you want to support, there are several websites that can help you decide upon a good charity that supports those efforts. These sites list whether the non-profit is organizationally sound, financially sound, and whether it uses the vast majority of the donated funds toward the stated cause.

Here are a few websites to help you: charitynavigator.com, charitywatch.org, givewell.org, give.org, and guidestar.org.

A Note on Financial Advisors

There is no perfect financial advisor, and financial advice from a professional certainly isn't free. Ideally all physicians would become educated enough to manage their own money to avoid ongoing fees, but not everyone has the time or is willing to spend their time learning how to manage their money. Some are perfectly content handing the reigns over to someone else. Even if you do choose the latter, you will still be much better off if you have the basic tenets of financial literacy (see the "Get Educated" section). Here are the things to look for in a financial advisor:

1. Fiduciary responsibility (ethical and legal responsibility to act in your best interests) and transparency when they stand to make a commission from a product, they are selling you.
2. Certification in finance (CFA (chartered financial analyst), CFP (certified financial planner), PFS (personal financial specialist – this is a CPA (certified public accountant) with financial planning expertise).
3. Physician clients, so they better understand your particular circumstances.
4. Reasonable fees: This is a vast topic that requires some investigation on your part. There are various fee models. Here are some of the most common: assets under management (AUM), flat yearly fee, hourly rate, fee per financial plan drafted. For those looking to primarily manage their own finances with intermittent advise, an hourly fee or fee for service arrangement may be best. For those looking to turn over their finances to an advisor, a flat annual fee is generally more favorable, especially as your portfolio nears seven digit range.

Work–Life Balance

You can't have everything you want, but you can have the things that really matter to you.
—*Marissa Mayer*, former president and CEO of Yahoo

Few topics engender as much interest as "work–life balance." Everyone is in search of work–life balance, though few seem to achieve it. An imbalance of work and life spheres is an important issue for many in academic medicine, but also for much of the U.S. professional workforce. The ever-increasing demands to be productive, prolific, and present in all parts of our lives fuels this imbalance. It is a long journey to become a practicing physician. As a student or trainee, there is often the hope that both your professional and personal lives will improve in the future, and they do in many ways. However, responsibilities accumulate over time, and professional and personal demands change. Achieving balance can be especially challenging for individuals caring for children and/or aging parents. Below are a few items that we, as parents working in academic medicine, have learned along the way that have helped us better balance our personal and professional lives.

A Few Key Points About Work–Life Balance

- There will be times when the various elements in your life are existing in harmony, and there will be other times when they are not. Work–life balance is not a destination, but a constant work in progress.
- The goal is not figuring out how to work less to live more; it is being fulfilled with what you are doing at work, at home, and with everything in-between. Work and personal life should not be competing choices, but rather complement each other in order to allow one to be fulfilled, both professionally and personally.
- A balanced life reduces stress and downstream stress-related complications, such as hypertension, obesity, anxiety, and other health issues.
- Greater balance allows for improved productivity in both your work and professional life.
- A good work–life balance allows for more personal connectedness in both your jobs and home life.
- Trying to find a harmonious balance on a day-to-day basis can be the small steps that you take so that when you look back over the years, you have slowly built a fulfilling and enjoyable life.

How Do You Know When Your Life Is Out of Balance?

If you are not effectively balancing your personal and professional priorities, you may start feeling or experiencing some of the following:

- Loss of interest
- Poor focus leading to inefficiency and/or procrastination
- Loss of confidence
- Feelings of depression, loneliness, irritability, and/or despair
- Decreased sense of well-being
- Fear of failure

- Feeling lack of control over your circumstances
- Intrusive feelings of guilt, worry, or anxiety

If you are experiencing a number of these symptoms, it may be helpful to speak to a professional, such as a counselor or psychiatrist. You can also usually easily and discretely access these resources through your institution's Employee Assistance Program (EAP).

How Do You Achieve Better Work–Life Balance?

There are some habits to develop and put into practice on a daily basis, and there are other more global themes that can help you to achieve better balance over the long run.

Macroscopic Goals

Goal Setting

First create and then document how you ideally envision your work and home life in 5 years, 10 years, and 20 years. This is critical in directing your efforts in the short term. When colleagues present you with opportunities, you will then be able to make deliberate decisions on which projects to take on, as opposed to just saying "yes" to everything. Pouring your efforts into these select items will help you achieve your long-term objectives. On a similar note, limit involvement in projects that are not contributing to your goals. Consider passing these on to colleagues for whom involvement would be applicable and boost their career trajectory. In turn, they are likely to do the same for you. Mentors who are familiar with your long-term goals may be helpful in guiding you through this process.

Reflection

You should engage in regular personal and professional reflection. Initially, this should ideally take place quarterly or biannually. Schedule a set amount of time in your calendar and most importantly, keep this appointment with yourself, in the same manner you would keep an appointment to attend a meeting with a colleague. During this time, identify your natural affinities and talents. Think about what topics you have knowledge on that others in your department may not. Are there platforms or situations that you have experience with that others do not? Most importantly, what are you passionate about professionally? What kind of tasks do you like to do? Building on your unique talents and affinities will help you bring value to your department/institution and allow you to carve out a niche for yourself. One way to stimulate these ideas and go through this process more objectively is to utilize available tools to identify your strengths (e.g., book/audiobook *Finding Your CliftonStrengths: StrengthsFinder 2.0* by Tom Rath).

At each subsequent reflection session, look back on the tasks that you have accomplished and those that remain a work in progress. What should you have planned for, but did not? What did not get accomplished and why not? What can you change moving forward to set yourself up for success? Is there a new opportunity on the horizon that you should consider allocating more time to? Document your thoughts and goals and put a new plan in place until your next reflection session.

Strategy

Once you have clearly stated your goals, build a smart strategy on how to get these items accomplished. Here are a few pointers:

- Everything is not equally important. Prioritize what is meaningful to you and what is not. Do the items that are meaningful to you and do them well.
- Focus on tasks that yield disproportionate results for time invested.
- Understand your natural work habits. This point straddles both reflection and strategy, but it is important to understand when and in what settings you are most focused and productive. Do you shine on individual or group projects? After identifying these things about yourself, arrange your work to be done during these times and in these settings.
- Be organized and plan ahead. Consider keeping running lists that contain tasks to accomplish on a daily, monthly, yearly, and long-term basis. To-do apps or other approaches such as the use of a Bullet Journal can facilitate this (see end of chapter resources).

Inspiration

Life isn't about finding yourself. Life is about creating yourself. – *George Bernard Shaw*

Here are a few pointers to find inspiration:

- *Focus on the positive and practice gratitude.* There may be days, weeks, or even months where things are not going so well, personally and/or professionally. You may wish things were different. When reflecting on these situations, if you can train your mind to pivot to the silver linings, in the end you may lessen down moods and feelings of discouragement. Your thoughts create your feelings and eventually your actions, so deliberately choosing how you frame situations can greatly alter your actions and thus your results. With a positive mindset, you will build resilience and the courage to tackle more projects and the momentum to see them through.
- *Secure regular blocks of uninterrupted time.* This is critical to allowing the mind to think deeply and creatively and to plan forward. See *Deep Work* book recommendation (below).

- *Celebrate your victories along the way (even if they are small).* Rewarding yourself and your supporting cast (both personally and professionally) will keep all of your spirits up and your momentum going. It also makes working through your upcoming tasks easier because as you will have something to look forward to after task completion.

Day-to-Day Goals

Several of the following habits, when implemented on a day-to-day basis, are the building blocks for achieving balance.

Approach each day in an organized way Plan ahead and set goals for what you want to accomplish in that day. Establish an opening routine for each day that involves reviewing your list and close the day by revisiting that list and composing your to-do list for the next day.

Set limits on what you agree to do This applies to tasks on a day-to-day and week-to-week basis. If you have thoughtfully and purposefully declined to do a task, do not look back or feel guilty. Making promises that you cannot keep can lead to constant worry and stress.

Aim to achieve more work-related tasks during your work hours Avoid the temptation to say, "I'll get that done at home." In the modern workplace, a clear separation between work and home does not often exist. That said, the more you can get done during work hours, the more you can unplug when you get home. Complete disconnection from your work-related tasks allows you to approach them the following day feeling recharged and with a fresh thought process. In order to accomplish this, you may need to rearrange your work schedule. Get rid of as many distractions and potential interruptions that you can. Group small packets of time together where "deep work" can be undertaken, allowing you to accomplish more and more meaningul work (see *Deep Work* under Additional Resources).

Do not excessively multitask To some degree, it impossible to avoid multitasking when in a clinical setting. For example, being called to check your films at the LINAC, while a patient is waiting in a clinic room and a colleague is paging you, is not an uncommon scenario. Because situations like this cannot be entirely avoided, make it a habit to look ahead at your schedule and reduce the chances of a traffic jam like this happening. The less often this occurs, the less derailed you will become. Allow time following each encounter for timely and efficient documentation, which obviates duplication of your thought process and other efforts later in the day.

Sometimes good enough is good enough Working on relatively unimportant things to the point of perfection wastes your time. Be comfortable with good work for the majority of tasks, and save perfection for select items that carry high importance. Apply this principle to decision-making. Refrain from treating all decisions as if they are critical decisions. If there are two reasonable options, and neither of which would lead to much difference in the outcome, pick one, and move along. If it turned out differently that you would have liked, then call it a learning experience and alter your choices the next time.

Take care of yourself If you are unwell physically, mentally or emotionally, nothing else matters. The following items can improve and help maintain your wellness:

- *Sleep:* Get regular and an adequate amount of sleep each night. This improves your focus and concentration while at work and allows to you to fully enjoy your leisure time.
- *Meditation:* This is an underused tool. It involves focusing the mind on a specific object or activity, such as breathing, for some period of time. It trains the mind to attain a state of calmness, attention, and awareness. Meditation, practiced regularly, facilitates clarity of thought and mental and emotional stability. There are a number of free or relatively inexpensive tools that can help you get started (see below).
- *Regular exercise*: Aside from keeping your body healthy, exercise builds your stamina and will allow you to better endure strenuous times that may occur in the future. Exercise also improves concentration and can set the stage for a good night's sleep.
- *Good nutrition:* "You are what you eat." Unplanned meals lead to hasty decisions (consumption of unhealthy/processed foods or skipping a meal altogether). Preparing meals ahead of time will allow you to eat healthier (and feel more energetic), and you will waste less of your precious work time procuring food.
- *Hobbies:* Take part in your hobbies. Some hobbies will also accomplish your goal of regular exercise. Utilizing different parts of your brain is enjoyable and can lead to fresh thoughts that may benefit you in other spheres of your life.
- *Vacation:* Utilize your allocated vacation days. Do not save them for years and use them all at once (unless you have to do this for a certain reason). Regular time away from work is healthy, and it allows you to come back to work feeling recharged and in good spirits.
- *Maintain meaningful relationships*: You may not be able to stay in regular contact with everyone in your life, but prioritize those relationships that are the most meaningful to you. Loving, positive relationships bring meaning to our lives.

Why Should an Employer Care About Their Employee's Work–Life Balance?

A culture supportive of work–life balance facilitates employees producing higher quality work with improved efficiency. Employee retention is higher amongst organizations that make accommodations allowing their employees to achieve this balance (e.g., flexible work hours, remote connection options, on-site childcare, access to flexible spending accounts that can be used toward childcare costs, paid maternity/paternity leave, wellness programs, allocated time for academic pursuits, lactation support/accomodations for new mothers, etc.). If employees are retained, there are decreased costs to the employer related to turnover (off-boarding, recruitment, credentialing, training, etc.). Happy and satisfied employees also contribute to a more positive work culture by having mutually encouraging and synergistic relationships. Working together, satisfied employees are more likely to take on larger projects that will help realize important departmental and/or institutional missions. Employees that feel well and fulfilled are less likely to have time away from work, again, allowing for improved productivity. Individuals who are happy in their workplace will spread the word to others. There are several national and local outlets that rate organizations on being "best places to work." Achieving this status improves an institution's reputation and thus its ability to recruit other top-notch employees.

Additional Resources

Books
1. *Off Balance: Getting Beyond the Work-Life Balance Myth to Personal and Professional Satisfaction* by Matthew Kelly
2. *The One Minute Manager Balances Work and Life* by Ken Blanchard
3. *Deep Work* by Cal Newport
4. *The Monk Who Sold His Ferrari* by Robin Sharma
5. *Enough: True Measures of Money, Business, and Life* by John C. Bogle
6. *Finding Your CliftonStrengths: StrengthsFinder 2.0* by Tom Rath
7. *The Bullet Journal Method: Track the Past, Order the Present, Design the Future* by Ryder Carroll

Podcasts
1. *Beyond the To-Do List* by Erik Fisher
2. *The Tim Ferriss Show* (author of *The 4-Hour Workweek)*
3. *The 5 A.M. Miracle with Jeff Sanders*
4. *WorkLife with Adam Grant*

Organizing (To-Do) Apps
1. *Todoist*
2. *Microsoft To Do*
3. *TickTick*
4. *Asana* (for large teams)

Meditation Apps
1. *Headspace*
2. *Calm*
3. *Buddhify*

Summary Points

Personal Finance:

1. Time is your greatest asset. Get educated and start making your financial plan early.
2. Unless considering Federal Public Student Loan Forgiveness, refinance to the lowest possible rate and pay off your student debt quickly.
3. Strongly consider protecting your assets and future income with insurance policies (disability, malpractice, life insurance, etc.), especially early in your career before you have reached relative financial security.
4. Figure out if you plan to manage your finances independently or with an advisor. Either is okay. Not having a plan is not okay.

Work–Life Balance:

1. Work–life balance is not a destination, but a constant work in progress.
2. Time is your greatest asset. Engage in regular goal setting to help you clearly articulate what you hope to achieve both personally and professionally. Take on tasks and engage in activities that help you achieve those ends.
3. Take care of yourself. If you are unwell physically, mentally, or emotionally, nothing else matters.

For Discussion with a Mentor or Colleague

Personal Finance:

- Do you manage your finances independently or with the help of a financial advisor?

    (a) If independently, what resources did you use to get started?
    (b) If with assistance of a financial advisor, how does that relationship work? What is their fee structure?

- What were the key steps you took early on that put you on a path toward financial success? Are there any financial pitfalls to avoid?

Work–Life Balance:

- What are some the key things that you did over the years that had the greatest positive impact on your work–life balance? Conversely, what were some of the things that negatively impacted this?
- Are there any tools or systems that you use on a regular basis to help you stay organized?

Paying It Forward: Being a Good Mentor, Steward, and Colleague

David T. Pointer Jr. and Sarah E. Hoffe

> *The delicate balance of mentoring someone is not creating them in your own image but giving them the opportunity to create themselves.*
>
> —Stephen Spielberg

Introduction

The term "mentor" was first introduced by Homer in his masterpiece *The Odyssey*. While away fighting the Trojan wars, Odysseus trusted his friend Mentor to oversee the upbringing of his son Telemachus [31]. This word, acquired from his namesake, is simply defined as a trusted counselor or guide. Mentorship, or the influence and guidance provided by a mentor, has played a pivotal role in the educational direction, personal growth, and professional development of most, if not all, successful individuals. Specifically defining mentorship is a challenge as the behavior is composed of a myriad of interactions utilized to achieve the goals of a designated mentee. For this reason, there is little consistency in the literature with upwards of 50 variations on the definition of mentoring described, from various perspectives and disciplinary backgrounds. Similarly, little consensus exists on specific methodology applicable to all subjects and disciplines[15, 17].

In medicine, mentoring has traditionally been important for graduate medical education and beyond into professional academic life, leading to productive faculty members who are promoted more quickly and more likely to stay at their home

D. T. Pointer Jr.
Department of Gastrointestinal Oncology, Moffitt Cancer Center and Research Institute,
Tampa, FL, USA

S. E. Hoffe (✉)
Department of Radiation Oncology, Moffitt Cancer Center and Research Institute,
Tampa, FL, USA
e-mail: sarah.hoffe@moffitt.org

© Springer Nature Switzerland AG 2021
R. A. Chandra et al. (eds.), *Career Development in Academic Radiation Oncology*, https://doi.org/10.1007/978-3-030-71855-8_31

institution [52]. The traditional mentor–mentee pairing is a dyad [44] that focuses on five major elements [37]. First, the relationship centers on the achievement of the mentee and the transfer of knowledge from the more experienced mentor. Second, the mentor offers emotional support with career goals and professional development while serving as a role model. Third, the relationship is reciprocal. Fourth, the mentor relationship involves direct interpersonal interaction. Finally, the dyad revolves around the mentor's greater experience, expertise, and influence. Descriptions by the National Institute of Health note that mentoring encompasses a wide variety of behaviors that may be appropriate at different times, such as teacher/guide/counselor/motivator/sponsor/coach/advisor/role   model/referral   agent   and   door opener [63].

Within radiation oncology, successful mentoring has led to improved mentee satisfaction, publication quality, and time to promotion with a positive correlation between the mentor's h index and the mentee's h index [34]. Yet junior faculty in our field do not experience uniform benefits. Recent reports indicate that only 49% of respondents were "very" or "somewhat" satisfied and only 51% reported having a primary mentor [40], with the majority of those indicating their derived benefit from sponsorship through support or invitation to present at national medical meetings. In this chapter, we will review the available literature on mentoring best practice to provide a roadmap on how to approach and structure mentoring relationships.

Mentoring in Academic Medicine

Within the last 20 years, the available literature on mentorship in academic medicine has been based largely on qualitative studies without any randomized trials reporting the effects of mentoring. Studies have indicated that mentors have significant impact on mentees with respect to specialty choice, academic career choice, research productivity (increased publications and grants), and promotion in rank [53]. Navigating the academic landscape to find appropriate mentors has been the subject of many papers as well [57, 58]. The degree of mentee benefit between assigned mentors versus chosen mentors remains unclear[51]. One recent study [54] explored various methods of mentor–mentee pairing at the medical student level, comparing personal matching by structured interviews with two online matching procedures where mentees could evaluate mentor profiles. No significant difference was found in the level of mentee satisfaction based on method of selection, but the personal method was superior in terms of the number of relationships that were formed.

Until recently, little data was reported on the outcomes of structured programs pairing a mentee with a selected mentor. In 2009, a prospective pilot study enrolled 23 junior faculty in the Radiation Oncology and the Anesthesia/Critical Care/Pain Management Departments at Harvard with long-term outcomes recently reported [23]. In this formal mentorship program, a mentor was paired with a junior faculty member after the mentee ranked the five areas of professional development they were looking for and the mentor ranked the five areas of mentorship they could provide. The pilot was structured with formal training sessions and regular meetings. The outcomes of the junior faculty mentees were compared with a control group, finding that mentees were more likely to be funded/promoted ($p = 0.03$) and more likely to hold senior faculty positions (47% vs. 13%, $P = 0.030$). Moreover, mentee satisfaction with work environment increased from 35% to 65% compared to the control group that noted no change in any domain other than a 9% increase in work environment. The study noted not only short-term but also long-term benefits, as the majority of mentees became mentors themselves and propagated a mentorship culture.

A similar mentoring pilot program has been reported from the surgery department at Massachusetts General Hospital [46] where all surgeons at the Instructor or Assistant Professor level were enrolled. The mentees were paired with mentors based on research interest and did not work in the same surgical division in order to avoid any conflicts of interest. The program was structured with at least three meetings per year. Results showed that over 75% of the mentees were invested in the program and wanted to continue, citing significant contributions to career plans and increased involvement in professional societies. Interestingly, the majority of the mentees had at least two other mentors in addition to the one assigned by the program.

Modern Mentoring: Beyond the Dyad

More than 20 years ago, Peter Drucker coined the phrase *you must be the CEO of your own life* [22]. Indeed, as your own CEO, you recognize you need a strong fund of expert knowledge coupled with valuable leadership skills to succeed in your career. Increasing interest in radiation oncology has recently focused on the importance of developing physician leadership potential and stewardship of cancer care resources [61]. Given the complexity of modern healthcare, obtaining all these traits from a single mentor can be elusive. With the flurry of changes in medicine promoting teams rather than silos and hierarchy, more recent mentoring models have been developed that transcend the dyad and involve a mentoring community [18]. This new mentoring Board of Directors (BOD) approach may allow each CEO to diversify their portfolio of human capital and learn from individuals with a broad array of talents, skills, and medical accomplishment [13]. Feedback from 90% of trainees in one recent study noted that team mentoring was helpful for their research and for their career development [32], with respondents noting that this diversity of thought and expanded networking transcended the scheduling conflicts and strife managing opposing opinions.

Working as a mentor on a team may have significant benefits in the current radiation oncology work environment where junior physicians must gain experience in procedures, clinical skills, and research. First, as departments are disease site specific, this model readily lends itself to multidisciplinary mentorship, such that the mentee with a particular subject matter interest can work with the matching experts in medical and surgical oncology as well. This multiple mentor relationship could enrich the mentee's experience and lessen the time demand for any one particular mentor as there could be delegation of roles. Second, with millennials comprising 25% of today's workforce and soon to be 75% by 2025 [62], there is already resonance with teamwork and collaboration better aligning this model with those novel learners [20]. Third, with multiple mentors, this could relax the pressure to maintain on-site relationships given time constraints of the more senior physicians and open up potential for more off-site mentoring with technology. For example, surgeons have been evaluating telementoring compared with traditional on-site mentoring, with one recent study reporting similar complication rates and operating times [4]. Applicable in our field, this suggests future radiation oncologists could utilize this strategy to mentor procedures such as brachytherapy using off-site technologies or even virtual reality [39].

Other models revolve around the concept of peer mentoring and peer networks [47], providing mentees with a safe and secure environment to obtain knowledge and ask questions. One such program involving 104 junior faculty noted improvements in clinical skills, attitudes, and self-reported knowledge [24]. Other variations of this include the creation of *a mastermind group*. Comprised from the mentee's peer network, this group meets regularly to provide feedback, share and fine-tune ideas, and hold each other accountable in their professional progression [13, 14].

Coaching

In distinction from mentoring, coaching is typified by one physician guiding the other to "find" the answer rather than "telling" them the answers directly [43]. Although some element of coaching may exist at various time points in the mentor–mentee relationship, another more tangible application of coaching may be in the peer setting of radiation oncology colleagues [19, 41]. With overall rates of 25–60% of physicians developing burnout, peer coaching can be an effective strategy to improve resilience [25]. As a work-related syndrome, burnout is steeped in emotional exhaustion, depersonalization, and a feeling that there is little meaning in work and low levels of accomplishment [64]. Indeed, higher levels of burnout can occur in female and younger physicians [65]. Studies have shown that interactions in the work environment can build community and foster a sense of connectedness which can decrease burnout [56].

Peer coaching is one practical way to "pay it forward" such that more junior physicians feel supported. Identifying peer coaches can help the junior physician develop a safe setting to explore some problematic issues that develop in the workplace. The more experienced physician can offer guidance and act as a confidential sounding board to facilitate the junior colleague's personal and professional development. This would foster a sense of connection for the junior physician that could increase resilience.

Mentoring: Best versus Worst

Objective outcome measures to evaluate the success of an individual mentor are still not well defined in academic medicine, although some investigators have sought to develop instruments to measure a mentee's satisfaction with the relationship [55] . There have been many publications that have enumerated the characteristics and responsibilities of the ideal mentor [3, 21, 49], but one of the most enlightening is a study that evaluated nomination letters for a Lifetime Achievement in Mentorship Award which highlighted common themes of 29 distinguished faculty recognized at UCSF [8]. Admirable personal qualities were commonly mentioned, rating enthusiasm, compassion, and selflessness as highly desirable. These features were joined by the nominees' dedication to acting as career guides and committing to high-quality mentoring sessions with set, scheduled times. The nominees were described as supportive, helping mentees learn to balance their work and personal lives. Finally, the nominees were outstanding role models who desired to leave a legacy by empowering mentees to forge academic success.

In practice, Tjan has recently described what the best mentors do [59]. First and foremost, those who excel put the relationship with the mentee before the mentorship. Indeed, there is no measurable difference between those mentored and those not unless there is a basic relationship based on mutual trust and respect [48]. Second, outstanding mentors do not tunnel vision competency but also focus on character to help shape the mentee's professional development. Third, the best mentors carefully consider the mentee's ideas with thoughtful intention before expressing negativity. Finally, those especially skilled in mentoring promote loyalty to the mentee and their career goals.

In addition to these characteristics, the best mentors commit to behaviors that reinforce to the mentee their responsibilities [3]. They show their commitment with timely, nonjudgmental feedback, providing critiques that challenge the mentee, encourage their ideas, and provide guidance. They acknowledge the mentee's contribution and provide resources. They are also talented communicators who practice active listening with mentees, capable of identifying their strengths and weaknesses in order to help mentees continue to improve and evolve [26].

Unfortunately, not all mentors place the best interest of the mentee before all other priorities. Chopra et al. describe six behaviors they term *mentorship malpractice* whereby the academic career of the mentee is at risk [9]. The authors describe mentoring sabotage that can occur by either active or passive means and they describe six behaviors for mentors to avoid. They label those mentors who usurp the mentee's ideas or projects as their own as *Hijackers*, noting that mentees in this situation develop a type of Stockholm Syndrome and think that by going along there will be a future reward that never comes. This is contrast to the *Exploiter* who uses the mentee to do their own work that serves them and is not in the mentee's best interest. The final type of active malpractice is called the *Possessor* and describes dominating behavior that isolates the mentee from others and increases mentee insecurity. In distinction, other types of mentoring behavior occur more obliquely but are nonetheless disruptive to the mentee's progress. With the actions of a *Bottleneck,* the mentor is so preoccupied with their own workload and priorities that they cannot perform their mentoring duties in a timely fashion, thus impeding the career development of the mentee. The *Country Clubber*, by contrast, is so focused on being the mentee's friend that they don't give the academic tasks the proper due diligence and the mentee's progress suffers. The last type of passive malpractice revolves around the actions of the *World Traveler* who is so busy with invited speaking engagements that they neglect the mentee.

Mentor Expectations

From the mentor perspective, the first consideration is how to choose a mentee. Many trainees will often email a potential mentor and ask if there are any projects in a desired area of research. At this point, some mentors request an in-person or telephone meeting with the potential mentee to discuss their goals and expectations to see if there is a potential fit. With this approach, mentors may be able to better assess if they or a colleague may be more aligned with the mentee and whether a multiple mentor approach may be more appropriate. Asking open ended questions of the mentee's vision of their future self at appropriate time points (1 year/5 year) can help both parties determine where the current gaps in professional/personal knowledge and competence exist. To bridge these gaps, the mentor may be better able to evaluate if these are compatible goals to accomplish with the mentor's skill set. Additional strategies of some mentors are to assign the possible mentee a short project such as reviewing an article in order to assess readiness and maturity for a formal relationship. This exercise will demonstrate the mentee's ability to manage time, communicate, and translate motivation into quality work [10, 11]. By investing time upfront in getting to know the goals and expectations of the mentee, the mentor can decide which relationships will offer the best academic returns for their time.

Once the mentee is accepted, defining the structure of the relationship helps ensure expectations on both sides. Explaining to the mentee that mentoring sessions are confidential helps foster mentee security. Ground rules for the flow of information and questions can help the mentee be prepared and show respect for the mentor's time. If in-person meetings with one mentor will be the norm, agreeing upon frequency and format at the beginning of the relationship can enhance role delineation so the mentee knows to drive the relationship [66]. Prior to such sessions, if the mentee sends an agenda of the items that need to be addressed, the mentor can ensure there is adequate time allotted to accomplish the requested tasks. Since a common pitfall of early relationship blunders can occur with project deadlines, establishing at the outset the timelines needed for various requests or projects can prevent miscommunication.

As the relationship progresses, ensuring mutual accountability is key. In the role of teacher, the mentor can help the mentee remain on task by reviewing the progress to date at each meeting and ensuring that the discussion points from the prior session are resolved. At each juncture, maintaining open and honest communication about performance helps the mentee stay on track. If issues do arise, by managing the conflict productively the mentor can help the mentee develop stronger interpersonal communication skills.

Part of mentorship involves difficult conversations when a mentee's work product is inferior or there are behavioral issues. Since the relationship can be like a parent to an adult child [10, 11], developing trust so that negative feedback can be accepted is important. Discussing how the feedback will be delivered by the mentor early in the relationship, ideally in a supportive and encouraging manner while also pointing out the areas requiring improvement, and how comfortable the mentee is receiving feedback, can ensure that both parties avoid rifts and reach their goals [36]. If receiving feedback is noted by the mentee to be difficult, desensitization toward neutral acceptance without undue stress or anxiety could become part of the mentee's personal goals, which could be improved with practice-based learning exercises.

Mentoring, Gender, and Underrepresented Minorities

The underrepresentation of faculty positions, the lower salaries, and the career advancement barriers of female physicians and those from underrepresented minorities (URM) are well delineated in the academic medicine literature [7, 38, 42]. Paralleling the lower rates of women in radiation oncology, with only 0.3% growth per year over the last 30 years [35], there has been a void in female leadership visibility. A recent study of 6030 faculty from 265 accredited US oncology programs reported that women were underrepresented in leadership, with rates of 31.4% in medical oncology, 17.4% in radiation oncology, 11.1% in surgical oncology, and only 11.7% of radiation oncology chairs were female [12]. Similarly, nonwhite faculty are less likely to be promoted, less likely to have early career mentoring opportunities [2], and are less likely to receive R01 grants [27]. Women are also less likely to have mentors or receive early formal mentoring [16]. Since studies have suggested that insufficient mentoring can be a major factor leading to gender inequity, strategies to improve and match appropriate mentors have received increasing attention [5]. Survey results of 3100 female faculty at 13 US medical schools revealed that same gender was more important for black female faculty, those at the rank of Instructor, and those without a current mentor while same race/ethnicity was more important for racial/ethnic minorities, those physicians who were foreign born or those who never had formal mentoring [6].

Thus, mentoring these populations requires special consideration. Access for these groups to create long-term mentoring relationships early in their career may be more limited and informal mentoring processes for the mentee to self-select may be more difficult. Often early career physicians in these categories may not yet see themselves as future leaders so they may not seek out roles to increase their status [50, 60]. In addition to the traditional mentorship roles, mentors should especially consider the role of sponsorship for these populations, a career advancement technique that medicine is now adopting after seeing it close the visibility gap in the business world for women and URM who were talented but whose contributions were not being harnessed [30]. In this context, sponsorship indicates advocacy on the part of the senior mentor for the mentee such that reputation is put at risk in order to use influence to create opportunities that the mentee would not otherwise have at that career point. When sponsoring, the focus is on advancing a junior faculty member's career and promoting visibility at a higher level whether inside the institution or externally [1]. Sponsorship programs at the national level have reported that mentees have higher self-confidence and an improved ability to advocate for themselves [50].

Emotionally Intelligent Mentoring

Central to mentorship is the nature of the relationship itself. Given the change in the physician relationship landscape from solo practitioners in silos to new models of teaming and collaboration, the relevancy of interpersonal skill models such as the Emotional Intelligence (EI) Model has increased [28, 45]. The model as described by Goleman and Boyatzis describes the four quadrants from self-awareness/self-management to social awareness/relationship management [29]. Within each quadrant, there are specific elements that form 12 core competencies (Table 1).

In the mentor toolbox, the first consideration is to examine self and understand one's own capacity for mentorship. Inventorying one's assets, both in the professional and personal categories, would be a first step to determine one's current level of readiness. First, take stock of your expertise in radiation oncology, your own

Table 1 Twelve core competencies forming the emotional and social competence inventory (ESCI)

SELF	OTHER
Self-awareness: Emotional self-awareness	**Social awareness:** Empathy, organizational awareness
Self-management: achievement orientation, adaptability, emotional self-control, and positive outlook	**Relationship management:** Coach and mentor, inspirational leadership, influence, conflict management, and teamwork

Reproduced and printed with permission from Applied Radiation Oncology, Anderson Publishing, Ltd. [33]

current level of achievement, and your level of security with your academic career. Then, evaluate your "soft" skills that may be of value to mentees such as interpersonal communication, negotiation, and conflict management skills with attention to how willing you would be to share this knowledge and help prepare the mentee to navigate the profession/department/institution. Once you are aware of your own capacity, you can then reflect on how you would manage yourself with a mentee. Analysis of these two quadrants allows a robust check in with yourself to assess your current level of mentor readiness. See Table 2 for questions to guide your assessment.

After analyzing yourself, you can then focus on social awareness. In academic medicine, one particular concern would be your department/institution and to what extent mentorship is valued. Reflect on the culture of the work environment where you practice to determine how you will balance a commitment to mentoring with your other academic responsibilities. The first three quadrants prepare you for the highly relevant EI quadrant for mentoring: relationship management. Before you agree to accept a mentee, spend some time to really evaluate the nature of the relationship you want to develop.

Table 2 A Guide to Mentor Readiness: Ask yourself these questions to identify the type of mentor you aspire to be and how you envision achieving that goal

Self-awareness	Social awareness
Am I secure in my own rank/position that I will not be threatened by a mentee? What are my expectations for what the mentee needs to contribute for a first author manuscript?	How much does your department/ institution value mentoring?
Could I have any areas of conflict of interest with a potential mentee such as authorship or intellectual property?	How does your Chair prioritize and value mentoring by the faculty?
What is my current stress level and workload?	What is the culture among your peers for devoting time to mentorship?
Do I have the time to be a good mentor? What motivates me to become a mentor?	How is mentoring success defined by the Promotion Committee at your center?
How do I define a successful mentor/mentee relationship?	How will you choose a mentee?
Do I consider myself open or guarded and how will that affect the mentoring relationship?	What attributes of a mentee would indicate that you would be a good "match"?
How comfortable am I to share my expertise and my experiences with a mentee?	What are the goals of my mentee and do they align with my professional and personal skills?
Do I feel prepared to be a mentor at present? If not, what can I do to become more prepared?	Can the mentee clearly define what they are looking for in a mentor? Would your mentorship style be the same regardless if your mentee was female or a member of an URM?

(continued)

Table 2 (continued)

Self-management	Relationship management
How will I set my expectations and make sure they match the mentee?	How will I role model positive behaviors and work ethic for the mentee?
How will I structure our meetings… will we meet in person or communicate electronically?	How will I resolve conflicts with my mentee?
How will I deliver feedback to the mentee and maintain emotional self-control?	If my mentee prefers a multiple mentor model, am I comfortable being on a team with other colleagues?
How will I carve out time for this relationship?	How will I influence the professional development of the mentee?
How will I prioritize mentoring?	Who will drive the relationship?
How adaptable am I if the needs/goals of the mentee change during the relationship?	How will I influence the personal development of the mentee?
If I am feeling more stress or anxiety with my own workload, how will I maintain a positive outlook and not let it affect the mentoring relationship?	How will I communicate my expectations to the mentee? What if the relationship is not working out, how will I set the rules for a "break up"?

The previous sections have enumerated the strengths of the best mentors and the sins of mentors who do not promote the best interest of the mentee. The questions below will help catalyze your assessment of what kind of mentor you aspire to be and how you envision that process. By having clarity of your goals and expectations, you will be poised to develop a career-enhancing relationship for your mentee. See Table 2.

Bullet Points

- Traditional mentoring in academic medicine has involved the dyad of a senior faculty member with a junior colleague but shifting paradigms now include team mentoring and peer mentoring.
- Coaching can be extremely valuable for enhancing the connectedness of colleagues to promote resilience and avoid burnout.
- Mentoring best practice is rooted in a sincere desire by the mentor to advance the career of the mentee by enhancing their skills and knowledge based on a mutually respectful personal and professional relationship.
- Avoid mentoring malpractice by knowledge of the worst behaviors of the Hijacker, Exploiter, Possessor, Bottleneck, Country Clubber, and World Traveler.
- Sponsorship is a technique whereby senior mentors risk reputation to advance the career of a mentee to create opportunities and may be especially important for mentees who are female or from URM.
- The EI Model can serve as a useful foundation to frame the mentor–mentee relationship.

Conclusion

Mentoring is important for junior physician professional development. Within academic medicine, best practice centers around the relationship an altruistic, supportive mentor can create with a motivated mentee, who drives the academic tempo to complete required tasks. Mentoring has an established role in radiation oncology but there are still issues with access at the most junior levels, leaving room for further study. Novel strategies such as Coaching or Sponsorship can be effective in the peer context with a professional colleague or in circumstances involving underrepresented populations. Using the EI Model as a foundation to pay it forward, physicians can not only foster the development of their mentees, but fine-tune their own personal growth and professional development. Using the strategies outlined in this chapter, one can be sure to leave a positive legacy of mentorship, leadership, and professional development in the field of radiation oncology.

References

1. Ayyala MS, Skarupski K, Bodurtha JN, et al. Mentorship is not enough: exploring sponsorship and its role in career advancement in academic medicine. Acad Med J Assoc Am Med Coll. 2019;94:94–100. https://doi.org/10.1097/ACM.0000000000002398.
2. Beech BM, Calles-Escandon J, Hairston KG, et al. Mentoring programs for underrepresented minority faculty in academic medical centers: a systematic review of the literature. Acad Med. 2013;88:541–9. https://doi.org/10.1097/ACM.0b013e31828589e3.
3. Berk RA, Berg J, Mortimer R, et al. Measuring the effectiveness of faculty mentoring relationships. Acad Med J Assoc Am Med Coll. 2005;80:66–71. https://doi.org/10.1097/00001888-200501000-00017.
4. Bilgic E, Turkdogan S, Watanabe Y, et al. Effectiveness of telementoring in surgery compared with on-site mentoring: a systematic review. Surg Innov. 2017;24:379–85. https://doi.org/10.1177/1553350617708725.
5. Blood EA, Ullrich NJ, Hirshfeld-Becker DR, et al. Academic women faculty: are they finding the mentoring they need? J Women's Health. 2002;21:1201–8. https://doi.org/10.1089/jwh.2012.3529.
6. Carapinha R, Ortiz-Walters R, McCracken CM, et al. Variability in women faculty's preferences regarding mentor similarity: a multi-institution study in academic medicine. Acad Med J Assoc Am Med Coll. 2016;91:1108–18. https://doi.org/10.1097/ACM.0000000000001284.
7. Chapman CH, Hwang W-T, Deville C. Diversity based on race, ethnicity, and sex, of the US radiation oncology physician workforce. Int J Radiat Oncol Biol Phys. 2013;85:912–8. https://doi.org/10.1016/j.ijrobp.2012.08.020.
8. Cho CS, Ramanan RA, Feldman MD. Defining the ideal qualities of mentorship: a qualitative analysis of the characteristics of outstanding mentors. Am J Med. 2011;124:453–8. https://doi.org/10.1016/j.amjmed.2010.12.007.
9. Chopra V, Edelson DP, Saint S. A piece of my mind. Mentorship malpractice. JAMA. 2016;315:1453–4. https://doi.org/10.1001/jama.2015.18884.
10. Chopra V, Saint S. 6 things every mentor should do. Harv Bus Rev. 2017.
11. Chopra V, Saint S. What mentors wish their mentees knew. Harv Bus Rev. 2017.
12. Chowdhary M, Chowdhary A, Royce TJ, et al. Women's representation in leadership positions in academic medical oncology, radiation oncology, and surgical oncology programs. JAMA Netw Open. 2020;3:e200708. https://doi.org/10.1001/jamanetworkopen.2020.0708.

13. Clark D. Your career needs many mentors, not just one. Harv Bus Rev. 2017.
14. Clark D. Create a "mastermind group" to help your career. Harv Bus Rev. 2015.
15. Crisp G, Cruz I. Mentoring college students: a critical review of the literature between 1990 and 2007. Res High Educ. 2009;50:525–45. https://doi.org/10.1007/s11162-009-9130-2.
16. Cross M, Lee S, Bridgman H, et al. Benefits, barriers and enablers of mentoring female health academics: an integrative review. PLoS One. 2019;14:e0215319. https://doi.org/10.1371/journal.pone.0215319.
17. Dawson P. Beyond a definition: toward a framework for designing and specifying mentoring models. Educ Res. 2014;43:137–45. https://doi.org/10.3102/0013189X14528751.
18. DeCastro R, Sambuco D, Ubel PA, et al. Mentor networks in academic medicine: moving beyond a dyadic conception of mentoring for junior faculty researchers. Acad Med J Assoc Am Med Coll. 2013;88:488–96. https://doi.org/10.1097/ACM.0b013e318285d302.
19. Deiorio NM, Carney PA, Kahl LE, et al. Coaching: a new model for academic and career achievement. Med Educ Online. 2016;21:33480. https://doi.org/10.3402/meo.v21.33480.
20. Desy JR, Reed DA, Wolanskyj AP. Milestones and millennials: a perfect pairing-competency-based medical education and the learning preferences of generation Y. Mayo Clin Proc. 2017;92:243–50. https://doi.org/10.1016/j.mayocp.2016.10.026.
21. Detsky AS, Baerlocher MO. Academic mentoring--how to give it and how to get it. JAMA. 2007;297:2134–6. https://doi.org/10.1001/jama.297.19.2134.
22. Drucker PF. Managing oneself. Harv Bus Rev. 1999;77(64–74):185.
23. Efstathiou JA, Drumm MR, Paly JP, et al. Long-term impact of a faculty mentoring program in academic medicine. PLoS One. 2018;13:e0207634. https://doi.org/10.1371/journal.pone.0207634.
24. Fleming GM, Simmons JH, Xu M, et al. A facilitated peer mentoring program for junior faculty to promote professional development and peer networking. Acad Med J Assoc Am Med Coll. 2015;90:819–26. https://doi.org/10.1097/ACM.0000000000000705.
25. Gazelle G, Liebschutz JM, Riess H. Physician burnout: coaching a way out. J Gen Intern Med. 2015;30:508–13. https://doi.org/10.1007/s11606-014-3144-y.
26. Geraci SA, Thigpen SC. A review of mentoring in academic medicine. Am J Med Sci. 2017;353:151–7. https://doi.org/10.1016/j.amjms.2016.12.002.
27. Ginther DK, Schaffer WT, Schnell J, et al. Race, ethnicity, and NIH research awards. Science. 2011;333:1015–9. https://doi.org/10.1126/science.1196783.
28. Goleman D, Boyatzis R, McKee A. Primal leadership: realizing the power of emotional intelligence. 7th ed. Boston: Harvard Business School Press; 2002.
29. Goleman D, Boyatzis RE. Emotional intelligence has 12 elements. Which do you need to work on? Harv Bus Rev. 2017.
30. Gottlieb AS, Travis EL. Rationale and models for career advancement sponsorship in academic medicine: the time is Here; the time is now. Acad Med J Assoc Am Med Coll. 2018;93:1620–3. https://doi.org/10.1097/ACM.0000000000002342.
31. Gough I. Mentoring: historical origins and contemporary value. ANZ J Surg. 2008;78:831–831. https://doi.org/10.1111/j.1445-2197.2008.04672.x.
32. Guise J-M, Geller S, Regensteiner JG, et al. Team mentoring for interdisciplinary team science: lessons from K12 scholars and directors. Acad Med J Assoc Am Med Coll. 2017;92:214–21. https://doi.org/10.1097/ACM.0000000000001330.
33. Hoffe SE, Quinn JF, Frakes J, et al (2017) Emotional-intelligence-centric leadership training for radiation oncologists 5.
34. Holliday EB, Jagsi R, Thomas CR, et al. Standing on the shoulders of giants: results from the radiation oncology academic development and mentorship assessment project (ROADMAP). Int J Radiat Oncol Biol Phys. 2014;88:18–24. https://doi.org/10.1016/j.ijrobp.2013.09.035.
35. Holliday EB, Siker M, Chapman CH, et al. Achieving gender equity in the radiation oncology physician workforce. Adv Radiat Oncol. 2018;3:478–83. https://doi.org/10.1016/j.adro.2018.09.003.

36. Jackson VA, Palepu A, Szalacha L, et al. "Having the right chemistry": a qualitative study of mentoring in academic medicine. Acad Med J Assoc Am Med Coll. 2003;78:328–34. https://doi.org/10.1097/00001888-200303000-00020.
37. Jacobi M. Mentoring and undergraduate academic success: a literature review. Rev Educ Res. 1991;61:505. https://doi.org/10.2307/1170575.
38. Jagsi R, Griffith KA, Stewart A, et al. Gender differences in the salaries of physician researchers. JAMA. 2012;307:2410–7. https://doi.org/10.1001/jama.2012.6183.
39. Jin W, Birckhead B, Perez B, Hoffe S. Augmented and virtual reality: exploring a future role in radiation oncology education and training. Appl Radiat Oncol. 2017:8, 808.
40. Lalani N, Griffith KA, Jones RD, et al. Mentorship experiences of early-career academic radiation oncologists in North America. Int J Radiat Oncol Biol Phys. 2018;101:732–40. https://doi.org/10.1016/j.ijrobp.2018.03.035.
41. Lovell B. What do we know about coaching in medical education? A literature review. Med Educ. 2018;52:376–90. https://doi.org/10.1111/medu.13482.
42. Mangurian C, Linos E, Sarkar U, et al. What's holding women in medicine Back from leadership. Harv Bus Rev. 2018.
43. Marcdante K, Simpson D. Choosing when to advise, coach, or mentor. J Grad Med Educ. 2018;10:227–8. https://doi.org/10.4300/JGME-D-18-00111.1.
44. Mayer AP, Files JA, Ko MG, Blair JE. Academic advancement of women in medicine: do socialized gender differences have a role in mentoring? Mayo Clin Proc. 2008;83:204–7. https://doi.org/10.4065/83.2.204.
45. Mintz LJ, Stoller JK. A systematic review of physician leadership and emotional intelligence. J Grad Med Educ. 2014;6:21–31. https://doi.org/10.4300/JGME-D-13-00012.1.
46. Phitayakorn R, Petrusa E, Hodin RA. Development and initial results of a mandatory department of surgery faculty mentoring pilot program. J Surg Res. 2016;205:234–7. https://doi.org/10.1016/j.jss.2016.06.048.
47. Pololi L, Knight S. Mentoring faculty in academic medicine. A new paradigm? J Gen Intern Med. 2005;20:866–70. https://doi.org/10.1111/j.1525-1497.2005.05007.x.
48. Ragins BR, Cotton JL. Mentor functions and outcomes: a comparison of men and women in formal and informal mentoring relationships. J Appl Psychol. 1999;84:529–50. https://doi.org/10.1037/0021-9010.84.4.529.
49. Rose GL, Rukstalis MR, Schuckit MA. Informal mentoring between faculty and medical students. Acad Med J Assoc Am Med Coll. 2005;80:344–8. https://doi.org/10.1097/00001888-200504000-00007.
50. Roy B, Gottlieb AS. The career advising program: a strategy to achieve gender equity in academic medicine. J Gen Intern Med. 2017;32:601–2. https://doi.org/10.1007/s11606-016-3969-7.
51. Sambunjak D, Marušić A. Mentoring: what's in a name? JAMA. 2009;302:2591–2. https://doi.org/10.1001/jama.2009.1858.
52. Sambunjak D, Straus SE, Marusic A. A systematic review of qualitative research on the meaning and characteristics of mentoring in academic medicine. J Gen Intern Med. 2010;25:72–8. https://doi.org/10.1007/s11606-009-1165-8.
53. Sambunjak D, Straus SE, Marušić A. Mentoring in academic medicine: a systematic review. JAMA. 2006;296:1103. https://doi.org/10.1001/jama.296.9.1103.
54. Schäfer M, Pander T, Pinilla S, et al. A prospective, randomised trial of different matching procedures for structured mentoring programmes in medical education. Med Teach. 2016;38:921–9. https://doi.org/10.3109/0142159X.2015.1132834.
55. Schäfer M, Pander T, Pinilla S, et al. The Munich-Evaluation-of-Mentoring-Questionnaire (MEMeQ)--a novel instrument for evaluating protégés' satisfaction with mentoring relationships in medical education. BMC Med Educ. 2015;15:201. https://doi.org/10.1186/s12909-015-0469-0.
56. Shanafelt TD, Noseworthy JH. Executive leadership and physician well-being: nine organizational strategies to promote engagement and reduce burnout. Mayo Clin Proc. 2017;92:129–46. https://doi.org/10.1016/j.mayocp.2016.10.004.

57. Straus SE, Chatur F, Taylor M. Issues in the mentor–mentee relationship in academic medicine: a qualitative study. Acad Med. 2009;84:135–9. https://doi.org/10.1097/ACM.0b013e31819301ab.
58. Straus SE, Johnson MO, Marquez C, Feldman MD. Characteristics of successful and failed mentoring relationships: a qualitative study across two academic health centers. Acad Med. 2013;88:82–9. https://doi.org/10.1097/ACM.0b013e31827647a0.
59. Tjan AK. What the best mentors do. Harv Bus Rev. 2017.
60. Travis EL, Doty L, Helitzer DL. Sponsorship: a path to the academic medicine C-suite for women faculty? Acad Med J Assoc Am Med Coll. 2013;88:1414–7. https://doi.org/10.1097/ACM.0b013e3182a35456.
61. Turner S, Seel M, Trotter T, et al. Defining a leader role curriculum for radiation oncology: a global Delphi consensus study. Radiother Oncol J Eur Soc Ther Radiol Oncol. 2017;123:331–6. https://doi.org/10.1016/j.radonc.2017.04.009.
62. Waljee JF, Chopra V, Saint S. Mentoring Millennials. JAMA. 2018;319:1547–8. https://doi.org/10.1001/jama.2018.3804.
63. Wasserman TH, Coleman CN. Mentors, mensches, and models. Int J Radiat Oncol. 2009;73:974–5. https://doi.org/10.1016/j.ijrobp.2008.10.078.
64. West CP, Dyrbye LN, Erwin PJ, Shanafelt TD. Interventions to prevent and reduce physician burnout: a systematic review and meta-analysis. Lancet Lond Engl. 2016;388:2272–81. https://doi.org/10.1016/S0140-6736(16)31279-X.
65. West CP, Dyrbye LN, Shanafelt TD. Physician burnout: contributors, consequences and solutions. J Intern Med. 2018;283:516–29. https://doi.org/10.1111/joim.12752.
66. Zerzan JT, Hess R, Schur E, et al. Making the most of mentors: a guide for mentees. Acad Med J Assoc Am Med Coll. 2009;84:140–4. https://doi.org/10.1097/ACM.0b013e3181906e8f.

Index

© Springer Nature Switzerland AG 2021
R. A. Chandra et al. (eds.), *Career Development in Academic Radiation
Oncology*, https://doi.org/10.1007/978-3-030-71855-8